Integrated Electronic Health Records

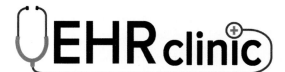

Fourth Edition

M. Beth Shanholtzer, MAEd, FAHIMA, RHIA

Director, HIM Program
Lord Fairfax Community College

Amy L. Ensign, MBA, BHSA, CMA (AAMA), RMA (AMT)

Baker College

INTEGRATED ELECTRONIC HEALTH RECORDS, FOURTH EDITION

Published by McGraw Hill LLC, 1325 Avenue of the Americas, New York, NY 10121. Copyright ©2021 by McGraw Hill LLC. All rights reserved. Printed in the United States of America. Previous editions ©2018, 2015, and 2012. No part of this publication may be reproduced or distributed in any form or by any means, or stored in a database or retrieval system, without the prior written consent of McGraw Hill LLC, including, but not limited to, in any network or other electronic storage or transmission, or broadcast for distance learning.

Some ancillaries, including electronic and print components, may not be available to customers outside the United States.

This book is printed on acid-free paper.

1 2 3 4 5 6 7 8 9 0 LMN 24 23 22 21 20

ISBN	978-1-260-08226-5 (bound edition)
MHID	1-260-08226-1 (bound edition)
ISBN	978-1-264-00465-2 (loose-leaf edition)
MHID	1-264-00465-6 (loose-leaf edition)

Executive Portfolio Manager: *William Lawrensen*
Senior Product Developer: *Michelle L. Flomenhoft*
Product Developer: *Erin DeHeck*
Learnsmart Product Developer: *Joan Weber*
Executive Marketing Manager: *James Connely*
Content Project Managers: *Laura Bies and Tammy Juran*
Buyer: *Susan K. Culbertson*
Design: *David W. Hash*
Content Licensing Specialist: *Melissa Homer*
Cover Image: *©alexskopje/Shutterstock*
Compositor: *MPS Limited*

All credits appearing on page or at the end of the chapters are considered to be an extension of the copyright page.

Library of Congress Cataloging-in-Publication Data

Names: Shanholtzer, M. Beth, author. | Ensign, Amy L., author.
  Title: Integrated electronic health records / M. Beth Shanholtzer, Amy L. Ensign.
  Description: Fourth edition. | New York : McGraw-Hill LLC, [2021] |
  Includes bibliographical references and index.
  Identifiers: LCCN 2020000409 (print) | LCCN 2020000410 (ebook) |
  ISBN 9781260082265 (bound edition ; alk. paper) | ISBN 1260082261
  (bound edition ; alk. paper) | ISBN 9781264004652 (loose-edition ; alk. paper) |
  ISBN 1264004656 (loose-edition ; alk. paper) | ISBN 9781264004676 (ebook)
  Subjects: MESH: Electronic Health Records | Software
  Classification: LCC R858 (print) | LCC R858 (ebook) | NLM WX 175 | DDC 610.285–dc23
  LC record available at https://lccn.loc.gov/2020000409
  LC ebook record available at https://lccn.loc.gov/2020000410

The Internet addresses listed in the text were accurate at the time of publication. The inclusion of a website does not indicate an endorsement by the authors or McGraw Hill LLC, and McGraw Hill LLC does not guarantee the accuracy of the information presented at these sites.

mheducation.com/highered

brief contents

contents

preface

Welcome to the fourth edition of *Integrated Electronic Health Records!*

Healthcare has made great progress in the use of electronic health records in the United States, which is creating even more opportunities for people who want to work in non-clinical health professions. From the front office staff to nurses, doctors, health information professionals, coders, and every worker in between, understanding how health information is transferred and how that information can improve the quality of healthcare is a valuable skill. Those working in healthcare settings will be impacted by electronic health records as they complete their daily tasks.

Developed as a comprehensive learning resource, this hands-on course for *Integrated Electronic Health Records* is offered through McGraw-Hill's *Connect. Connect* uses the latest technology and learning techniques to better connect professors to their students, and students to the information and customized resources they need to master a subject.

Integrated Electronic Health Records complements the online *Connect* course and is written by authors with extensive backgrounds in health information management/health information technology in the case of M. Beth Shanholtzer, MAEd, FAHIMA, RHIA, and clinical/administrative medical assisting in the case of Amy Ensign, MBA, BHSA, CMA (AAMA), RMA (AMT).

Both the worktext and the online course include coverage of EHRclinic, an education-based EHR solution for online electronic health records, practice management applications, and interoperable physician-based functionality. EHRclinic will be used to demonstrate the key applications of electronic health records. Attention is paid to providing the "why" behind each task, so that the reader can accumulate transferable skills. The coverage is focused on using an EHR program in a doctor's office, while providing additional information on how tasks might also be completed in a hospital setting.

Electronic health records impact a variety of programs in the health professions; thus, this content will be relevant to health information management, health information technology, medical insurance, billing and coding, and medical assisting programs.

New to the Fourth Edition

In the fourth edition of *IEHR*, new key terms have been added to chapters as needed. The EHR used to demonstrate common electronic health record applications in the fourth edition is EHRclinic. EHRclinic combines the features of simulated exercises within a sandbox environment, providing students with the opportunity to master their practical EHR skills. As with the first three editions, the applications will be described, including why each step is necessary; students will observe a demonstration; they will be given a chance to practice; and then they will be graded on their attempts to successfully complete the exercise. For the fourth edition, we have added instructional notes in the eBook to various exercise steps to help students as they work through the exercises. These notes and the steps can also be downloaded from www.mhhe.com/iehr4.

While content updates have been made to all of the chapters, here are the highlights:

Chapter 5

In the fourth edition, the use of medication databases within EHR software has been expanded upon.

Chapter 6

In the fourth edition, ICD-9-CM is briefly mentioned as the legacy coding system, and ICD-10-CM/PCS is the coding system highlighted in this edition. Code linkage as part of the billing process, patient payments such as co-pays and coinsurances, adjudication, and the medical billing and documentation cycle are also discussed in greater detail. There are new exercises using EHRclinic in the fourth edition.

Chapter 8

Several exercises have been changed in EHRclinic relating to internal communication, keeping track of tasks, workflow, and patient reminders.

Chapter 9

The fourth edition goes into more detail about Stage 3 updates that are in effect as of 2019.

Chapter 10

The fourth edition includes an update of the acceptance of the EHR and ancillary technologies now that the EHR has been adopted on a wide scale for the last five or so years. Upcoming technologies are also covered.

Chapter 11

Chapter 11 also has new and different exercises using EHRclinic to give students practice in the use of an electronic health record.

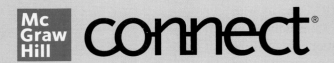

You're in the driver's seat.

Want to build your own course? No problem. Prefer to use our turnkey, prebuilt course? Easy. Want to make changes throughout the semester? Sure. And you'll save time with Connect's auto-grading too.

65%
Less Time Grading

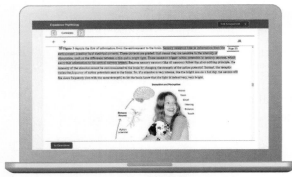

Laptop: McGraw-Hill; Woman/dog: George Doyle/Getty Images

They'll thank you for it.

Adaptive study resources like SmartBook® 2.0 help your students be better prepared in less time. You can transform your class time from dull definitions to dynamic debates. Find out more about the powerful personalized learning experience available in SmartBook 2.0 at **www.mheducation.com/highered /connect/smartbook**

Make it simple, make it affordable.

Connect makes it easy with seamless integration using any of the major Learning Management Systems— Blackboard®, Canvas, and D2L, among others—to let you organize your course in one convenient location. Give your students access to digital materials at a discount with our inclusive access program. Ask your McGraw-Hill representative for more information.

Padlock: Jobalou/Getty Images

Solutions for your challenges.

A product isn't a solution. Real solutions are affordable, reliable, and come with training and ongoing support when you need it and how you want it. Our Customer Experience Group can also help you troubleshoot tech problems— although Connect's 99% uptime means you might not need to call them. See for yourself at **status. mheducation.com**

Checkmark: Jobalou/Getty Images

SUPPORT AT every step

FOR STUDENTS

Effective, efficient studying.

Connect helps you be more productive with your study time and get better grades using tools like SmartBook 2.0, which highlights key concepts and creates a personalized study plan. Connect sets you up for success, so you walk into class with confidence and walk out with better grades.

Study anytime, anywhere.

Download the free ReadAnywhere app and access your online eBook or SmartBook 2.0 assignments when it's convenient, even if you're offline. And since the app automatically syncs with your eBook and SmartBook 2.0 assignments in Connect, all of your work is available every time you open it. Find out more at **www.mheducation.com/readanywhere**

"I really liked this app—it made it easy to study when you don't have your text-book in front of you."

- Jordan Cunningham, Eastern Washington University

Calendar: owattaphotos/Getty Images

No surprises.

The Connect Calendar and Reports tools keep you on track with the work you need to get done and your assignment scores. Life gets busy; Connect tools help you keep learning through it all.

Learning for everyone.

McGraw-Hill works directly with Accessibility Services Departments and faculty to meet the learning needs of all students. Please contact your Accessibility Services office and ask them to email accessibility@mheducation.com, or visit **www.mheducation.com/about/accessibility** for more information.

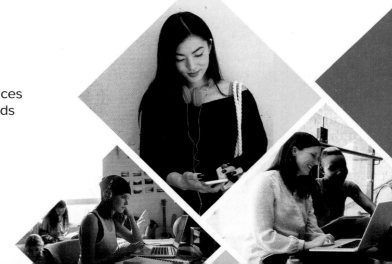

Top: Jenner Images/Getty Images, Left: Hero Images/Getty Images, Right: Hero Images/Getty Images

A one-stop spot to present, deliver, and assess digital assets available from McGraw-Hill: McGraw-Hill Connect Integrated EHR

Nearly 70 hands-on simulated EHRclinic exercises are available through *Connect*:

- EHRclinic exercises appear in Chapters 3–9 and 11. The exercises in Chapters 3–9 are correlated to Learning Outcomes, while the exercises in Chapter 11 include references back to earlier chapters.
- EHRclinic exercises include the following modes (with the instructor deciding which modes to assign to the students):
  - *Demo Mode—watch a demonstration of the exercise (includes optional audio of the steps)*
  - *Practice Mode—try the exercise yourself with guidance (includes optional audio of the steps)*
  - *Assessment Mode—complete the exercise on your own*
- Students receive a score from *Connect* after completing each mode. They receive 100% for completing all steps in Demo Mode and again in Practice Mode. They receive a percentage based on how many steps they execute correctly in Assessment Mode.
- For each EHRclinic exercise, the same data is used for all of the modes in order to reinforce the skill being taught in that exercise.

- Each EHRclinic exercise is labeled with
  - *HIM (health information management)*
  - *PM (practice management)*
  - *EHR (electronic health records)*
  - *Or some combination of the above three*

Much more information on how to complete the exercises in *Connect* can be found in the Library tab in *Connect* (instructor access only).

Instructor Resources

You can rely on the following materials to help you and your students work through the material in the book; all are available in the Instructor Resources under the Library tab in *Connect* (available only to instructors who are logged in to *Connect*).

Supplement	Features
Instructor's Manual (Organized by Learning Outcomes)	Each chapter has • Lesson Plans and Teaching Tips • Outline of PowerPoint Presentations • Answer Keys for Check Your Understanding Questions and End-of-Chapter Questions
PowerPoint Presentations (Organized by Learning Outcomes)	• Key Terms • Key Concepts • Created using MHE Accessible Template

Supplement	Features
Electronic Test Bank	- Computerized and *Connect* - Word Version - Questions are tagged with learning outcomes, level of difficulty, level of Bloom's taxonomy, feedback, ABHES, CAAHEP, and CAHIIM competencies.
Tools to Plan Course	- Transition Guide, by chapter, from Shanholtzer, 3e, to Shanholtzer, 4e - Correlations by learning outcomes to ABHES, CAAHEP, CAHIIM, and NHA - Sample Syllabi and Lesson Plans - Certificate of Completion - Asset Map—a recap of the key Instructor Resources, tied to the Learning Outcomes, as well as information on the content available through *Connect*
Tips for EHRclinic Exercises	- Multiple documents to help you and your students implement the EHRclinic exercises in your course through *Connect*

Want to learn more about this product? Attend one of our online webinars. To learn more about them, please contact your McGraw-Hill learning technology representative. To find your McGraw-Hill representative, go to www .mheducation.com and click "Get Support," select "Higher Ed," and then click the "Get Started" button under the "Find Your Sales Rep" section.

Need help? Contact the McGraw-Hill Education Customer Experience Group (CXG). Visit the CXG website at www.mhhe.com/support. Browse our frequently asked questions (FAQs) and product documentation and/or contact a CXG representative.

Walkthrough of EHRclinic Exercises in *Connect*

EHR Matters . . . Be Prepared!

Complete nearly 70 simulated EHRclinic exercises, organized into the following modes (the instructor will determine which modes are assigned to the students):

DEMO: Watch a demonstration of the exercise. Note the Path Window on the right of the screen, which can be expanded, collapsed, or hidden to allow full view of the exercise screen. Audio is available with this mode. This mode is autograded based on completion of the entire exercise.

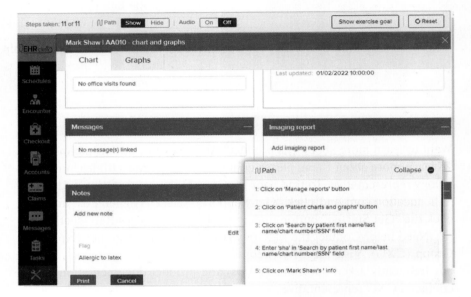

PRACTICE: Try the same exercise yourself with guidance. The Path Window and audio are also available with this mode. This mode is also autograded based on completion of the entire exercise.

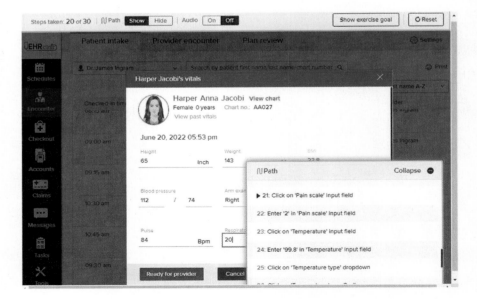

ASSESSMENT: Complete the same exercise on your own, without on-screen steps for guidance. This mode is graded on the data submitted, rather than the correct order of steps, so you are able to use critical thinking skills to complete exercises and correct errors prior to submission, with no point penalty.

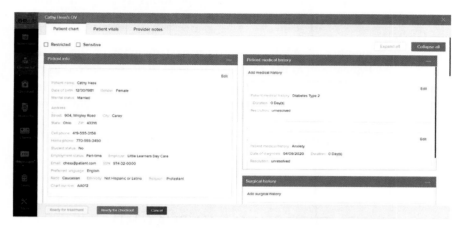

about the Authors

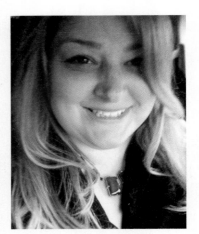

M. Beth Shanholtzer, MAEd, FAHIMA, RHIA
Courtesy of Beth Shanholtzer

M. Beth Shanholtzer, MAEd, FAHIMA, RHIA, has been in the health information management field for 39 years. Her experience has included HIM department management positions within hospitals in New Jersey, Pennsylvania, West Virginia, and Maryland. She has been in academics for 27 years and is currently the program director for a HIM associate degree program, a medical billing and coding certificate program, and a medical administrative assistant certificate program at Lord Fairfax Community College in Middletown, Virginia. She previously held positions as program director and instructor of associate degree programs at Kaplan University (now Purdue Global).

She is a member of AHIMA and is a past member of the AHIMA Assembly on Education (AOE). On the state level, Beth has served as president, education chair, and legislative chair of the West Virginia Health Information Management Association; and is currently a member of the Virginia Health Information Management Association.

Beth lives in Martinsburg, West Virginia, with her husband, Neil; they have three children.

Amy Ensign, MBA, BHSA, CMA (AAMA), RMA (AMT), has been in the medical field for over 20 years, working clinically, administratively, and in higher education. Beginning her career as a medical assistant with one of Michigan's major healthcare organizations, she moved into a leadership role working with senior management and supervising medical assistants. During this time, she began teaching as an adjunct instructor for Baker College and 10 years ago moved into her current position as medical assistant and medical administrative specialist program director for Baker College of Clinton Township. She is also active in the AAMA as treasurer of Michigan's Macomb Chapter. Amy lives in Sterling Heights, Michigan, with her husband; they have two children.

Amy Ensign, MBA, BHSA, CMA (AAMA), RMA (AMT)
Courtesy of Amy Ensign

acknowledgments

Suggestions have been received from faculty and students throughout the country. This vital feedback is important for product development. Each person who has offered comments and suggestions has our thanks. The efforts of many people are needed to develop and improve a product. Among these people are the reviewers and consultants who point out areas of concern, cite areas of strength, and make recommendations for change. In this regard, the following instructors provided feedback that was enormously helpful.

Textbook Reviewers

Multiple instructors reviewed the book prior to publication, providing valuable feedback that directly impacted the book.

Erika Bailey, MBA, RHIA
Grand Valley State University

Lorraine U. Brown, MSPH, RHIA, CCS, CCS-P
College of Southern Nevada

Kelsey Brunner, CPC, CPMA, CRC, CCS-P, CMRS
University of Rochester

Denese Davis, RN, MED, RHIT
Wiregrass Georgia Technical College

Savanna Garrity, CPC, MPA
Madisonville Community College

Janis A. Klawitter, AS, CPC, CPB, CPC-I, Provider Audits/Analytics
Bakersfield Family Medical Center

Tracey A. McKethan, MBA, RHIA, CCA
Springfield Technical Community College

Victoria L. Mills, MBA, RHIA
Gordon State College

Corina Miranda, CMPC-I, CMRS, CPC, CIC, CPCO
Alamo Community Colleges

Samuel P. Newberry, DC
Bryant & Stratton College

Donna Pritchard, RHIA LPN
Ozarks Technical Community College

Patricia Saccone, MA, RHIA, CDIP, CCS-P, CPB
Waubonsee Community College

Special thanks to the instructors who helped with the development of *Connect* and the EHRclinic Exercises. These include:

Julie Alles, DHA, RHIA
Grand Valley State University

Angela M. Chisley, AHI, RMA, CMA, AMCA
Gwinnet College

Laura Diggle, CMA (AAMA)
Independence University

Terri Fleming, EdD
Ivy Tech Community College

Savanna Garrity, CPC, MPA
Madisonville Community College

Corina Miranda, CMPC-I, CMRS, CPC, CIC, CPCO
Northwest Vista Community College

Janna Pacey, DHA, RHIA
Grand Valley State University

Kristi Perillo-Okeke, DC, CMRS
Bryant & Stratton College

Donna Pritchard, RHIA LPN
Ozarks Technical Community College

Patricia Saccone, MA, RHIA, CDIP, CCS-P, CPB
Waubonsee Community College

Acknowledgments from the Authors

From Beth Shanholtzer: This text is dedicated to my family, who are always supportive and patient when I ask "How's this sound?" over and over again; to my colleagues, who are encouraging and give great advice; and to my students, who remind me every day why I love being an educator. As always, a special thank you to the McGraw-Hill Health Professions team for guiding this project along so smoothly—particularly Michelle Flomenhoft, Erin DeHeck, Laura Bies, and Bill Lawrenson—and for giving me the opportunity to share my years of practical and academic experience through this text. And finally, to Amy Ensign; collaborating with you has been a joy—thank you!

From Amy Ensign: I would like to say a special thank you to the McGraw-Hill Health Professions Team, namely Michelle Flomenhoft, Bill Lawrensen, and all of the folks who work behind the scenes to make the magic happen. Thanks to Erin DeHeck, Product Developer, and Laura Bies, Senior Content Project Manager at McGraw Hill for their skillful work on this project.

I would also like to thank a very special friend, Liz Hoffman, and Baker College for providing me with the opportunity many years ago to blend my medical background with academia. It has been a wonderful experience to reach out to the medical community and touch the lives of patients exponentially through my students. I am grateful!

A final thank you to my family, Jason, Ryan, and Brandon, who have been patient and supportive champions of every endeavor I undertake. You are the foundation of all of my successes!

From All: Much appreciation goes to the McGraw-Hill staff for bringing this product to life: Bill Lawrensen, Executive Portfolio Manager for Health Professions; Roxan Kinsey, Executive Marketing Manager for Health Professions; Yvonne Lloyd, Business Product Manager for Health Professions; Michelle Flomenhoft, Senior Product Developer for Health Professions; Laura Bies, Senior Content Project Manager, Tammy Juran, Lead Content Project Manager, Sue Culbertson, Senior Buyer; David Hash, Lead Designer, and Melissa Homer, Senior Content Licensing Specialist. Additional thanks go to Karen Jozefowicz for the support on the digital end, as well as to Joan Weber, Senior Product Developer, for managing SmartBook.

We would also like to thank our partners at Tricon for their continued support of this project, especially Hima Bindu and her team.

An Overview of

EHRclinic's Practice Management and Electronic Health Record Software

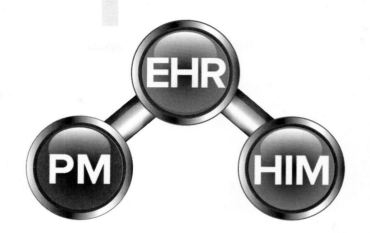

Learning Outcomes

At the end of this chapter, the student should be able to

1.1 Describe practice management applications.

1.2 List the advantages and disadvantages of an electronic health record.

1.3 Describe EHR applications.

1.4 Chart the flow of information from registration through processing of the claim.

1.5 Use the Help feature in EHRclinic.

Key Terms

Application

Care provider

Clearinghouse

Current Procedural Terminology (CPT®)

Demographic (identifying) data

Electronic claims submission

Electronic health record (EHR)

Electronic medical record (EMR)

Encounter form (Superbill or routing slip)

HIPAA Transactions and Code Set Rule (TCS)

International Classification of Diseases, 10th revision, Clinical Modification/Procedure Coding System (ICD-10-CM/PCS)

Interoperability

Master Patient Index (MPI)

Patient List

Point of care

Practice management (PM)

Routing slip (encounter form or Superbill)

Speech recognition technology

Superbill (encounter form or routing slip)

The Big Picture

What You Need to Know and Why You Need to Know It

The purpose of this worktext is to introduce students to software used to gather, track, and store the clinical and administrative information of patients seen in the medical facility. This information is used for coordinating patient care; for filing claims for reimbursement; for reporting practice information to insurance carriers as well as government and nongovernment agencies; and for gathering statistics about the types of patients treated at the facility. We will be using EHRclinic practice management (PM) and electronic health record (EHR) software throughout the text. This worktext is not meant to teach all the functionality of EHRclinic; instead, it is meant to demonstrate the most common electronic functions carried out in a medical office, hospital, or other healthcare facility.

This first chapter is an introduction and overview. The concepts in this chapter will be further explained throughout the text.

Practice management (PM) Software used in physicians' offices to gather data on every patient and perform administrative functions from the time an appointment is made through the time the bill for each visit is paid.

Electronic health record (EHR) Comprehensive record of all health records for a patient, which is able to be shared electronically with other healthcare providers as necessary.

Electronic medical record (EMR) The legal patient record that is created within any healthcare facility (hospital, nursing home, ambulatory surgery facility, physician's office, etc.). The EMR is the data source for the electronic health record (EHR).

for your information

A healthcare facility is a hospital, physician's practice, dental practice, outpatient diagnostic center, outpatient rehabilitation, outpatient psychological services, hospice, home healthcare, long-term care, or ambulatory surgery center.

for your information

The length of an office visit is based on the reason for the patient's visit. For example, a follow-up appointment for an earache might be assigned a 10-minute appointment, whereas a physical exam might be allotted 30 minutes or more, depending on the practice's policies.

1.1 Practice Management Applications

Typically, software (computer programs that carry out functions or operations) used in a medical office for administrative functions is known as **practice management (PM)** software. Filing an insurance claim for a patient is an example of an administrative function. Through the use of PM software, data are gathered on every patient from the time an appointment is made through the time the bill for each visit is paid. **Electronic health (medical) record (EHR/EMR)** software includes the clinical documentation of patient care. The patient's chief complaint, record of vital signs, results of physical examination, past medical history, and documentation of any therapy or procedures performed are all examples of clinical data.

EHRclinic software provides both a PM and an EHR solution using a single database. The use of this single database to document the administrative and clinical aspects of patient care allows the provider to concentrate on the care of the patient, improve the quality of the documentation collected, and share that documentation with other healthcare providers as appropriate, with the result of better coordination of the patient's overall care.

We will first look at the applications typically found in practice management software, including EHRclinic. *Practice management* is a term used in physicians' practices. In other healthcare facilities, including hospitals, these functions will also be computerized but are referred to as Registration, Admission, Discharge, Transfer (RADT); billing systems; or something similar.

The main applications of practice management include

- Entering each patient seen into a master list
- Scheduling appointments/registering an inpatient
- Assigning ICD-10-CM/PCS and CPT® codes after the visit is complete
- Completing a billing claim form for each visit
- Sending the insurance claims to insurance carriers

More details on each of these applications follow.

Entering Each Patient Seen into a Master Patient Index

Each patient seen, whether in a physician's office or a hospital, is only entered once into what is known as the **Patient List** or **Master Patient Index (MPI)** (listings of all patients seen in an office or hospital). These will be further discussed in a future chapter. This is done during the registration process. The first time a patient is registered, the patient is entered into the Master Patient Index/Patient List; on subsequent visits, the Master Patient Index/Patient List is searched for that patient, and any changes in demographic information, such as a change in address, phone number, or insurance coverage are made. The current encounter appears once the registration is complete as well.

It is during the registration process that consent forms to treat as well as to bill insurance are typically signed.

Scheduling Appointments

To maintain efficiency in an office, it is important that appointment times are entered accurately. Think of it this way—if a patient were told to come to the office for an appointment at a particular date and time, but the appointment book showed another date and time for that patient to be seen, the end result would be disorganization for the office as well as unhappy patients and staff. Computerizing this function allows sufficient time to be allotted to each patient based on the reason for his or her visit, and it allows for more efficient scheduling of the provider's time. In a hospital setting, appointments are only made if the hospital runs clinics, for instance orthopedic or cardiac clinics where patients are seen by care providers on an outpatient basis. These are common in Veterans Hospitals.

Assigning ICD-10-CM/PCS and CPT® Codes

You may have noticed during a visit to your own physician's office that you are given a piece of paper when you leave the examining room. This is referred to as an **encounter form**, a **Superbill**, or a **routing slip**. For our purposes throughout this worktext, we will refer to this as a Superbill. There are many numbers, known as codes, on the Superbill. Every diagnosis made by a care provider is written in narrative form in a patient's health record and then carried over to the Superbill. These narrative diagnoses are converted into alphanumeric form with a coding system known as **International Classification of Diseases, 10th revision, Clinical Modification (ICD-10-CM)**. In a hospital setting, *procedures* are coded using **International Classification of Diseases, 10th revision, Procedure Coding System (ICD-10-PCS)**. In a physician's practice or other outpatient setting, the same occurs for each procedure performed, but the coding system used is **Current Procedural Terminology (CPT®)**. Since CPT® codes represent procedures (or in some instances, services), the amount of money charged for that service is also connected with each CPT® code, and will be transferred to the bill for the encounter. The Superbill and coding functions will be covered in detail in the chapter on insurance and billing functions of this worktext. Most likely, you will have a separate course or courses in billing and coding as well.

Master Patient Index (MPI)/Patient List A permanent listing of all patients who have received care in a hospital (inpatient or outpatient). In physicians' offices often referred to as a Master Patient List or Patient List. May also be known as a Master Person List or Master Person Index.

Superbill A document (paper or electronic) that is used in medical offices to capture the diagnoses and services or procedures performed and from which the CMS-1500 billing form is completed. Also known as a routing slip or encounter form.

International Classification of Diseases, 10th revision, Clinical Modification (ICD-10-CM) and Procedure Coding System (ICD-10-PCS) ICD-10-CM is the classification system used to convert narrative diagnoses into alpha-numeric codes in all healthcare settings.

ICD-10-PCS is the classification system used to convert narrative procedures into alphanumeric codes in hospital settings.

Effective October 1, 2015, these classification systems replaced ICD-9-CM.

Current Procedural Terminology (CPT®) Coding system used to convert narrative procedures and services into numeric form. CPT® is used to code procedures and services in a physician's office; in a hospital setting, it is used for outpatient coding (emergency room, outpatient diagnostic testing, or ambulatory surgery, for example).

Completing a Billing Claim Form for Each Visit

In order to submit bills to health insurance carriers, a claim form must be generated for each visit. This is done by compiling the patient's identifying data, his or her insurance data, and the ICD-10-CM/PCS and/or CPT® codes into claim forms such as the CMS-837P (electronic) or CMS-1500 (paper), which are used by physicians' practices and other outpatient settings, or the UB-04, which is used to bill hospital, rehabilitation, end-stage renal facility, and other long-term care–type settings.

Sending the Insurance Claims to Insurance Carriers

Once the claim form is generated, it is submitted to the insurance carrier for payment. Some hard-copy claim forms are still mailed to the insurance carrier, but the majority of forms are sent by **electronic claims submission**. If filed electronically, it is done so using a set of standards that are mandated by the **HIPAA Transactions and Code Set Rule (TCS)**. Electronic filing is faster and more accurate, and it is actually less expensive for the healthcare facility. Filing a claim electronically means that the information is sent by wire to a **clearinghouse** or directly to the insurance carrier. A clearinghouse is a service that processes data into a standardized billing format and checks for inconsistencies or other errors in the data. Filing claims electronically reduces billing errors and processing time, which results in faster payment.

The patient's **demographic (identifying) data** are collected as part of the administrative (non-clinical) information, as well as information needed for the business processes that take place in a healthcare facility—for instance, gathering insurance information, completing a claim form, and submitting a claim.

Administrative data include insurance and financial data, authorization to bill the insurance company, correspondence related to billing matters, and the like. Demographic data identify the patient—name, address, phone numbers, sex, race, and so on. The demographic data are specific administrative data that help differentiate one patient from another with the same name.

Electronic claims submission
Submitting insurance claims via wire to a clearinghouse or directly to the insurance carrier.

HIPAA Transactions and Code Set Rule (TCS) Adopted in fiscal year 2003, a set of rules that standardized the electronic exchange of patient-identifiable, health-related information. This rule set is based on electronic data interchange (EDI) standards, and its purpose is to simplify the processes and decrease the costs associated with payment for healthcare services.

Clearinghouse A service that processes data into a standardized billing format and checks for inconsistencies or other errors in the data.

Demographic (identifying) data Data that identify the patient. Consist of name, date of birth, sex, race, and Social Security number (may vary by facility policy).

Check Your Understanding

1. Would EHRclinic be described as a practice management tool, an electronic health record, or both? Explain your answer.
2. List the types of data gathered during the registration process that eventually appears on the insurance claim form for that encounter.

1.2 Why Adopt Electronic Health Record Applications?

The widespread acceptance of an electronic health record has lagged behind other industries such as banking or retail. Healthcare administrators and care providers have long been leery of electronic health records. Security concerns, the lengthy implementation process, and the high cost of implementing an EHR headline the reasons for a culture of uncertainty and a "let's wait and see" attitude. The perception has been that paper records are more secure—not as susceptible to loss, theft, or tampering—since there is a tangible object that can be seen or carried from place to place by a human being. In reality, paper records are potentially more susceptible to loss or tampering than an electronic record. A paper record cannot be "followed," whereas every entry, change, or view of an electronic record can be tracked and reported. With proper backup procedures, EHRs cannot be lost or misfiled, which is not the case with paper records. Of course, if a patient's name is misspelled or if a patient used a different name on a previous registration, then location will be difficult, but there are other ways to search for the record such as by date of birth, which is not possible with a paper record. Security will be discussed in more detail in the chapter on privacy and security.

The initial purchase and implementation costs of an EMR/EHR are high—much higher than the cost of file folders and filing equipment in a paper system. The research and development of an electronic system by service providers (software companies), the allocation of human resources for planning and training, and the cost of hardware and additional software all contribute to these costs. There is an ongoing cost of maintaining any system, paper or electronic. The return on investment of an electronic system is in enhanced patient safety and improved quality of care, less duplication of effort, a more efficiently run office, instant access to patient health records, and the data needed for reporting purposes. Though for a time the paper system will still be maintained, gradually the costs of filing supplies, the physical space needed for paper records, and long-term storage (archiving) will lessen once the electronic system is in place.

For care providers, there is a high learning curve, and they must be willing to devote time to the new system before it is second nature to them. Now that it has been approximately six years into fairly widespread use of the EHR, many physicians are turning to the use of medical scribes to document in the EHR as the physician dictates his or her findings while examining the patient. Medical scribes will be discussed in a later chapter.

As for administrative staff, learning an EHR system is more time consuming and has a higher learning curve than the manual processes associated with paper records. After all, filing, whether alphabetic or numeric, is more intuitive than searching a computer database or knowing which screen a particular piece of data resides on; and again, a piece of paper or a folder full of papers is tangible, whereas an electronic system is not.

Sharing information has also been a sticking point. Though patients have had access to their records for many years, they were not well informed about how to gain that access, and many did not know that they could even request an amendment to their health records. Healthcare providers have been fearful of releasing patients' health records to others, including other healthcare providers, because there is a sense of loss of control over the information and lack of confidentiality.

This sharing of health information with other healthcare providers or entities is possible because of **interoperability**. It means that many different functions can take place and information can be shared between computer systems, or within applications of the same computer system, which is not possible with a manual or paper record system. For instance, in her physician's practice, Alicia Matthews' medical information is readily accessible and just a couple of clicks away regardless of whether a pharmacy needs a list of her allergies before refilling a prescription or the practice's billing staff needs her policy number. Also, let's say Alicia is a patient of Dr. Ingram. She has been seen for repeated bouts of strep throat. Dr. Ingram has referred her to Dr. Johnson, an otorhinolaryngologist (ear, nose, and throat specialist). Her appointment with Dr. Johnson is set up for July 2. When she arrives for her appointment, Dr. Johnson already

Interoperability Many different functions can take place and information can be shared between computer systems, or within applications of the same computer system, which is not possible with a manual or paper record system.

has her records from Dr. Ingram, and rather than having to take all of Alicia's information over again, the doctor can spend the time examining Alicia and determining a plan of care. Because the computer systems at the two offices are interoperable, the information can be shared seamlessly.

A January 2019 article by the U.S. Department of Health and Human Services Patient Safety Network noted that research has shown a decrease in medical errors, improved guideline adherence, enhanced safety attitudes and job satisfaction among physicians (after the implementation phase was complete); however, this study did uncover other issues with EHR use—for instance, ease of usability, which will be covered throughout the text as necessary. EHRs do support an increase in timeliness of diagnosis and treatment due in large part to timely access to information—for instance, a patient's allergy to penicillin or the fact that a patient has already had her gallbladder removed, thus there are care providers and administrators who are more open-minded and are pushing for totally paperless systems within their facilities. Increasingly, healthcare providers are accepting that an informed patient is a more compliant patient and that patients should have a say in their medical care.

Compliance with government regulations and accreditation standards is also made easier and more efficient through the use of an electronic health record. Additionally, report-writing capabilities available in electronic systems allow for fast, reliable data submission and retrieval.

Table 1.1 shows a comparison of issues encountered in paper record-keeping versus electronic record-keeping.

From a more global perspective, the use of electronic medical records will allow for the collection of incredible amounts of clinical data for use in medical research and epidemiology, which will have a profound effect on healthcare worldwide.

TABLE 1.1	Comparison of Paper to Electronic Health Records
Paper Health Records	**Electronic Health Records**
Security concerns include theft and tampering with documentation.	Security concerns include loss of data and computer hackers.
Individual records are easily lost or misfiled.	Misfiling is not an issue as long as the patient's name is spelled correctly.
Startup costs are relatively inexpensive.	Startup costs are relatively high.
Operating costs are relatively inexpensive, as the system does not change drastically from year to year.	Operating costs are dependent on the level of support from the software vendor, maintenance costs, and cost of upgrades.
Records take up a great deal of space.	They do not take up physical space other than desktop computers.
Archiving costs are high.	Archiving costs are for disk or server space.
Training staff is a relatively short and inexpensive process.	Staff and physician training is time-consuming.
Physicians perceive that writing or dictating is easier than typing into a computer.	Once learned, documentation is easily done by point and click or voice recognition systems.
Documentation by care providers tends to be less detailed.	Documentation by care providers tends to be more detailed.
Sharing health information with other care providers or healthcare facilities is a time-consuming process and may delay diagnosis or treatment.	Sharing health information with other care providers or healthcare facilities is done in a timely manner and may assist in timely diagnosis and treatment.

Check Your Understanding

1. Is a paper-based system of records more secure than an electronic one? Explain your answer.
2. Why are startup costs significantly higher with EHRs versus paper-based records?

1.3 Electronic Health Record Applications

Now, let's take a look at common functionality of an electronic health record.

It is through the EHR functionality that clinical information is collected and includes the patient's medical history, the patient's current condition(s), the treatment rendered, the results of treatment, the prognosis, the plan of care, the diagnosis, and any instructions given by the provider.

Individual functions of an electronic health record (or any computer system) are referred to as **applications** and often include

- Clinical documentation of a patient's visit (the progress note) by the **care provider**
- The prescribing of medications and their electronic submission to the patient's pharmacy of choice through the use of electronic prescribing (sometimes referred to as ePrescribing)
- Electronic exchange of clinical information between medical providers or other entities with a need to know
- The ability to access clinical trials, evidence-based medicine, and pharmaceutical research to improve patient care, as well as access to clinical and financial benchmarking services to enhance financial management
- Mobile EHR applications available on personal digital assistants (PDAs) or smartphones to allow providers instant access anytime and anywhere
- **Point of care (POC)** dictation of progress notes by the provider using **speech recognition technology**. Speech recognition technology allows documentation to occur on the computer screen as the care provider dictates notes. *Point of care* refers to the dictation that occurs at the very time the patient is being seen.

Application Software that has a special purpose, such as word processing or spreadsheet, or is for a particular industry such as practice management or electronic health record software.

Care provider Term used to refer to a physician, physician's assistant, dentist, psychologist, nurse practitioner, or midwife.

Point of care (POC) Documentation, dictation, and ordering of tests and procedures that occur at the same time the patient is being seen.

Speech recognition technology Software that recognizes the words being said by the person dictating and digitally converts the speech to text; as it is used it "learns" the dictator's voice, and therefore improves the accuracy of the transcription.

Check Your Understanding

1. Documentation done as care is being given is known as_____ —for instance, dictating while examining the patient.
2. Dr. Smith uses her smartphone to document a phone call she made from home to a patient. She used _____ EHR technology to do this.
3. Dr. Harrison's office uses EHRclinic as its practice management (PM) and electronic health record (EHR) solution. For each of the following, which application within EHRclinic would be used? Would it be ePrescribing, EHR, electronic exchange of information, voice recognition technology, or scheduling? Select the *best* answer. (An application may be used more than once or not at all.)

(continued)

a. Elaine Verados is a patient of Dr. Harrison, and he has referred her to Dr. Smithton, an otorhinolaryngologist, for an opinion on treating a persistent problem with her right ear. Dr. Harrison documents the patient's history, the results of the physical examination, and his diagnosis in her _____.

b. As Dr. Smithton concludes his examination of Elaine Verados, he dictates a letter to Dr. Harrison, giving his opinion of Elaine Verados' condition using _____.

c. Carl Pike calls the office of Dr. Harrison because he wishes to establish care at that office. Dr. Harrison is taking new patients, so a mutually agreed-upon time is set up for Carl to have a physical exam by Dr. Harrison. The application used to do this is _____.

d. Dr. Harrison documents Carl Pike's known drug allergies. This is done in which application? _____

e. Dr. Harrison dictates the results of Carl Pike's physical examination, and his words appear on the computer screen as he is speaking. This application is _____.

1.4 The Flow of Information from Registration through Processing of the Claim

If you think about your past experiences visiting a physician's office, you will recognize many of the steps in the processes described below, and how similar they are to your experience. Of course, not every step is exactly the same in every office, but the basic premise is the same.

In step one (Figure 1.1) an appointment is made. Of course, if the patient is going to an urgent care center or an emergency room, this step is not necessary. Once the appointment is made, the patient arrives at the

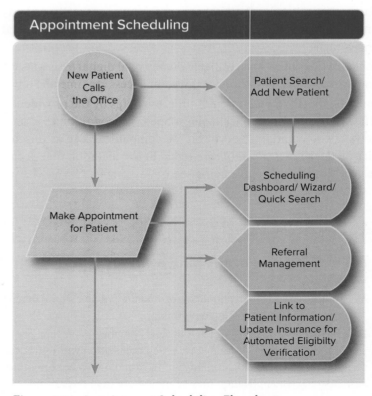

Figure 1.1   Appointment Scheduling Flowchart

office on the day and time of the appointment and is "checked in." This is known as "registration"— some of the patient's administrative data may have been taken over the phone, but the data may be verified and more may be collected when the patient arrives for the appointment. Also, if new authorization forms or other administrative forms need to be signed, that is done at this point.

After the patient has checked in, he or she waits to be seen by the care providers (Figure 1.2). First, the patient is called back to the exam room by a healthcare professional (Figure 1.3); his or her height, weight, and vital signs (temperature, pulse, blood pressure) are taken; and a series of questions are asked about why the patient is being seen today, the patient's medical history, and medications the patient is currently taking. Once those are complete, the care provider steps in for the actual exam (Figure 1.4).

Once the care provider has completed the exam, assessed the patient's condition, and determined a plan of care, including instructions to the patient, the business functions begin (Figure 1.5 and Figure 1.6). These include the check-out and billing procedures. Some of these procedures are repeated or continue for several weeks or months until the claim is paid and the patient's account reflects a zero balance.

In cases where the care provider has ordered diagnostic procedures such as x-rays or laboratory tests, the clinical documentation steps are repeated (Figure 1.7).

for your information — fyi
The term *care provider* will be used to refer to any physician, physician's assistant, dentist, psychologist, nurse practitioner, or midwife.

for your information — fyi
The medical assistant, nurse, receptionist, health information technician, medical biller/coder, and office administrative personnel will be referred to as *healthcare professionals* throughout the text.

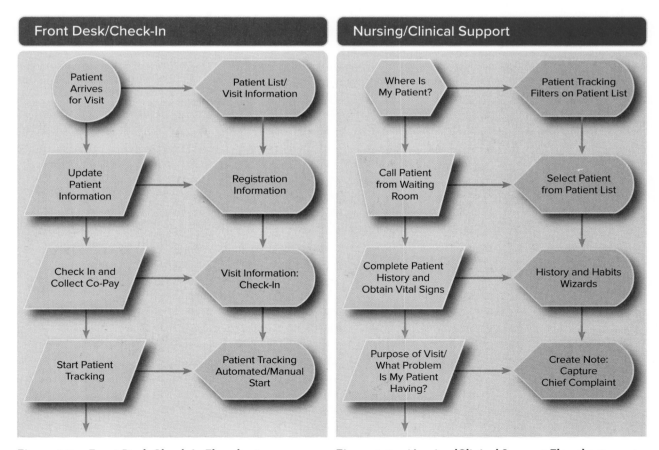

Figure 1.2   **Front Desk Check-In Flowchart**

Figure 1.3   **Nursing/Clinical Support Flowchart**

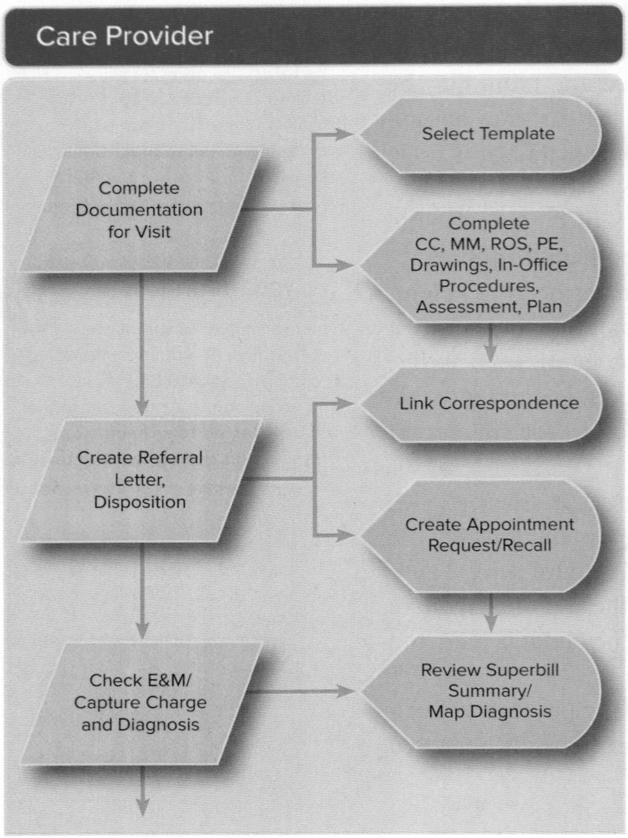

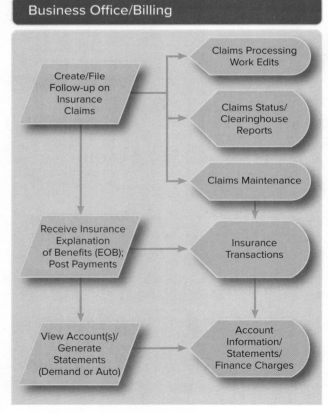

Figure 1.4   Care Provider Flowchart

Figure 1.6   Business Office/Billing Flowchart

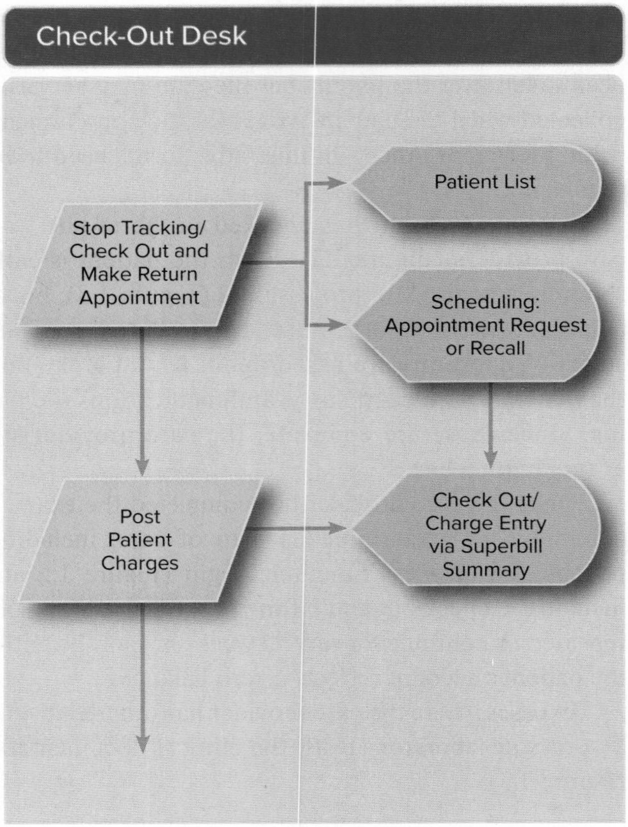

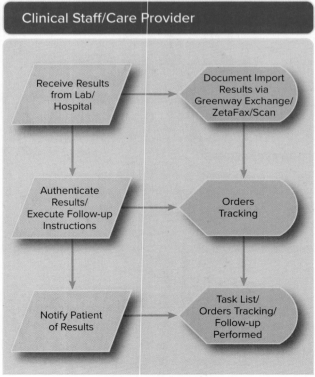

Figure 1.5   Check-Out Desk Flowchart

Figure 1.7   Clinical Staff/Care Provider Flowchart

Check Your Understanding

1. Put the following steps in the flow of information into the correct order: front desk checks in the patient; business office/billing processes charges; the patient is processed at check-out desk; appointment scheduling personnel make patient's appointment; nursing/clinical support sees patient; clinical staff/care provider examines patient.

2. Under what circumstances would clinical documentation steps need to be repeated?

1.5 Use of the Help Feature

The use of Help text or of a Help function is standard in most software applications. You have no doubt used it from time to time when preparing word processing or spreadsheet applications. EHRclinic is no different.

EHRclinic Help text can be accessed through any screen, as you can see in Figure 1.8.

The care provider or healthcare professional can gain access to the entire User's Guide or just the topic needed at that time. For instance, if you want to know more about vocabulary reconciliation, locating that section of

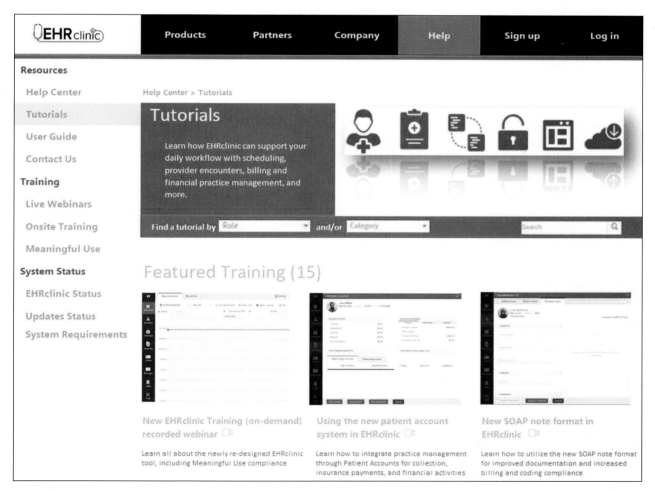

Figure 1.8   EHRclinic Help Feature

the User's Guide is easily found by doing a keyword search, where the system begins to predict what you are searching for based on the first few characters typed in the search field. You have probably done something similar in other software when using an online dictionary or glossary.

The important thing about Help is that it is there for just that—to help you learn to use EHRclinic, to assist you when you are unsure of the steps you need to complete, and to keep you up to date with changes or new functionality added to the software.

Check Your Understanding

1. You are a new employee and you are registering a patient. You have a question, but no one is nearby to ask. What can you do within EHRclinic to find your answer?
2. Why might someone need to use the Help feature?

chapter 1 **summary**

LEARNING OUTCOME	CONCEPTS FOR REVIEW

1.1 Describe practice management applications.	– What is practice management?
	– Practice management applications
	  • Master Patient Index/Patient List
	  • Schedule appointments
	  • Assign ICD-10-CM/PCS and CPT® codes
	  • Complete billing claim form
	  • Send insurance claims to carriers

1.2 List the advantages and disadvantages of an electronic health record.	– Disadvantages
	  • Increased security concerns
	  • High cost of implementation
	  • Training requirements
	– Advantages
	  • Possibly more secure than paper records
	  • High return on investment
	  • All information in one place
	  • Interoperability
	  • Assures regulatory compliance
	  • Exchange of information with those who have a need to know

1.3 Describe EHR applications.	– Clinical documentation – Electronic prescribing – Exchange of clinical information – Research evidence–based medicine, pharmaceutical research, clinical and financial benchmarking studies – Speech recognition

1.4 Chart the flow of information from registration through processing of the claim.	– Appointment scheduling
	– Front desk check-in
	  • Verify demographic information
	  • Sign authorization/administrative forms, if necessary
	– Patient taken to examining room
	  • Height, weight, vital signs taken
	  • Patient states the reason for today's visit (chief complaint)

(continued)

LEARNING OUTCOME	CONCEPTS FOR REVIEW	

	- Care provider meets with the patient
	  • Provider verifies reason for visit, updates history
	  • Provider examines patient
	  • Provider makes referrals, if necessary
	  • Prescriptions electronically sent to pharmacy, if necessary
	  • Provider completes the chart, which then starts the coding and claims process
	  • Provider completes the visit and provides patient with a Superbill, routing slip, or encounter form
	- Patient stops at the check-out desk
	  • Superbill/routing slip/encounter form given to staff member at the check-out desk
	  • Patient pays co-pay, if not paid during check-in process
	  • Patient leaves the office
	- Business office/billing
	  • Insurance claim form completed electronically
	  • Insurance claim submitted electronically
	  • Insurance payment (or notice of denial) received
	  • Payment entered in the system
	  • Patient's account updated
	  • Statement sent, if necessary
	- Follow-up
	  • Results of diagnostic tests received, if applicable
	  • Record updated with results
	  • Provider reviews results
	  • Patient contacted, if necessary	

1.5 Use the Help feature in EHRclinic.	- Understand the use of the Help feature - Name the help features available in EHRclinic	

MATCHING QUESTIONS

Match the terms on the left with the definitions on the right.

_____ 1. **[LO 1.2]** interoperability

_____ 2. **[LO 1.3]** application

_____ 3. **[LO 1.3]** care provider

_____ 4. **[LO 1.1]** clearinghouse

_____ 5. **[LO 1.1]** electronic claims submission

_____ 6. **[LO 1.1]** encounter form

_____ 7. **[LO 1.3]** point of care (POC)

_____ 8. **[LO 1.1]** practice management software

_____ 9. **[LO 1.3]** speech recognition

_____ 10. **[LO 1.1]** demographics

a. form generated at the completion of an office visit, a portion of which details the patient's diagnosis, the procedures and services performed, and the charge for each procedure/service

b. filing of a healthcare claim using a computer rather than paper

c. technology that digitally transcribes spoken words

d. specialized computer software that performs administrative and billing procedures in medical offices

e. documented patient information such as age, sex, and race

f. procedures that take place at the time of care, rather than at a remote location or at a point in time after care is complete

g. person, usually a physician, who performs healthcare services requiring specialized education and training

h. software with a unique purpose, such as word processing, or used for a specific industry

i. allows syncing of multiple, unrelated functions or systems

j. service that assists in claims processing by standardizing billing and performing error checks

MULTIPLE-CHOICE QUESTIONS

Select the letter that best completes the statement or answers the question:

1. **[LO 1.1]** EHR/EMR software is more comprehensive than practice management software because it
   a. is computerized.
   b. contains more menu options.
   c. includes clinical documentation.
   d. submits insurance claims.

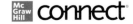

Enhance your learning by completing these exercises and more at https://**connect.mheducation.com**!

2. **[LO 1.3]** EHR applications typically
   a. allow for ePrescribing.
   b. have mobile applications.
   c. assist in information exchange.
   d. all of these.

3. **[LO 1.1]** A patient is entered into the Patient List/Master Patient Index
   a. once.
   b. twice.
   c. after a procedure.
   d. each time he or she is seen.

4. **[LO 1.2]** When transitioning from a paper to an electronic health record, healthcare facilities can expect the costs associated with health records to
   a. increase.
   b. decrease.
   c. stay the same.
   d. disappear.

5. **[LO 1.4]** The patient's demographic information (for instance, his or her address or phone number) is typically updated at what point in the information cycle?
   a. patient history
   b. physical exam
   c. registration (check-in)
   d. check-out

6. **[LO 1.3]** Clinical documentation of a patient's visit is known as the
   a. Superbill.
   b. progress note.
   c. medical claim.
   d. point of care.

7. **[LO 1.1]** An encounter form is also known as a/an
   a. EHR.
   b. history.
   c. claim form.
   d. Superbill.

8. **[LO 1.1]** The _____ is a form used to bill patient claims in physicians' offices.
   a. CMS-1500
   b. ICD-10
   c. CPT®
   d. UB-04

9. **[LO 1.2]** One factor that might contribute to slow acceptance of EHRs is
    a. security fears.
    b. laziness.
    c. fear of change.
    d. space concerns.

10. **[LO 1.3]** Which of the following illustrates clinical information collected through an EHR?
    a. insurance policy
    b. plan of care
    c. research effects
    d. regulatory guidelines

11. **[LO 1.2]** _____ is not easily attained when using a manual record system.
    a. Communication
    b. Data capture
    c. Interoperability
    d. Maintenance

12. **[LO 1.5]** EHRclinic's User's Guide is accessed through the _____ feature.
    a. Accounts
    b. Help
    c. Tools
    d. Schedules

SHORT-ANSWER QUESTIONS

1. **[LO 1.4]** List the steps included in a patient's flow of information.

2. **[LO 1.2]** Outline at least three advantages to electronic health records as discussed in the text.

3. **[LO 1.1]** What functions are performed in practice management software?

4. **[LO 1.4]** What is the first step in the patient flow of information?

5. **[LO 1.1]** Why is a claim form completed for every patient visit?

6. **[LO 1.3]** Mobile EHR applications are currently available on which mobile devices?

7. **[LO 1.2]** Define interoperability and give an example of how it might be used in the healthcare field.

8. **[LO 1.1]** What is electronic claims submission? Why is this the preferred method of claims submission?

9. **[LO 1.1]** List at least three main applications found in a typical practice management program.

10. **[LO 1.4]** What is the final step in the front desk/check-in process?

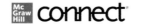 Enhance your learning by completing these exercises and more at https://**connect.mheducation.com**!

APPLYING YOUR KNOWLEDGE

1. **[LO 1.2]** Your medical office is preparing to transition from a paper-based office to an electronic one; you are really excited about this change. One day you receive an email from one of your colleagues, Sari Murray, negatively discussing the change and wondering why things cannot stay how they are now. Your colleague is looking to you and asking your opinion on the upcoming transition. Write an email back to Sari, discussing your thoughts on the change to electronic records.

2. **[LOs 1.1, 1.2, 1.3]** The physician partners in your practice have asked you to write up a justification for purchasing a PM/EHR software package such as EHRclinic. Write a thorough justification for their review.

3. **[LO 1.4]** Denise Cruz arrives at your office for her annual check-up appointment with Dr. Smith. Discuss what will happen with Denise as she moves through each step of patient flow.

4. **[LOs 1.2, 1.3]** A patient is seen in a hospital emergency department after experiencing constant, severe abdominal pain for the past three hours. After numerous tests, no cause for abdominal pain can be determined. Discuss how EHRs might help diagnose this patient.

5. **[LOs 1.1, 1.2, 1.3]** Compare and contrast a typical day in a paper-based office with a day at an office that uses practice management software.

6. **[LOs 1.1, 1.2, 1.3, 1.4, 1.5]** The medical office you work in recently transitioned into an electronic office and is implementing practice management software. You are excited about this change and are learning all you can about the new technology. However, some of your coworkers are having trouble grasping the basics and are now saying they don't want to use the software at all. What steps could you take to assist your struggling coworkers?

chapter references

U.S. Department of Health and Human Services. Agency for Healthcare Research and Quality: Patient Safety Network. *Patient Safety Primer. Electronic Health Records*. Retrieved from https://psnet.ahrq.gov /primers/primer/43/Electronic-Health-Records. January 19, 2019.

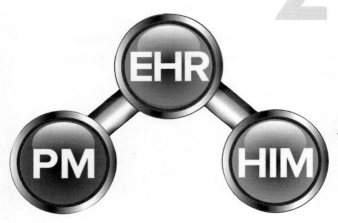

chapter **two**

Health Data Structure, Collection, and Standards

Learning Outcomes

At the end of this chapter, the student should be able to

2.1 Describe the roles of six healthcare professionals who maintain or use practice management and electronic health record applications.

2.2 Explain the difference between data and information.

2.3 Define information governance and the HIM and healthcare administrative professionals' role in it.

2.4 Identify computer-based health information media.

2.5 Relate how screen-based data collection tools are used in healthcare.

2.6 Demonstrate how individual data elements are collected.

2.7 Describe electronic health record applications.

2.8 Identify laws, regulations, and standards that govern electronic health information.

2.9 Distinguish between practice management software and hospital health information software.

Key Terms

Advancing Care Information Reporting Standards
American Recovery and Reinvestment Act of 2009 (ARRA)
Certification Commission for Health Information Technology (CCHIT)
Clinical decision support (CDS)
Data
Health and Medicine Division
Health information exchange (HIE)
Health Information Technology for Economic and Clinical Health (HITECH) Act
Health Insurance Portability and Accountability Act (HIPAA)
Healthcare administrator
Healthcare systems administrator
Information
Information governance
Institute of Medicine (IOM)
Meaningful Use (MU)

Merit-based Incentive Payment System (MIPS)
National Academies of Sciences, Engineering, and Medicine (the National Academies)
National Provider Identifier (NPI)
Nationwide Health Information Network (NHIN)
Office of the National Coordinator for Health Information Technology (ONC)
Personal health record (PHR)
Picture Archiving and Communication System (PACS)
Promoting Interoperability Program
Protected health information (PHI)
Qualitative analysis
Quantitative analysis
Regional extension center (REC)
Regional Health Information Organization (RHIO)
Structured data
Unstructured data

20

What You Need to Know and Why You Need to Know It

As a healthcare professional you will be one of many who will be selecting, maintaining, and using electronic health record and management software. Knowing who within the organization is using the software and how he or she is using it is important to selecting a system that meets the needs of the organization. The collection of data must be done efficiently while meeting the documentation requirements of licensing and accrediting agencies, as well as private insurance carriers, Medicare, and Medicaid, while conforming to the legal definition of an electronic health record. We will begin this chapter by reviewing the professionals involved and the positions they hold within the organization. Then, the concepts of data structure, collection, and standards will be introduced in preparation for a more detailed level of instruction in the remaining chapters of the text. We will also cover how data is collected; the tools used to collect the data; how data are transformed into information; and the regulations and standards that dictate the collection, maintenance, use, and storage of health information in an electronic form.

Health information management spans a wide range of functions and processes within a healthcare organization. Just about every decision is based on statistics that are largely collected from the health records of a facility or medical practice. The data that are captured will result in information used by care providers to make decisions regarding patient care and to justify reimbursement. In addition, various levels of administrators will use information in risk management activities, budgeting, strategic planning, quality assessment, and financial reporting. Report writing will be discussed in greater detail in the chapter covering decision and compliance support.

Table 2.1 depicts many of the medical professions within healthcare, the education or certifications they may hold, and the responsibilities they may have as they pertain to the collection and use of data. This is not an exhaustive list, as there are many other positions such as therapists, laboratory technicians, and radiology technicians, just to name a few. Those listed are the positions held by individuals who are more likely to be involved in selecting, implementing, maintaining, and using the electronic systems in a healthcare facility.

During the process of selecting the system, it is imperative that people with knowledge of health information standards, structure, and content be involved. In hospital settings, the health information professional fulfills this role. In addition, administrative staff who are responsible for the effective operation of the entire organization, including facility- or enterprise-wide information systems, are key to the process as well. That is not to say that individual department managers (laboratory, nursing, radiology, etc.) do not have a say—but the administrators responsible for those departments may be the key players in the early stages of system selection.

In physicians' practices, there is typically an office manager or other administrative staff member, known as health administrative professionals, with health information knowledge or credentials who will oversee the process. In smaller offices, the services of a consultant may be used, or the EHR vendor may have the health information expertise to oversee the process.

| TABLE 2.1 | Medical Professions within Healthcare |

Profession	Certifications	Description/Positions Held
Health information and informatics	• Registered Health Information Administrator (RHIA®) • Registered Health Information Technician (RHIT®) • Certified Health Data Analyst (CHDA®) • Certified in Healthcare Privacy and Security (CHPS®) • Certified Professional in Health Information and Management Systems (CPHIMS) • Clinical Documentation Improvement Specialist (CDIS)	• Work in any healthcare setting, but most often in acute care or specialty hospitals • Work in healthcare-related professions such as consultants, software trainers and installers, and employees of government agencies, and staff of insurance companies and law offices • Associate's, bachelor's, and master's degrees available • Many healthcare facilities, particularly hospitals, require certification. • Performs concurrent and/or retrospective review of documentation and suggests improvement of documentation of all conditions, treatments, and care plans to ensure highest quality of care is provided to the patient. Educates clinical staff in appropriate documentation criteria. Positions held in the following areas: • Health information department management • Information technology and systems management • Project management • Software analysis • Implementation support • Information system design • EHR implementation and management • Data analysis • Documentation management • Privacy/security assurance • Release of healthcare information oversight • Risk management • Compliance management • Utilization management • Quality assessment/assurance • Cancer registry management • Medical staff coordination • Nursing
Health information specialty areas (AHIMA Certified Healthcare Technology Specialist [CHTS] credentials)	Require completion of non-degree educational programs that prepare students for competency in • Assessing workflows • Selecting hardware and software • Working with vendors • Installing and testing systems • Diagnosing IT problems • Training practice staff on systems	• The most recent health information/informatics roles • May work in any healthcare facility, inpatient or outpatient • Each competency exam is specific to a particular role that plays a part in meaningful use of the electronic health record (EHR). • Registration/scheduling staff within healthcare facilities, particularly hospitals
Coding professionals	• Certified Coding Associate (CCA®) • Certified Coding Specialist (CCS®) • Certified Coding Specialist-Physician-based (CCS-P®) • Certified Professional Coder (CPC®) • Certified Outpatient Coder (COC®) • Certified Inpatient Coder (CIC®) • Certified Interventional Radiology Cardiovascular Coder (CIRCC®) • Specialty coding designations	• Work in all healthcare settings • Work in healthcare-related settings such as consulting firms, software vendors, insurance companies • Certificate or associate's degree Positions held in the following areas: • Medical coder • Reimbursement specialist • Insurance biller • Chargemaster specialist • Insurance claims specialist

Profession	Certifications	Description/Positions Held
Medical assistants	• Certified Medical Assistant (CMA) • Registered Medical Assistant (RMA)	• Typically employed in physician's office or other outpatient setting • Requires associate's degree or certificate • Perform clinical duties such as prepping patients, taking vital signs, taking medical histories, assisting physician during exams, explaining minor procedures and giving instructions based on physician's orders, and collecting specimens • Perform administrative duties such as answering phone, making appointments, registering patients, maintaining health records, handling correspondence, filing health insurance claims, scheduling outpatient services, arranging referrals, and managing the office in general • May hold positions as office managers or business managers within a medical practice
Healthcare administrators	• Certified Healthcare Facility Manager (CHFM) • Fellow of the American College of Healthcare Executives (FACHE) • American College of Medical Practice Executives (ACMPE) certification • Certified Practice Manager (CPM) • Certified Medical Practice Compliance Specialist (CMPCS) • Certified Physician Practice Manager (CPPM®) • Certified Healthcare Administrative Professional (CHAP®)	• Work in all healthcare organizations • Bachelor's or master's degree typically required • Plan, organize, coordinate, and direct facility or department operations Positions held with the following titles: • Hospital administrator • Chief information officer/manager • Project manager • Department manager • Office manager • Office administrator • Compliance officer
Care providers	• Physicians—Doctor of Medicine (MD), Doctor of Osteopathy (DO) • Physicians' assistants (PA, PA-C) • Certified Nurse Practitioner (CNP) • Certified Registered Nurse Midwife (CRNM)	• Work in any healthcare setting • Requires advanced education, licensure, and possibly certification • The only medical professionals who can diagnose a patient and order diagnostic testing and therapeutic (including medications) measures
Nursing	• Registered Nurse (RN) • Licensed Practical Nurse (LPN)	• Provide direct care to patients • May also hold non–direct care positions in utilization management, risk management, quality assessment, and general management within a healthcare facility • Nursing informatics • Requires associate's or bachelor's degree at a minimum; management positions and informatics positions may require a master's degree

2.1 The Professionals Who Maintain and Use Health Information

In the inpatient setting, the **healthcare administrator** may be a chief executive officer (CEO), chief operating officer (COO), chief financial officer (CFO), or chief information officer (CIO). These individuals typically have

Healthcare administrator A leadership position within a healthcare facility, including chief executive officer, chief operating officer, chief financial officer, chief information officer, or other higher-level management positions. May also be referred to as healthcare manager or health systems manager.

Healthcare systems administrator A leadership position specifically responsible for the information technology (IT) functions within an organization or facility. May also be known as a chief information officer.

a bachelor's or master's degree (preferred) in healthcare administration and are responsible for overseeing several departments (or the entire organization, in the case of the CEO). Their degree is most likely in healthcare administration, healthcare management, or health systems administration. These individuals concentrate on the big picture—the operation of the organization as a whole. **Healthcare systems administrators** are concerned with how all automated systems, including the electronic health record, affect individual departments. For example, will all the information needs of the board of directors and administration for adequate, easily obtainable decision support data be met by the current (or proposed) electronic health record system? Will the clinicians have fast, easily accessible, accurate clinical information? Is the system secure and does it meet all standards and regulations? The healthcare systems administrator may be known as the chief information officer and typically has a great deal of knowledge and experience related to the technical aspects of automated systems.

In a hospital setting, the director of the health information department and the chief information officer work closely. Each plays a key role in the selection of the product. Health information professionals have basic clinical knowledge, technical knowledge of automated systems, and expertise in record-keeping practices, putting them in a position to lead automation of health information efforts. Depending on the level and content of his or her education, a health information management professional may hold the position of chief information officer. Traditionally, the data stored in health records (once patients have been discharged) have been the health information manager's main concern, and the actual use of the technology has been the chief information officer's domain. The staff of the health information department will need to maintain and retrieve data from electronic health records and may be certified by the American Health Information Management Association (AHIMA). Various certifications are listed in Table 2.1, as well as other certifications for health information professionals. The most recent development in health information careers and competencies is the recognition of competency exams in specialty areas, which are also explained in Table 2.1.

In a medical office or other outpatient setting, healthcare administrators may have the same titles as those used in the inpatient setting, or they may be called office manager, office administrator, business manager, and the like. These individuals are keenly aware that electronic systems can greatly enhance the efficiency of an office or can just as easily be a negative force that causes inefficiencies; therefore, these hospital administrators are at the forefront of selecting and maintaining electronic systems that meet the needs of the practice and its practitioners. Certification of professionals in the outpatient setting is just as important as in the inpatient setting.

Healthcare professionals such as medical assistants, medical administrative assistants, health information managers, nurses, medical coders and billers, and other administrative professionals will be using the software in a medical practice, hospital, or other outpatient healthcare setting and will want it to be "user friendly," since they will be required to enter and retrieve data quickly yet accurately. The office administrator, also known as the office manager, will be gathering information from the practice management and EHR systems to ensure that claims are filed and paid accurately and in a timely manner, to ensure that the requirements of managed care organizations are met, and to ensure compliance with the **Promoting Interoperability Program** and **Merit-based Incentive Payment System (MIPS)** requirements, which include the **Advancing Care Information Standards**. These standards replaced the Medicare Electronic Health Records (EHR) Incentive Program for eligible clinicians, known previously as **Meaningful Use (MU)**.

Both the Promoting Interoperability Program and MIPS require the use of certified EHR technology that meets the standards and criteria established by the Office of the National Coordinator of Health Information Technology (ONC). Effective in 2019, changes were made that shifted the focus of the regulations to patient access and high-quality care as opposed to duplicate and outdated regulations that had been imposed on providers.

Participation in the Centers for Medicare & Medicaid Services (CMS) performance categories of MIPS gave providers incentives in the form of performance-based payment adjustments. In other words, providers will receive increased payments if they are able to demonstrate compliance with these incentives.

The American Health Information Management Association (AHIMA), the American Association of Medical Assistants (AAMA), the American Medical Technologists (AMT), the Healthcare Information and Management Systems Society (HIMSS), and the Physician Office Management Association of America (POMAA) are all professional associations offering certifying exams; providing members with up-to-date, relevant information about their respective fields; and offering continuing education opportunities, networking opportunities, publications, and career assistance. Each has an extensive website accessible by a search of the name.

Check Your Understanding

1. What roles might be held by a healthcare administrator in an inpatient or outpatient setting?
2. What is the difference between a medical assistant and an office administrator?
3. Explain the Merit-based Advancing Care Information Reporting system.

2.2 Data versus Information

Throughout this worktext you will see the terms **data** and **information**. They are often used interchangeably, but they are not entirely the same. Look up each term in a dictionary, and you will see within the definitions that the terms are almost interchangeable, or synonymous. Think of it this way, though: Data are single facts, such as *the patient is 60 years old* or *the patient is female* or *the patient is African American*. Single facts come together to form information. For example, the fact that Elena Jones is allergic to penicillin is a piece of data. But add to that piece of data the fact that she breaks out in hives, has difficulty breathing, and required an emergency room visit for her last allergic reaction and we have information about Elena and her allergy to penicillin. It is vital that each piece of data is accurate, valid, and timely to ensure that the information resulting from the data is also accurate, valid, and timely and is in a usable format to ensure quality medical care.

Promoting Interoperability Programs Formerly known as Meaningful Use, now referred to as Promoting Interoperability, this name change and the provisions of the program were made as a result of the 21st Century Cures Act and the Bipartisan Budget Act of 2018. The goal continues to be the use of certified electronic health record technology to improve quality, safety, and efficiency, as well as to reduce health disparities within the Medicare population.

Merit-based Incentive Payment System (MIPS) A reimbursement system that replaces the Sustainable Growth Rate formula previously used by Medicare Part B with a value-based system. The value-based system is called the Quality Payment Program (QPP).

Advancing Care Information Standards Part of the Merit-based Payment Incentive System's (MIPS), the Advancing Care Information performance category supports the **secure exchange** of health information and **encourages use of certified EHR technology**.

Meaningful Use The use of certified electronic health record technology with the purpose of improving quality, safety, and efficiency, as well as reducing health disparities within healthcare. Meaningful Use is now known as Promoting Interoperability.

Data A raw fact, or group of facts, such as a patient's name, height, or weight. A health record contains hundreds or thousands of pieces of data. The term *data* is used both as a singular term and a plural term. When pieces of data come together in a meaningful way, information results; thus, the word *data* is often used interchangeably with the word *information*, though they are not synonymous terms.

Information Raw facts that, when viewed as a whole, have meaning. Example: a report of all patients treated in the emergency department of Memorial Medical Center with a primary diagnosis of streptococcal pharyngitis (strep throat), sorted by patients' age.

Unstructured data Data in the form of words or audio files that cannot be tracked. Examples include emails, written narratives, and audio files from speech recognition technology.

Structured data Data that fit a particular model or format, which can be tracked and may be part of a database. Examples include ICD-10-CM/PCS codes, CPT® codes, a patient's temperature, or a patient's age.

Data may be **unstructured** or **structured**. Unstructured data are written in narrative form, such as in a sentence. Structured data are in a specified format such as numeric, alphabetic, or alphanumeric and are of a specified length and format. Examples of unstructured data are a transcribed report based on a physician's dictation, a written progress note, voice files, and scanned images of original documents. In this unstructured format, it is difficult, if not impossible, to track or trend statistics or to share information with healthcare agencies, public health agencies, or insurance carriers. Structured data—such as standard templates that are used to collect the elements of a dictated report or progress note, bar codes to identify types of reports or individual files, and numeric codes that equate to a written diagnosis or procedure—allow computers to process the data into usable information.

Check Your Understanding

1. Define data.
2. Differentiate between structured and unstructured data. Give an example of each.

2.3 Information Governance

Information governance As defined by AHIMA, "the enterprise-wide framework for managing information throughout its lifecycle and supporting the organization's strategy, operations, regulatory, legal, risk and environmental requirements."

Information governance is not a new concept; however, since the electronic collection, maintenance, and storage of health information are relatively new to healthcare, so is the concept of **information governance**. The acceptable protocol and structure for electronically preserving health information is at the core of information governance.

The American Health Information Management Association (AHIMA) defines information governance as "an organization-wide framework for managing information throughout its lifecycle and for supporting the organization's strategy, operations, regulatory, legal, risk and environmental requirements" (AHIMA information governance glossary at http://www.ahima.org/topics/infogovernance/ig-glossary).

In Section 2.2, you learned that data come together to form information. The gathered data are used for a myriad of reasons throughout healthcare: to diagnose a patient's condition; for financial reasons; to show compliance with various rules, regulations, and standards; for quality assessment activities and risk management; to defend the legal interests of the facility, healthcare practitioners, and providers; and to carry out administrative responsibilities at all levels.

One of the principal responsibilities of health information management (HIM) and office management professionals is the capture, handling, and storage of data. Not only does data have to be captured and stored, it must be accurate, timely, credible, and secure—all attributes of information governance, and thus logical responsibilities for the HIM professional. Though HIM and office management staff capture the non-clinical data, remember that the clinical data captured by nurses, technicians, medical administrative assistants, and physicians are part of the medical record, for which HIM and office management staff are responsible. There are rules surrounding the capture and storage of the data (which becomes information). The rules come from licensing agencies, accrediting agencies, private insurers, government agencies, and internal bylaws or policies. HIM professionals or medical administrative assistants analyze health records to ensure that these rules are met, and the health record is the source document to ensure that the rules are being followed. These administrative professionals make sure that required content is present in health records; for instance, the surgery schedule for the day may be reviewed by a member of the medical transcription staff to ensure that all scheduled surgical patients have had a history and physical examination dictated, transcribed, and posted to the patients' health records prior to their posted surgery start time. After discharge, records are analyzed to ensure that all entries are authenticated (signed), that the records of all patients who have undergone surgery include a dictated operative report, and that all inpatient records include a discharge summary by the patient's attending physician. This is known as **quantitative analysis**.

HIM staff or medical administrative assistants may review health records qualitatively as well, known as **qualitative analysis**—for instance, the medical history of a 60-year-old patient being seen with a chief complaint of a persistent cough should reflect whether that patient has been a smoker, the patient's current and past occupations, and whether there is a family history of lung cancer. And finally, these professionals code diagnoses and procedures, which allows for the collection of data that will be used not only for reimbursement purposes but also for public health initiatives—to collect statistics on mortality and morbidity locally, nationally, and globally—and for decision making in healthcare facilities to allocate resources for purchases of equipment, staffing, and expansion (or decrease) of services.

Quantitative analysis Review of the health record to ensure that all required documentation is present. Examples include history and physical exam, all entries authenticated (signed) by providers, and operative report present when a procedure has been performed.

Qualitative analysis Review of documentation in the health record to ensure the quality of the clinical documentation, that it is timely, not contradictory, complete, and clear.

Check Your Understanding

1. Why is information governance important in a field such as health information?
2. Dr. Smith saw Carol Brady in the emergency department of Memorial Hospital on January 5. Dr. Smith dictated the results of the physical exam performed on the patient on January 7. Should that be of concern to the individual responsible for information governance at Memorial Hospital? Why or why not?

2.4 Computer-Based Health Information Media

Prior to there being an electronic health record system, clinicians relied on one medium—paper—to collect and access information about patients. Many pieces of paper make up a health record, and paper records are often several inches thick. Paper records are contained in a folder, which is filed numerically by a medical record number or alphabetically by the patient's last name. Paper is still in use to some degree, and there are still providers who do not want to give up paper records, but electronic media are gaining acceptance in the healthcare community. As of 2017 the electronic health record is a requirement rather than a choice, thanks to the **Health Information Technology for Economic and Clinical Health (HITECH) Act**, which will be covered more thoroughly later in this chapter. In addition, many health

Health Information Technology for Economic and Clinical Health (HITECH) Act A portion of the American Recovery and Reinvestment Act (ARRA) that is meant to increase the use of an electronic health record by hospitals and physicians through a monetary incentive program.

Personal health record (PHR) A record, kept by the patient, that contains a person's health history, immunization status, current and past medications, allergies, and instructions given by a care provider; it often includes patient education materials as well.

Clinical decision support (CDS) An electronic application that allows access to current treatment options for a disease, through electronic or remote methods. Alerts the care provider to possible medication interactions, gives treatment options based on results of clinical trials or research, and alerts the provider that a patient may have a particular diagnosis based on the data found in the patient's electronic record.

insurance plans are making electronic **personal health records (PHRs)** available to their subscribers and have been doing so for the past few years. Some patients keep their own PHRs in a folder, in paper form, or in computerized form—for instance, in a spreadsheet. When a patient maintains his or her own PHR, it often contains the patient's health history, immunization status, current and past medications, and allergies; instructions given by a care provider; and patient education materials. The PHR—whether kept by the patient on paper, in a spreadsheet, or on the patient's insurer's software—does not replace the legal health record kept by the patient's care provider or hospital.

In addition to being the repository for all the clinical data about individual patients, electronic health records provide physicians with **clinical decision support (CDS)** software as well, which is used to access current information about a disease or condition. This technology alerts the care provider to possible medication interactions, gives treatment options based on results of clinical trials or research, and alerts the provider that a patient may have a particular diagnosis based on the data found in his or her electronic record. Not so long ago, physicians were opposed to this technology, thinking it was "cookbook medicine"; this is no longer the case, since great advances in the diagnosis and treatment of illnesses occur so quickly, making it very difficult or impossible to keep up with the most recent studies, findings, and recommended treatments. Thus, decision support applications in an EHR software package help keep physicians up to date as well as improve the quality of patient care.

Physicians can use computerized models within the EHR to show where a patient's rash is located, for example, rather than a crudely drawn picture of a patient's back (Figure 2.1 and Figure 2.2).

Streaming videos, podcasts, and DVDs are not new technologies, though they are used more often to educate patients about the procedure or treatment they are about to undergo than are handouts or educational booklets. The care provider may choose to show patients a video while they are in the office or to provide a link to a video for patients to view from their home computer. Using this type of media ensures that the information used to educate patients is consistent. Other types of presentation software, such as graphs or anatomy images like the one seen in Figure 2.2, are also used to educate patients or to capture a more succinct representation of the patient's problem.

Most EHRs now provide embedded educational materials, which can be specific to a particular patient's conditions, including treatment options and medications. The educational materials may be printed out for the patient or provided through a secure portal the patient accesses from home.

Physicians and administrators may want to visually present the findings of a study or to consult with another physician and show a patient's disease progression. This can be done through the use of software that has been available for years—presentation software such as Microsoft PowerPoint® or OpenOffice Impress™. Spreadsheets are often useful in making a point as well. EHR software

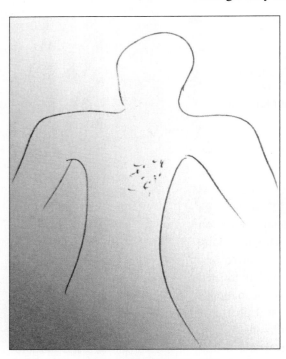

Figure 2.1 **Drawing of Placement of a Rash on a Patient's Back as It Would Have Appeared in a Paper Health Record** Source: Beth Shanholtzer

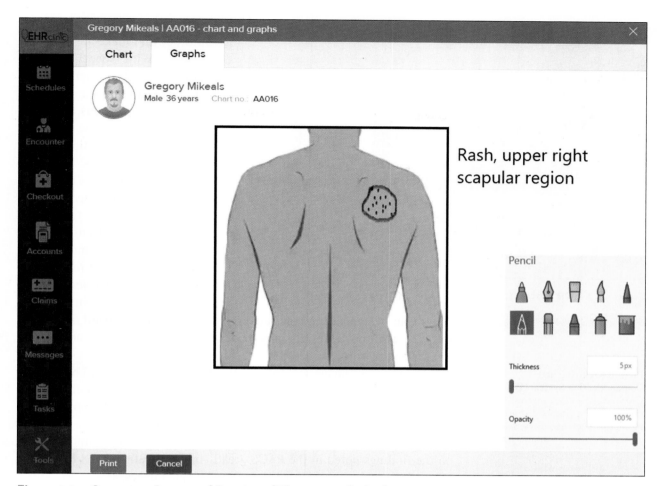

Figure 2.2   Computer-Generated Drawing of Placement of a Rash on a Patient's Back

provides the ability to visually chart changes in a patient's vital signs, for example, and show trends or statistical changes. Patient care and treatment are greatly enhanced with the ability to track vital signs over time, thus alerting the care provider to changes in a patient's condition.

Let's look at a particular scenario. Patti Wolfe has been seeing Dr. Raszkowski for the past five years. She has been faithful about having a yearly physical exam. For the past four years, her blood pressure has increased on each visit. In 2015, her blood pressure was 130/80; in 2016, it was 135/82; in 2017, it was 130/83; and in 2018, it was 140/88. Seeing this steady climb, Dr. Raszkowski explained the situation to Mrs. Wolfe and started her on a treatment regimen. Without this quick visual of her blood pressures, the physician may not have picked up the subtle changes, and her high blood pressure might have gone untreated.

Speech recognition technology is a medium that has been available for many years and has steadily gained in popularity. This software translates what a provider is saying and types those words into text. Whereas physicians used to dictate into a microphone and a medical transcriptionist typed the words using word processing software, through the use of speech recognition software the physician still dictates, but the software captures his or her words, then converts speech into text. The software is not 100% accurate, however, and in the world of medicine, it needs to be. Thus, a human being

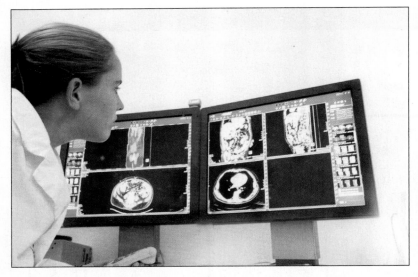

Figure 2.3   DR Systems, Inc., PACS Sigrid Gombert/Getty Images

must still review the final document for accuracy and make all necessary corrections. With speech recognition, the medical transcriptionist's role has changed from transcriber to editor. As the corrections are made, the software "learns" the dictator's voice so that future dictations do not reflect those same errors. Let's look at an example: Dr. Curtis dictates the sentence "There is no further medical history of note," but the speech recognition software translates that sentence as "There is no murmur history of note." The word *further* may have been heard as *murmur* because of a particular inflection in the physician's voice The next time the same physician dictates the word *further*, the software will understand the physician's tone and voice inflection and will transcribe the word correctly.

Picture Archiving and Communication System (PACS)
Computerized system for enhanced viewing and sharing of images such as x-rays, scans, ultrasounds, and mammograms.

A **Picture Archiving and Communication System (PACS)** allows providers to view images such as x-rays, scans, and ultrasounds. Originally used as a means to store x-ray film, a PACS makes it possible for providers to remotely view x-ray film to aid in clinical decision support. The improved image quality using a PACS and the ability to add alerts or reminders based on the findings noted in the PACS greatly improve patient care. Figure 2.3 illustrates a typical PACS used to view radiologic images.

Check Your Understanding

1. In the past, physicians marked the location of a patient's pain by drawing on a picture of a body. With the advantage of EHRs, what are they now able to do?
2. What does PACS stand for?
3. What does PACS allow providers to do?

2.5   Screen-Based Data Collection Tools

Members of the healthcare team who are entering (also known as capturing) data typically do so on a computer screen. It may be done on a desktop computer, a laptop, a notebook computer, or a personal digital assistant (PDA). On all these devices, data are entered and then retrieved using a computer screen. Think of the screen as the replacement for paper. Advantages include the portability of the handheld devices used to enter the data, the ability to have multiple monitors showing different images at the same time, and the ability to customize a screen based on user preference if supported by the software. In EHRclinic the facesheet categories can be expanded and collapsed, but not re-ordered. Figure 2.4 is an example of an EHRclinic facesheet; notice that Patient Information,

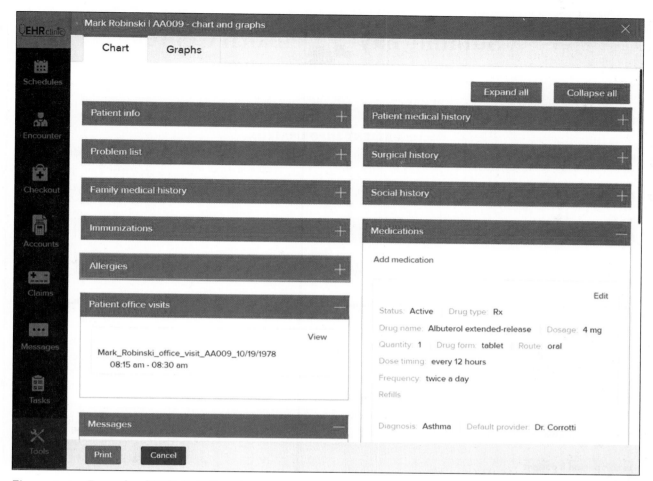

Figure 2.4   Example of EHRclinic Facesheet

Allergies, and Immunizations, for example, are still collapsed (the information within these sections is not visible), but the Patient's Office Visits and the Medications areas have been expanded so that the information within them is visible to the care provider.

Check Your Understanding

1. What types of computers are used for data capture?
2. What are some advantages of screen-based data collection tools?

2.6   Collecting Data Elements

So, we have this data, but how did we get it in the first place? It all starts when the patient makes an appointment with a physician's office or goes to the hospital for an emergency department, outpatient diagnostic, outpatient therapy, or outpatient surgery encounter or an inpatient admission. We collect identifying information verbally from the patient (or representative), or we ask the patient to complete a form (or a combination of both). See Figure 2.5 for an example of a patient registration form.

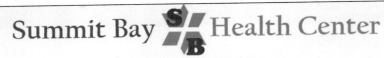

REGISTRATION FORM
(Please Print)

Today's date:	Care Provider:

PATIENT INFORMATION

Patient's last name:	First:	Middle:	☐ Mr. ☐ Mrs.	☐ Miss ☐ Ms.	Marital status (circle one) Single / Mar / Div / Sep / Wid

Is this your legal name? ☐ Yes ☐ No	If not, what is your legal name?	(Former name):	Birth date:	Age:	Sex: ☐ M ☐ F

Street address:		Social Security no.:	Home phone:	Cell phone:

P. O. Box:	City:	State:	ZIP Code:

Occupation:	Employer:	Employer phone no.:

E-mail address:

Race:	Ethnicity:	Primary language:	Religion:

Other family members seen here:

INSURANCE INFORMATION
(Presentation of Insurance Card is required at time of each visit)

Person responsible for bill:	Date of birth:	Address:	Home phone:	Cell phone:

Is this person a patient here?	☐ Yes ☐ No

Occupation:	Employer:	Employer address:	Employer phone no.:

Is this patient covered by insurance?	☐ Yes ☐ No

Please indicate primary insurance

☐ McGraw-Hill Healthmark Insurance ☐ BlueCross/ Blue Shield ☐ [Insurance] ☐ [Insurance] ☐ [Insurance]

☐ [Insurance] ☐ Workers' Compensation ☐ Medicare ☐ Medicaid *(Please provide card)* ☐ Other

Subscriber's name:	Subscriber's S.S. no.:	Date of birth:	Group no.:	Policy no.:	Co-payment: $

Patient's relationship to subscriber:	☐ Self ☐ Spouse ☐ Child ☐ Other	Effective Date:

Name of secondary insurance (if applicable):	Subscriber's name:	Group no.:	Policy no.:

Patient's relationship to subscriber:	☐Self ☐ Spouse ☐ Child ☐ Other

IN CASE OF EMERGENCY

Name of local friend or relative (not living at same address):	Relationship to patient:	Home phone no.: ( )	Work phone no.: ( )

The above information is true to the best of my knowledge. I authorize my insurance benefits be paid directly to the physician. I understand that I am financially responsible for any balance. I also authorize [Name of Practice] or insurance company to release any information required to process my claims.

_____
Patient/Guardian signature

Date

Figure 2.5   Patient Registration Form

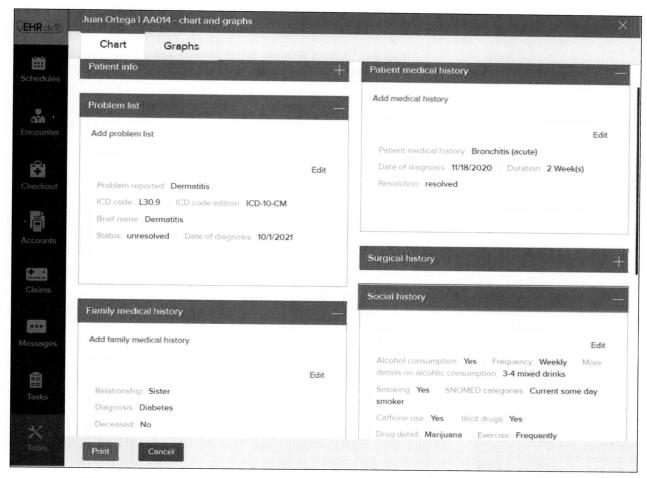

Figure 2.6 **EHRclinic Documentation of Patient's Past Medical History**

The patient's past medical, surgical, social, and family histories are collected and entered into the EHR as well. Figure 2.6 illustrates documentation in EHRclinic; each of the areas, when clicked on, includes more detailed information about the patient. Medication allergies, current medications, and immunization history are typically captured as part of the past medical history. The history is taken from a history form and/or the patient is asked questions in order to capture those data elements in the EHR. Remember, attention to detail is essential when documenting in the EHR.

The care provider then documents the history of present illness (HPI) and performs and documents a physical exam. He or she views all of this information to make an assessment of the patient (to diagnose the patient's conditions) and then determines a treatment plan (also called a plan of care).

In addition, the patient's previous health records are often used as a source of data. This information may be sent to the facility in a paper format, which is later scanned into the patient's health record, or the information can be retrieved electronically, eventually becoming part of the patient's record.

Check Your Understanding

1. Besides a patient's medical, social, surgical, and family histories, what other data are entered into his or her EHR?

2. Can a patient's previous health records be used as a source of data? Explain your answer.

3. Name two ways that identifying information is collected from a patient.

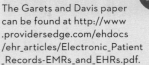

The Garets and Davis paper can be found at http://www .providersedge.com/ehdocs /ehr_articles/Electronic_Patient _Records-EMRs_and_EHRs.pdf.

Health Insurance Portability and Accountability Act (HIPAA) Passed in 1996, this act includes regulations that afford people who leave their employment the ability to keep their insurance or obtain new health insurance even if they have a pre-existing medical condition. Also sets standards for storing, maintaining, and sharing electronic health information while ensuring its privacy and security.

Regional Health Information Organization (RHIO) Group of healthcare organizations in a geographic area that exchange health information with the goal of improving patient care, reducing duplication, and reducing unnecessary costs.

Health information exchange (HIE) The movement or sharing of information between healthcare entities in a secure manner and in keeping with nationally recognized standards.

Institute of Medicine (IOM) An independent, nonprofit, nongovernmental organization that works to provide unbiased and authoritative advice to decision makers and the public. Beginning in March 2016, the IOM is the Health and Medicine Division (HDM) of the National Academies of Sciences, Engineering, and Medicine (the National Academies).

2.7 Electronic Health (Medical) Records (EHRs) (EMRs)

A health record that is in electronic form is referred to as an electronic health record (EHR) and sometimes an electronic medical record (EMR). The Office of the National Coordinator for Health Information Technology (ONC), however, differentiates between the two, based on a white paper by Garets and Davis. According to Garets and Davis, the EMR is the legal patient record that is created within any healthcare facility (hospital, nursing home, ambulatory surgery facility, physician's practice, etc.). The information in that EMR relates solely to one episode of care, and the EMR is the data source for the EHR. The individual records feed into the EHR so that healthcare providers, patients, employers, and insurance carriers can access a patient's health records as appropriate and in accordance with **Health Insurance Portability and Accountability Act (HIPAA)** regulations. Only those who have a need to know should access the information found in a patient's record.

Let's look at an example. Alison Holt was seen in the emergency room of Memorial Hospital on July 15, 2016. An EMR was compiled for that visit. She also has an EMR for an inpatient stay in Memorial Hospital from October 5 to October 10, 2017. There are additional EMRs for Alison Holt that pertain to various physician office visits and outpatient diagnostic testing. Then, in April 2019, Ms. Holt sees a pulmonary specialist, who needs to review her previous health records. Her providers and the hospitals she has been admitted to are able to share information through a **Regional Health Information Organization (RHIO)**, which includes healthcare organizations in her area that exchange patient information in order to improve care. This **health information exchange (HIE)** results in the quick and easy sharing of her medical history with the pulmonary specialist. Her individual records thus become part of an EHR. In effect, an EHR allows for the exchange of information among caregivers and others (insurance, employers, etc.) who have a need to know, but in a secure environment and according to certain standards. In the years since the establishment of health information exchanges, some have been successful but some have not; thus, many are still working to share data efficiently, effectively, and privately and to achieve true interoperability of healthcare data.

In 2003, the **Institute of Medicine (IOM)** defined the functions of an EHR. The eight core functions are

- Health information and data
- Result management

- Order management
- Decision support
- Electronic communication and connectivity
- Patient support
- Administrative processes and reporting
- Reporting and population health

We will no doubt continue to use the terms *EMR* and *EHR* interchangeably, but it is important to remember that in order for the benefits of the EMR to be realized, an EHR must exist. Without an EMR, the EHR, by definition, would not exist.

In 2016 the Institute of Medicine was renamed. It is now the **Health and Medicine Division (HMD)** of the **National Academies of Sciences, Engineering, and Medicine (the National Academies)**. The HMD is continuing the work of the IOM but has enlarged its focus to a broader range of health-related issues.

for your information fyi

To avoid any confusion caused by use of the acronyms EMR and EHR, throughout this worktext we will use the term *electronic health record (EHR)*.

Health and Medicine Division As of 2016, Health and Medicine Division is the new name of the Institute of Medicine. The full name is the Health and Medicine Division of the National Academies of Sciences, Engineering, and Medicine.

National Academies of Sciences, Engineering, and Medicine (the National Academies) Replaced the Institute of Medicine and provides healthcare-related data at a national level. The specific division of the National Academies that is related to healthcare is the Health and Medicine Division (HMD).

Check Your Understanding

1. The legal patient record created for one episode of care is known as the _____.
2. Who is allowed to access the information contained in a patient's record? Explain your answer.

2.8 Laws, Regulations, and Standards

Health Insurance Portability and Accountability Act (HIPAA)

As a healthcare professional, you will get used to the fact that many outside influences affect how and why you do your job. We will start our journey through the agencies, regulations, and laws that govern the keeping and exchange of health information with HIPAA, although many laws and standards came before it. As mentioned previously, HIPAA stands for Health Insurance Portability and Accountability Act. HIPAA was passed on August 21, 1996, with a multifaceted purpose. It included regulations that afforded people who left their employment the ability to keep their health insurance or obtain new insurance, even with a pre-existing medical condition. It also set standards for several aspects of storing, maintaining, and sharing electronic health information while ensuring the privacy and security of health information.

Several rules are addressed in HIPAA, including the Privacy Rule, with an effective compliance date of April 14, 2003. Part of its intent is to ensure the privacy of health information and the use of **protected health information (PHI)**, which is information that identifies the patient. The Office of Civil Rights enforces compliance with the Privacy Rule. All healthcare facilities and providers are required to comply with HIPAA. The specifics of the Privacy Rule will be covered in more detail in the privacy, security, confidentiality, and legal issues chapter; however, it is important to know that electronic data collection, maintenance, use, and storage are

for your information fyi

To learn fast facts about HIPAA privacy and security, go to http://www.hhs.gov/hipaa/index.html.

Protected health information (PHI) HIPAA defines protected health information (PHI) as "individually identifiable information related to the present, past, or future health status of an individual that is created, collected, or maintained by a HIPAA-covered entity in relation to the provision of healthcare, payment of healthcare services, or use in healthcare operations (PHI business uses)."

all governed by standards, and many of these come from HIPAA. Health records are legal documents and must be compliant with state and federal regulations, as well as with standards set forth by accrediting agencies and insurance carriers.

In February 2003, the HIPAA Security Rules were published. The deadline for facilities to implement the Security Rules was April 20, 2005. These security standards require healthcare organizations to implement safeguards (administrative, physical, and technological) to ensure that health information is protected, that it is kept private, and that it is retrievable in the event that the integrity of the electronic system is compromised.

The HIPAA Electronic Healthcare Transactions, Code Sets, and National Identifiers Rules require that medical providers who submit claims electronically be compliant with regulations requiring standardization of electronic collection and exchange of health information. Hospitals, physicians' offices, and clearinghouses (entities that process medical claims prior to payment) are required not only to submit claims (and diagnosis and procedure codes) electronically but also to receive information, such as remittance advices, from insurance companies electronically. Compliance was required by October 23, 2003. On January 1, 2012, HIPAA version 5010 of the Code Set Rule went into effect and is part of the electronic transaction standards of HIPAA. This is an upgrade from version 4010, which had been in use since 2000. Like any other software, it had become outdated and was in need of upgrading. The driving force behind the effective date, though, was the impending change from ICD-9-CM to ICD-10-CM/PCS, used to code diagnoses (CM) and procedures (PCS). In order to accept and transmit codes that are alphanumeric and that vary in length, new software was necessary; 4010 could not accommodate the new coding structure. In addition, version 5010 includes improved instructions for use of the **National Provider Identifier (NPI)** number, which is a unique identifier that must be used on insurance claims to identify the care provider and/or group practice that rendered care to the patient. The NPI implementation was the last of the original HIPAA regulations to take effect.

Health Information Technology for Economic and Clinical Health (HITECH) Act

The Health Information Technology for Economic and Clinical Health (HITECH) Act is part of the **American Recovery and Reinvestment Act of 2009 (ARRA)**, which was signed into law by President Obama on February 17, 2009. The HITECH portion of ARRA is meant to increase the use of an EHR by hospitals and physicians. The incentive program, made possible through HITECH, included $18 billion in funding for this purpose. Physicians and hospitals that show meaningful use of the information collected through the use of an EHR will benefit from HITECH. The incentives can be used to implement new EHR systems or to upgrade those that are already in place. Later in this text, we will demonstrate the meaningful use of data. There are three stages of Meaningful Use; the first stage is the collection and use of data (including submission of public health data, even when not required by state/local law), the second stage is the secure exchange of information in the form of electronic messaging and an electronic medication administration record, and the third stage is the use of patient data to improve patient outcomes, including a full electronic health record with

National Provider Identifier (NPI) A unique 10-digit identifier, issued by the Centers for Medicare & Medicaid Services (CMS), that must be used on insurance claims to identify the care provider and/or group practice that rendered care to the patient.

American Recovery and Reinvestment Act of 2009 (ARRA) Signed into law by President Obama on February 17, 2009; this economic "stimulus plan" includes provisions for the Health Information Technology for Economic and Clinical Health (HITECH) Act.

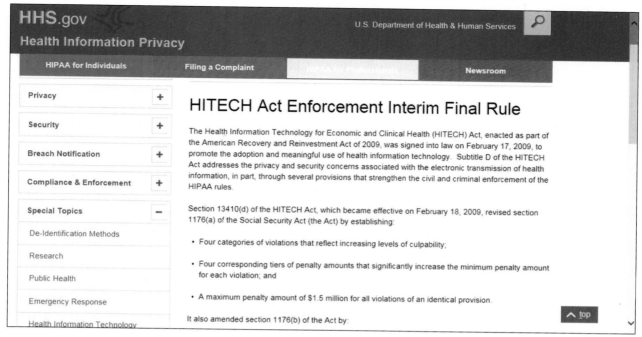

Figure 2.7 HITECH Act Enforcement Interim Final Rule Source: HHS.gov

the functionality, mentioned previously as well as computerized physician order entry, summary care records, and patient-specific educational materials. Figure 2.7 depicts the HITECH interim final rule from the Health and Human Services (HHS) website.

Office of the National Coordinator (ONC)

From ARRA also came the **Office of the National Coordinator for Health Information Technology (ONC)**. The ONC was created in 2004 through a presidential order but was later mandated by legislation (HITECH). According to the ONC website, "ONC is the principal Federal entity charged with coordination of nationwide efforts to implement and use the most advanced health information technology and the electronic exchange of health information."

Office of the National Coordinator for Health Information Technology (ONC) The principal federal entity charged with coordination, implementation, and use of health information technology and the electronic exchange of health information.

Nationwide Health Information Network (NHIN)

The ultimate goal of using EHR technology is to improve patient care—sharing information to improve diagnosis, treatment, and prognosis—while doing so in an economically efficient manner. In order to share health information electronically, though, standards must be set, and policies must be adhered to. According to the ONC website, the **Nationwide Health Information Network (NHIN)** is "a set of standards, services, and policies that enable the secure exchange of health information over the Internet" (National Health) The activities of the NHIN include the following:

Nationwide Health Information Network (NHIN) A set of standards, services, and policies that enable the secure exchange of health information over the Internet.

Nationwide Health Information Network (NHIN)—"a set of standards, services, and policies that enable the secure exchange of health information over the Internet" (HealthIT.gov)

National eHealth Collaborative (NeHC)—created through a grant from the ONC, a public-private partnership that enables secure and interoperable nationwide health information exchange to advance health and improve healthcare. "The broad mission of NeHC is three-fold: consumer engagement in eHealth, health IT education, and HIE" (National eHealth Collaborative).

Direct Project—a project aimed at developing standards and services that will enable the secure exchange of information on a local level among trusted providers to support stage 1 of the Meaningful Use incentives, which went into effect on January 1, 2011

CONNECT—free, open-source software that supports health information exchange

Changes continue in the eHealth spectrum. The electronic keeping of patients' health records is not perfect and continues to have its critics. There has been progress as well as setbacks in healthcare reform since the first edition of this worktext was written. With the vast number of treatment modalities and pharmaceuticals and the sheer volume of information in the 21st century, it is virtually impossible to keep health records in a manual format and have them be useful to anyone other than one health provider at a time, however. In addition, new reimbursement models have been launched, and with them has come more of an emphasis on competitiveness in providing healthcare, as well as more of a shared risk/shared reward system (Berry). Data is required in order to measure healthcare quality, and the resulting quality measures are necessary to roll out these new models of reimbursement; therefore, the exchange of health information also becomes a necessity.

Certification Commission for Health Information Technology (CCHIT) and Other Certifying Agencies

Certification Commission for Health Information Technology (CCHIT) A nonprofit, nongovernmental agency whose purpose was to certify electronic health records for functionality, interoperability, and security.

In the first several years of HITECH, to ensure that health information was shared securely and that the shared information was used for its intended purpose, the **Certification Commission for Health Information Technology (CCHIT)** was founded to develop certifying criteria for the functionality, interoperability, and security of EHRs. A non-governmental, nonprofit organization, CCHIT began certifying EHR systems in 2004 and ended operations in November 2014. Since then, certification of EHR systems has been the responsibility of the Office of the National Coordinator for Health Information Technology (ONC).

The Healthcare Information and Management Systems Society (HIMSS), a nonprofit organization that focuses on the use of information technology (IT) and management systems needed to improve healthcare, provides important information regarding the EHR on its website, found at http://www.himss.org/ASP/topics_ehr.asp.

The Medicare and Medicaid EHR incentive programs require the use of certified EHR technology; a listing of certified EHR technologies can be found at https://chpl.healthit.gov/#/search.

Regional Extension Centers

As part of HITECH, extension centers are funded by the federal government. Their purpose is to lend technical assistance and guidance regarding best practices in the selection, implementation, and maintenance of an EHR that will satisfy the Meaningful Use requirements. Each **regional extension center**, or **REC** (pronounced R-E-C), is responsible for a geographic region in the United States and is a nonprofit entity. An overview of RECs can be found at https://www.healthit.gov/topic/regional-extension-centers-recs. Now that the EHR and HITECH have been in existence for several years and goals have been achieved, many RECs have either changed their emphasis or have closed completely.

Regional extension center (REC) An organization that assists healthcare providers with the selection and implementation of electronic health record systems.

Thus, many entities exist to ensure that health information is shared so that safe, effective, quality medical care is provided in a manner that allows for the security and privacy of that information exchange.

Check Your Understanding

1. The original agency/organization responsible for developing the criteria for and then certifying EHR systems was _____.
2. Name the four subcategories of HIPAA.
3. What does PHI stand for?
4. The organization currently responsible for certifying EHR systems is _____.
5. What office ensures compliance with the Privacy Rule?
6. Explain the necessity behind upgrading to HIPAA 5010.

2.9 Similarities and Differences between a Physician's Office and Hospital Information Systems

Regardless of the healthcare setting—inpatient or outpatient—every patient seen must have a health record that includes his or her history of present illness, past medical and surgical history, record of physical exam, record of treatment rendered, results of diagnostic tests, plan of care, and diagnoses. In a physician's office setting, the patient schedules an appointment, which is part of the registration process. In a hospital setting, a patient may arrive without an appointment for an emergency department visit or outpatient lab work; in either case, an appointment is typically unnecessary or impossible. In other instances, such as for a CT scan, which requires a significant amount of time and specially trained staff, an appointment is necessary. And in a hospital setting, a patient may be scheduled for elective surgery such as a cholecystectomy (removal of the gallbladder), which would also be a scheduled (planned) visit.

The steps taken to capture the fact that a patient was seen, no matter what the setting, are most easily (and accurately) done using computerization. In a physician's office, this is done using practice management (PM) software. In a hospital, these captured records are called the Master Patient Index (MPI), and the MPI is part of the Registration, Admission, Discharge, Transfer (RADT), or just ADT, functions of the hospital's automated information system. Each patient is entered only once into the MPI, although there may be several visits (encounters) for each patient as a subset of the main entry. This allows the documentation of each individual visit to be filed in one place within the MPI.

Increasingly in the past 15 years or so, single hospitals and physician practices have been purchased by large hospital systems. The single hospitals/offices then become part of an "enterprise." In some cases, the individual institutions or offices maintain their own records and operate autonomously. In others, the MPI is shared (an enterprise-wide MPI) and more than likely will result in duplicate patient records and an increase in incorrect data. Obviously, correct data in the MPI is always a priority, but when an enterprise-wide MPI is used, it becomes even more imperative to have staff that continually monitor for and clean up any inaccurate, duplicate, erroneous, or unreliable data. It also becomes more important for registration staff to do a thorough check of the MPI before adding a patient as new or before selecting an existing patient.

Practice management software is used to handle office administrative functions such as listing all patients who have been seen in that practice; capturing insurance and demographic information; entering charges and diagnosis and procedure codes; filing, maintaining, and following up on medical claims and collections (billing procedures); running statistical reports about the practice; and scheduling patients' appointments.

The capture of the identifying information and clinical documentation discussed earlier in this chapter is part of the electronic health record in both hospitals and physicians' offices.

All the various functions performed have different names in different settings, but their goals are the same: registration of the patient and then compilation of a health record for every encounter the patient has in that facility or office.

Table 2.2 compares common jargon used in a hospital to that used in a physician's office. For instance, "SOAP" stands for Subjective (the patient's complaint in his or her own words), Objective (a description of what the care provider observes or measurable findings), Assessment (the diagnosis), and Plan (the treatment) and is a format used to document

TABLE 2.2	Comparison of Outpatient to Inpatient Setting	
Action	**Physician's Office or Other Outpatient Setting**	**Hospital**
Patient seeks care	Schedule patient or make an appointment	Register or admit a patient
Health record compiled	Documentation in a SOAP note format, narrative progress note, or "chart"	End product is a health (medical) record
Listing of all patients seen by the facility	Once the patient is registered one time, he or she appears in the Patient List	Once the patient is registered one time, he or she appears in the Master Patient Index (MPI)
Patient has outpatient care	Each is called an encounter or a visit	Each is called an encounter
Patient stays overnight	n/a	Patient is an admission or inpatient
Patient is finished with the encounter	Patient checks out	Patient is discharged

progress notes in any setting, but it is most often used in outpatient settings such as physicians' offices. SOAP notes are equivalent to progress notes in inpatient settings.

The objective of an EMR/EHR is to capture timely, accurate, usable health information to ensure quality medical care; provide for coordination of care; support the medical necessity for diagnostic testing; protect the legal interests of the patient, provider, and hospital; collect data used in statistical reporting; and file insurance claims.

In order to select, implement, maintain, and use practice management software or the electronic health record, a team of professionals is typically assembled to investigate several software options. Those on the team should include individuals who understand not only how to use the software but also what to look for when selecting software that will meet the stiff regulations that govern the keeping of health information. It is vital that this health information be maintained in a way that is private, confidential, and secure yet readily available when needed. In addition, the information must be accurate, reliable, and valid. Over the past several years, the federal government has affirmed that there is an urgent need for an electronic health record that will provide for more efficient, effective, and safe healthcare for Americans.

Check Your Understanding

1. The SOAP note format of writing progress notes is generally used in a/an _____ setting.
2. Could a patient ever have outpatient care in a hospital setting? Explain your answer. If so, what is an episode of outpatient care called?
3. What term refers to a hospital's historical list of patients?

APPLYING YOUR SKILLS

You have learned much about how healthcare is structured in the United States and the professionals who manage various aspects of healthcare, and you have been introduced to the organizations that govern the electronic systems used in healthcare facilities. To tie all of these together, you will set out on a virtual scavenger hunt. Use the Internet to answer the following questions about your region of the country.
1. Find the website for a hospital near you. Who is the CEO?
2. By searching the Web or reading a newspaper or magazine article, find information related to healthcare, such as current cancer rate, death rate for a particular region, or proven treatment for a particular disease. What makes this information rather than data?
3. Find the regional extension center for your state.
4. Find the health information exchange for your state.
5. Find three hospitals or physician practices within a 100-mile radius of your home. For each, is the hospital or practice stand-alone or part of an enterprise system?

chapter 2 **summary**

LEARNING OUTCOME	CONCEPTS FOR REVIEW

2.1 Describe the roles of six healthcare professionals who maintain or use practice management and electronic health record applications.	– Healthcare professionals, their educational background, their certifications, and how they use health information:
	  • Chief information officer
	  • Health information professionals
	  • Chief financial officer
	  • Healthcare administrators/managers/office administrators
	  • Care providers
	  • Nurses, medical assistants

2.2 Explain the difference between data and information.	– Often used interchangeably – Data are single facts – Single facts come together to form information – Structured vs. unstructured data
2.3 Define information governance and the HIM and healthcare administrative professionals' role in it.	– Define information governance – List the uses of healthcare data – List the attributes of data

2.4 Identify computer-based health information media.	– Role of the Health Information Technology for Economic and Clinical Health (HITECH) Act in the adoption of an electronic health record
	– Define personal health record (PHR)
	– Electronic health record includes
	  • Decision support technology
	  • Computerized models and images
	  • Presentation aids
	  • Speech recognition technology
	  • Picture Archiving and Communication System (PACS)

2.5 Relate how screen-based data collection tools are used in healthcare.	– Hardware used to collect health information:
	  • Desktop computers
	  • Laptop computers
	  • Notebook computers
	  • Personal digital assistants (PDAs)
	– Advantages include portability and customization

LEARNING OUTCOME	CONCEPTS FOR REVIEW
2.6 Demonstrate how individual data elements are collected.	– Data collected through use of forms or in person – Registration forms used as method of collecting patient identifying and demographic information – Patient history form used as method of collecting past medical, surgical, family, and social histories; allergies; and medication history
2.7 Describe electronic health record applications.	– Differentiate between electronic medical record (EMR) and electronic health record (EHR) – Role of the Office of the National Coordinator for Health Information Technology (ONC) – Differentiate between Regional Health Information Organization (RHIO) and health information exchange (HIE) – List the functions of the EHR as detailed by the Institute of Medicine (IOM)/ Health and Medicine Division of the National Academies (HMD)
2.8 Identify laws, regulations, and standards that govern electronic health information.	– Identify the Privacy, Security, Transactions, and Code Set Rules of HIPAA – Define protected health information (PHI) – Define National Provider Identifier (NPI) number – Describe the Health Information Technology for Economic and Clinical Health (HITECH) Act and its role in requiring electronic health records – Define Meaningful Use of data collected through use of an EHR – Describe the purpose of the Office of the National Coordinator for Health Information Technology (ONC) – Explain the Nationwide Health Information Network (NHIN) – Explain the Certification Commission for Health Information Technology (CCHIT) – Relate the purpose of regional extension centers (RECs)
2.9 Distinguish between practice management software and hospital health information software.	– Describe the functions of practice management software – Differentiate between RADT (ADT) systems and EHR systems in a hospital setting – Discuss the use of a Master Patient Index and Patient List – Articulate the purpose of an EHR

chapter review

MATCHING QUESTIONS

Match the terms on the left with the definitions on the right.

_____ 1. **[LO 2.2]** data

_____ 2. **[LO 2.7]** health information exchange

_____ 3. **[LO 2.2]** unstructured data

_____ 4. **[LO 2.1]** healthcare systems administrator

_____ 5. **[LO 2.1]** Meaningful Use

_____ 6. **[LO 2.4]** clinical decision support

_____ 7. **[LO 2.9]** Master Patient Index

_____ 8. **[LO 2.8]** protected health information

_____ 9. **[LO 2.8]** Office of the National Coordinator (ONC)

_____ 10. **[LO 2.7]** Institute of Medicine (IOM)

_____ 11. **[LO 2.3]** information governance

a. any piece of identifying or clinical information about a patient

b. organization that is responsible for certifying electronic health records for viability

c. staff member whose responsibilities include management of a facility's IT functions

d. use of health information in an effective and efficient manner to improve patient care

e. single facts often used interchangeably with information

f. original entity to define the functions of an EHR; now known as the Health and Medicine Division of the National Academies

g. method of accessing current treatment options for a disease, through electronic or remote methods

h. sharing of health information among various entities, using standardized and secure processes

i. record of the names of all patients seen in a hospital setting

j. details that cannot be tracked, such as emails and speech recognition technology audio files

k. organization-wide framework for managing information throughout its lifecycle and for supporting the organization's strategy, operations, regulatory, legal, risk, and environmental requirements

MULTIPLE-CHOICE QUESTIONS

Select the letter that best completes the statement or answers the question:

1. **[LO 2.7]** The acronym HIE stands for
   a. health information exchange.
   b. hospital information exchange.
   c. health information electronically.
   d. hospital institutional exchange.

2. **[LO 2.5]** An advantage of using screen-based data collection tools is that the layout of the information can be
   a. printed.
   b. deleted.

   c. shredded.

   d. customized.

3. **[LO 2.7]** The _____ defined the eight core functions of an EHR.

   a. National Institutes of Health

   b. American Recovery and Reinvestment Act

   c. Institute of Medicine

   d. HITECH Act

4. **[LO 2.8]** Which of the following is a goal of HIPAA?

   a. establish standards for keeping health information

   b. ensure that patients receive timely treatment

   c. allow a person's insurance to transfer from one job to another

   d. guide how Picture Archiving and Communication Systems are used

5. **[LOs 2.6, 2.9]** In a physician's office, patient data collection begins when

   a. the patient exam begins.

   b. the patient calls to make an appointment.

   c. the medical assistant takes the patient's vital signs.

   d. the patient signs in at the front desk.

6. **[LO 2.4]** An advantage of EHRs is that patients are now able to _____ about procedures they are undergoing from their own homes, on their own schedules.

   a. negotiate charges with insurance representatives

   b. see diagrams

   c. ask questions

   d. view patient education videos

7. **[LO 2.2]** "Jim Smith had a heart attack when he was 53" is an example of

   a. data.

   b. information.

   c. support.

   d. technology.

8. **[LO 2.9]** When patients are finished with their encounter at a hospital, they

   a. are admitted.

   b. check out.

   c. complete a SOAP note.

   d. are discharged.

9. **[LO 2.8]** If a hospital uses information gathered through its EHR to justify the purchase of state-of-the-art equipment to improve patient care, it is

   a. violating the Privacy Rule.

   b. engaging in Meaningful Use.

   c. abusing protected health information.

   d. following CCHIT.

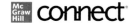

Enhance your learning by completing these exercises and more at https://connect.mheducation.com!

SHORT-ANSWER QUESTIONS

1. **[LO 2.1]** List six healthcare professionals (clinical and non-clinical) who use the contents of an EHR and explain the role of each.

2. **[LO 2.8]** Explain the evolution of CCHIT.

3. **[LO 2.1]** Explain the differences among a healthcare administrator, a healthcare manager, and a health systems administrator.

4. **[LO 2.9]** List the six objectives of an EHR.

5. **[LO 2.8]** HIPAA is an acronym for _____.

6. **[LO 2.7]** Contrast an EHR with an EMR.

7. **[LO 2.2]** Explain the difference between data and information and give an example of each.

8. **[LO 2.4]** Why might physicians be opposed to clinical decision support functionality?

9. **[LO 2.5]** List and explain the four types of histories entered into a patient's electronic record.

10. **[LO 2.5]** Name two advantages of using screen-based data collection tools.

11. **[LO 2.1]** If someone has the letters "RHIA" after his or her name, what does that mean?

12. **[LO 2.9]** What does the RADT (also seen as R-ADT) acronym mean in a hospital setting? Explain its purpose.

13. **[LO 2.8]** Explain the purpose of a regional extension center (REC).

14. **[LO 2.4]** Discuss at least one way that speech recognition technology can be used in a medical setting.

15. **[LO 2.3]** In a physician's practice, which staff position is likely to be responsible for functions of information governance?

APPLYING YOUR KNOWLEDGE

1. **[LOs 2.4, 2.5, 2.7, 2.8]** Discuss any potential drawbacks to the full-scale use of EHRs and explain what precautions or regulations have been put in place to deal with each drawback.

2. **[LO 2.8]** Incentives are a significant part of the HITECH Act. Discuss the advantages and potential disadvantages associated with using incentives as a tool for implementing EHRs.

3. **[LOs 2.2, 2.6]** In the following case study, determine what would be considered data and what would be considered information: New patient Alice Jones is a 32-year-old female who presents with chest pains. She tells you that in the past she has been diagnosed with rosacea and is allergic to latex. In addition, she has had surgery for a broken arm. She does not smoke, is a social drinker, and has no family history of heart problems.

4. **[LO 2.9]** A physician's office and a hospital use different terminology and process flow when maintaining records and monitoring patient flow. Why is there no set protocol that is used by all healthcare settings?

5. **[LO 2.4]** Describe a scenario where presentation software might be used in a physician's practice.

6. **[LO 2.9]** Think about the six main objectives of an EHR. Which of the six do you feel would be most useful for care providers? For patients? For office managers? Explain your answers.

7. **[LO 2.8]** Visit the HIPAA Fast Facts website located in the FYI box in Section 2.8. Summarize the information found on the website and write a brief scenario that illustrates how the information could be put into practice at a physician's office or a hospital.

8. **[LO 2.1]** Choose one of the professional associations listed in Section 2.1. Locate the association's website and create an outline for a sample presentation you might give to your office staff that highlights the important aspects of that association's influence on health information management.

9. **[LO 2.3]** One of the physicians in your practice thinks it is a waste of time to review the quality of documentation of the health records in this three-physician practice. You are the office manager. Explain to the physicians why the quality, thoroughness, and timeliness of documentation are so important.

chapter references

Berry, Kate. (2013, March). HIE Quality Check. *Journal of AHIMA, 84*(3): 28–32.

Certification Commission for Health Information Technology. (2013). *About the Certification Commission for Health Information Technology.* Retrieved from http://www.cchit.org/about.

Department of Health and Human Services, Centers for Medicare & Medicaid Services. (2016). *Administrative Simplification Overview.* Retrieved from https://www.cms.gov/Regulations-and-Guidance /Administrative-Simplification/HIPAA-ACA/.

Department of Health and Human Services, Centers for Medicare & Medicaid Services. Medicare Learning Network. (2014). *The National Provider Identifier (NPI): What You Need to Know.* Retrieved from http:// www.cms.gov/MLNProducts/downloads/NPIBooklet.pdf.

Garets, D., and Davis, M. (2005, October). Electronic Patient Records: EMRs and EHRs. *Healthcare Informatics.* Retrieved from http://www.providersedge.com/ehdocs/ehr_articles/Electronic_Patient_Records -EMRs_and_EHRs.pdf.

Health Careers Center. (2004). *Health Care Administrator.* Retrieved from http://www.mshealthcareers.com /careers/healthcareadmin.htm.

Interoperability Portfolio: Nationwide Health Information Network. (2013). Retrieved from http://www.healthit .gov/policy-researchers-implementers/nationwide-health-information-network-nwhin.

Marron-Stearns, Michael. "MACRA 2019 Update: What to Know." *Journal of AHIMA 90,* no. 2 (February 2019): 26–33.

National Academies of Sciences, Engineering, and Medicine. Health and Medicine Division. *About Our Division and Website.* Retrieved from http://www.nationalacademies.org/hmd/.

National Academies: Health and Medicine Division (HMD). (2013). *Key Capabilities of an Electronic Health Record System.* Retrieved from http://nationalacademies.org/hmd/reports/2003/key-capabilities-of-an- electronic-health-record-system.aspx.

Newby, Cynthia. (2009). *HIPAA for Allied Health Careers.* New York: McGraw-Hill.

SmartData Collective. (2014). *A Quick Guide to Structured and Unstructured Data.* Retrieved from http:// www.smartdatacollective.com/michelenemschoff/206391/quick-guide-structured-and-unstructured-data.

U.S. Department of Health and Human Services, Office of the National Coordinator for Health Information Technology. (2011). *National Health Information Network: Overview.* Retrieved from http://www.healthit .gov/policy-researchers-implementers/nationwide-health-information-network-nwhin.

U.S. Department of Health and Human Services, Office of the National Coordinator for Health Information Technology. Retrieved from http://www.healthit.gov/newsroom/about-onc.

U.S. Department of Health and Human Services, Office of the National Coordinator of Health Information Technology. Retrieved from https://www.healthit.gov/topic/regional-extension-centers-recs.

U.S. Department of Health and Human Services, Office of the National Coordinator for Health Information Technology. *HITECH and Funding Opportunities.* Retrieved from http://www.healthit.gov /policy-researchers-implementers/hitech-programs-advisory-committees.

chapter **three**

Content of the Health Record— Administrative Data

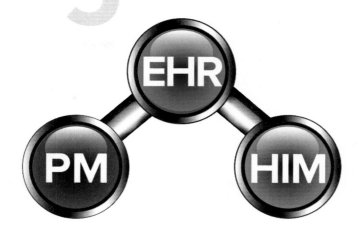

Learning Outcomes

At the end of this chapter, the student should be able to

3.1 Identify administrative data elements.

3.2 Explain the administrative uses of data.

3.3 Explain the use of EHR data in an Accountable Care Organization (ACO).

3.4 Explain the use of the Master Patient Index (MPI).

3.5 Apply procedures to register a new patient in EHRclinic.

3.6 Apply procedures to schedule a patient's appointment in EHRclinic.

3.7 Apply procedures to edit demographic information in EHRclinic.

3.8 Identify the steps performed upon patient check-in.

3.9 Apply procedures to capture insurance information in EHRclinic.

3.10 Locate the User's Guide and Help feature in EHRclinic.

Key Terms

Account (billing) number
Accountable Care Organization (ACO)
Administrative data
Chief complaint
Clinical Documentation Architecture (CDA)
CMS-1500
Continuity of Care Document (CCD)
Data dictionary
Default value
Demographic (identifying) data

Health Level Seven (HL7)
Interoperability
Library
Master Patient Index (MPI)/Patient List
Medical record number
Medicare Access and CHIP Reauthorization Act (MACRA)
Merit-based Incentive Payment System (MIPS)
Quality Reporting Document Architecture (QRDA)
UB-04

The Big Picture

What You Need to Know and Why You Need to Know It

In previous chapters we talked about the importance of each patient having only one record in the EHR of that facility. Remember, though, that one record may have many individual encounters attached to it, one for each visit to a healthcare facility as a patient. In this chapter we will discuss the administrative data, including demographic (identifying) data, that are collected about each patient, thus forming the master record or Master Patient Index for each patient.

Administrative data Identifying information, insurance-related information, authorizations, and business correspondence found in a patient's health record.

Demographic (identifying) data Data that identify the patient. Consists of name, date of birth, sex, race, and Social Security number (may vary by facility policy).

CMS-1500 The form used by physicians' offices and other outpatient settings to submit insurance claims.

UB-04 The form used to submit insurance claims for hospital patients.

Medical record number (MRN) A unique number assigned to a patient that links to all account numbers for that patient in a given healthcare facility or office. Example: A patient is seen for the first time at Memorial Hospital and is assigned medical record number 50801. In the next 10 years the patient has 10 encounters for care at Memorial Hospital. All 10 of those records can be located under medical record number 50801, though all have different account numbers.

Account (billing) number A unique number assigned to every new encounter (emergency department visit, outpatient visit, ambulatory surgery visit, inpatient stay, or physician's office visit).

3.1 | Administrative Data Elements

Administrative data refers to nonclinical data and does not include data relative to the diagnosis, prognosis, treatment, or plan of care. A subset of administrative data is **demographic (identifying) data** and includes data collected to identify a particular patient. These data elements include the patient's full name, date of birth, race, ethnicity, gender, marital status, address, and phone number. The Social Security number used to be an additional identifier that was widely used; however, because of identity theft concerns, that practice is now not as common, or some practices request only the last four digits of the patient's Social Security number. Additional information that is typically collected includes employed/student status, employer name and address, next of kin, and insurance policy name, policy number, and group number. In addition to identifying patients, many administrative data elements are required to complete insurance claim forms such as the **CMS-1500** and the **UB-04**, as required by HIPAA. The CMS-1500 form is used to bill outpatient encounters, and the UB-04 is used to bill hospital admissions/encounters. Examples of the CMS-1500 and the UB-04 are available in the Appendix.

Identifying information for inpatients and outpatients, as included in the core health data elements recommended by the National Center for Vital and Health Statistics in 1996, should include the data elements listed here:

- Patient's full name
- Previous name (maiden name or previous married name)
- **Medical record number**, also referred to as personal/unique identifier or chart number
- **Account (billing) number**
- Date of birth
- Gender
- Race
- Ethnicity
- Residence (address)
- Marital status
- Current or most recent occupation (employer)
- Type of encounter (inpatient, emergency room visit, physician's office visit, ambulatory surgery, outpatient diagnostic visit, etc.)
- Admission date (inpatient) or date of encounter (outpatient)
- Discharge date (inpatient)

- Facility identification (unique identifier of the medical office, hospital, outpatient surgery center, etc.)
- Type of facility/place of encounter (hospital, physician's office, surgi-center, etc.)
- Healthcare practitioner identification number (outpatient)
- Provider location or address of encounter (outpatient)
- Attending physician identification (inpatient)
- Patient's expected sources of payment (Medicare, Medicaid, insurance, self-pay, etc.)
- Whether injury is related to employment or accident
- Total billed charges

These data elements are also included in the **Health Level Seven (HL7)** standards. HL7 allows different software packages to interface with one another, that is, it allows them to share data. Many different companies develop healthcare applications and systems, and by writing the software according to HL7 standards, the applications "talk to each other"; if they did not, the data would have to be entered separately in each application. Hospitals and medical practices may have different vendors for different systems. For instance, there may be one service provider for the laboratory system, one for the pharmacy system, one for tracking incomplete records, and so on. Through use of HL7 standards, if a piece of data is changed in one application system (say, the patient's telephone number), the change will be reflected in each system. This is a very important requirement, because without this standard language, **interoperability** (sharing data through a single database) would not be possible.

HL7 has been the most widely used and recognized standard in the healthcare industry. HL7 now recognizes new, more specific standards, which include **Clinical Documentation Architecture (CDA)** and **Quality Reporting Document Architecture (QRDA)**. The CDA is used for an important piece of the Meaningful Use legislation in preparing a **Continuity of Care Document (CCD)**, and the QRDA is important for quality reporting purposes as well as for sharing information between providers or facilities. The Continuity of Care Documents tie directly to one of the major goals of an electronic health record—that is, improving patient care and patient outcomes through information. The ability to electronically share important clinical data among caregivers, even those from different or even competitive healthcare facilities, is a step toward improving overall quality of care. Service providers (EHR and PM software vendors) are finding it more beneficial to work together to form new partnerships, resulting in collaborative relationships, than to concentrate on selling their product(s) alone.

Commonwell Health Alliance is an example of how health information technology vendors are working together to collaborate toward the ultimate goal of true interoperability of healthcare electronic systems. According to Commonwell's website, "The Alliance intends to be an independent, not-for-profit trade association that will support and promote the seamless interoperability of and access to patient data across the healthcare system."

Meaningful Use (now known as Promoting Interoperability) will be covered in more detail in the chapter on decision and compliance support in this worktext. A detailed explanation about the protocols themselves for HL7 is not necessary in this text, but they will be covered in a more advanced information technology course.

Health Level Seven (HL7) A set of standards that makes sharing of data between or among health-care entities possible.

Interoperability Many different functions can take place and information can be shared between computer systems, or within applications of the same computer system, which is not possible with a manual or paper record system.

Clinical Documentation Architecture (CDA) Developed by HL7, a document markup standard that specifies the structure and semantics of clinical documents such as discharge summary, operative report, etc.

Quality Reporting Document Architecture (QRDA) Based on HL7's approved Clinical Documentation Architecture (CDA), QRDA is a data standard used for reporting quality measure data and that is EHR compatible across different health IT systems.

Continuity of Care Document (CCD) A document exchange standard used to share patient summary information, such as in the case of a patient being referred from one healthcare provider to another.

One of the data elements listed earlier in this section is previous name (maiden name or previous married name). Collecting this data element allows for cross-referencing of files. If a woman was previously seen at a facility under her maiden name but is being seen for the first time using her married name, she should be listed only one time in the master list of patients (Master Patient Index).

In an outpatient setting, the data elements listed previously are collected on a patient registration form, which is completed at the time care is established with that facility or office. The information should be verified with the patient each time he or she is seen to ensure that there has been no change in information, and that there have been no additions or deletions to the information. Examples include changes in address, telephone number, marital status, or expected source of payment. In a hospital setting, the information may be required prior to a patient's undergoing an elective admission, or it may be collected face-to-face in the registration department when the patient presents for care.

Equally important when collecting sufficient identifying information is that each data element is consistently defined by the facility. Use of a **data dictionary**, as seen in Figure 3.1, will ensure that each member of the registration staff has defined the data element correctly, and that only valid entries are made in a particular data element.

Let's look at a few examples. First, consider the possible data dictionary choices for marital status. The typical choices are single, married, separated, widowed, divorced, and unknown. If that is the definition of marital status in your facility, then those are the *only* choices available in the practice management system. Data dictionaries should be very specific. An example is the definition of "separated." Some facilities may consider a patient to be separated only if she presents a legal document stating such, and if she cannot do that, she is considered married for data collection purposes, even though she considers herself to be separated in the legal sense. Another example is the patient's full name. In the facility's data dictionary, the full name may be defined as the patient's last name, first name, middle name. Or it may be defined as the last name, first name, middle initial. Thus, when a patient is registered, the name should be collected exactly as defined in that facility's data dictionary. Failure to follow the data dictionary definitions will result in unreliable data.

For consistency of wording and to save time, many fields in EHRclinic have a **library** of possibilities from which to choose. These are commonly referred to as drop-down menus. Examples of libraries are employers, medications, religions, ethnicities, medical conditions, and elements of a physical exam. Clinical templates are also found in libraries (Figure 3.2).

Data dictionary A document that specifies the format of each data field as well as a detailed explanation or definition for that field, which allows for consistency of data collection.

Library In computer software, a listing or choice of entities, for instance, employers, insurance plans, ICD-10-CM codes, or CPT® codes.

Field Name	Data Type	Field Length	Description
Last name	Alphabetic	18	Patient's legal surname
First name	Alphabetic	10	Patient's first name
Middle name	Alphabetic	10	Patient's middle name
DOB	Numeric	08	Date of birth as it appears on birth certificate
Phone number	Numeric	10	Preferred phone number including area code

Figure 3.1   **Excerpt from a Data Dictionary**

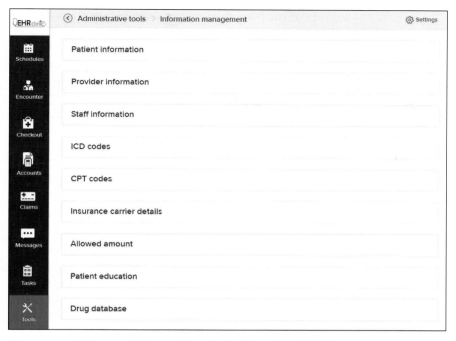

Figure 3.2   **Library of Clinical Templates Found in EHRclinic**

3.2	**Administrative Uses of Data**

In addition to identifying a particular patient, administrative data are also used to satisfy HIPAA data requirements, which in turn are used to file electronic health claims for reimbursement. The CMS-1500 form is used to submit claims electronically for outpatient encounters, and the UB-04 is used to submit hospital claims. There are five major sections or levels on the claim form (refer to the CMS-1500 and UB-04 forms found in the Appendix).

1. Provider information

The name, address, National Provider Identifier (NPI) number, and telephone number of the provider

2. Subscriber and patient information

This section includes information about the policyholder (subscriber) of the insurance and the patient identifying information. These may be one and the same if the patient is the policyholder (the primary insured). Following is a partial list of information collected but it is not limited to

- Policyholder's (subscriber's) name
- Group or insurance plan name
- Identification (policy) number
- Patient's relationship to the policyholder

3. Payer information

- Group or insurance plan name
- Plan identification
- Address
- Assignment of benefits authorization (allows payment to be made directly to the provider)
- Release of information authorization (allows clinical information to be released to the insurance company)

- Referral number (if the patient was referred by another provider)
- Prior authorization number (obtained when insurance plan requires procedures to be approved for payment in advance)

4. Claim details—a partial list of data includes
   - Individual account number or identification for that particular encounter
   - Total charges submitted
   - Place of service code
   - Provider signature
   - Details about the onset of the illness/accident
   - Date(s) of service
   - Amount collected from the patient
   - Unique identifier (medical record number or chart number)
   - The International Classification of Diseases, 10th revision contains diagnosis codes. With it, written diagnoses are converted to alpha-numeric codes. It is published and maintained by the World Health Organization (WHO). In the United States, it has been "clinically modified" and is known as ICD-10-CM.

     It is the classification system required by the Centers for Medicare and Medicaid Services (CMS) to bill Medicare and Medicaid services in all healthcare settings. For example, the ICD-10-CM code for a patient with type 2 diabetes mellitus with diabetic nephropathy is E11.21.
   - Whether the encounter was due to an auto or other accident or was a work-related injury

5. Services
   - Procedures performed as indicated by Current Procedural Terminology (CPT®) codes. CPT® codes convert written procedures and services into numeric form. This code set is published by the American Medical Association (AMA) and is the required code set for submitting procedures and services for outpatients. An example of a CPT® code is 82247, which is the code for a total bilirubin test. HCPCS (Healthcare Common Procedure Coding System) codes are level 2 codes required by Medicare and Medicaid to document equipment, supplies, and patient transport. For example, code J0135 would be assigned for a 20 mg injection of the drug adalimumab. For hospital inpatients, ICD-10-PCS is used only in the United States and converts written descriptions of procedures into coded format and is used only in the inpatient setting. For example, the ICD-10-PCS code for a left heart catheterization is 4A023N7.
   - Date(s) of service

Information collected in each of these major sections may overlap. For instance, the place of service code or the dates of service code would be collected only once but satisfies the claim details as well as the services section requirements.

Administrative data, as well as clinical data, which describe the patient's diagnosis and procedures, may also be used to satisfy reporting requirements. For instance, capturing the race and ethnicity of all patients and then completing a report requested by the state department of health regarding race and ethnicity distribution is an example of the administrative use of data and an example of the meaningful use of data. Other administrative data elements that are required to satisfy Meaningful Use/Promoting Interoperability requirements are the patient's gender, preferred language, and date of birth. An example of a clinical data element that is collected from within the provider's documentation or in the health history is the patient's smoking status (if the patient is 13 years of age or older). A report that includes the total number of patients living in a particular ZIP code with a diagnosis of COPD (chronic obstructive pulmonary disease) is an example of a report that uses both administrative and clinical data. Another is the total number of patients between the ages of 13 and 50 years who are smokers and have a diagnosis of asthma. Either of these reports may be used by public health agencies or in educational materials for a smoking cessation class.

3.3 Accountable Care

The Patient Protection and Affordable Care Act (ACA) is part of the healthcare reform legislation passed in 2010. Included in that piece of legislation is the formation of the **Accountable Care Organization (ACO)**. An Accountable Care Organization is a healthcare model whereby a group of physicians, hospitals, and/or other healthcare providers (e.g., home health agencies) form a partnership that provides high-quality, coordinated care to a population of patients. The payment for the care is based on quality measures, as opposed to the traditional fee-for-service model. Data are necessary to report the results of each quality measure (Washington). ACO models include the Centers for Medicare & Medicaid Services (CMS) models and various commercial payer models.

The ACO models rely on the data gathered from individual providers' EHR systems. The exchange of health information that we discussed earlier is critical to the success of ACOs, since the point is coordination of care and the reduction of redundant or unnecessary treatments or diagnostics. Though this may result in a decrease in revenue for providers, it is essential if healthcare costs are to be contained. Health information professionals and practice managers play a major role in the ACO model, since quality data in the form of diagnosis and procedure codes, patient identification, and so on is essential in ensuring accurate, quality measurement and data integrity. ACOs will remain important as healthcare organizations prepare for the Medicare Access and CHIP Reauthorization Act of 2015 (MACRA).

Medicare Access and CHIP Reauthorization Act of 2015 (MACRA)

The **Medicare Access and CHIP Reauthorization Act (MACRA)** is also known as the "Doc Fix Act." It ended the Sustainable Growth Rate formula that had been used to determine payments to providers for healthcare services billed to Medicare beneficiaries. MACRA provides a framework that rewards care providers who give better (not necessarily more) care to Medicare beneficiaries and combines existing quality reporting systems into one new system. The point of MACRA is to reward providers for value rather than volume of care. It streamlines various quality programs under the **Merit-based Incentive Payment System (MIPS)** and gives bonus payments for providers who participate in alternative payment models, or APMs. In addition, MACRA required the removal of Social Security numbers from all Medicare cards by April 2019.

Accountable Care Organization (ACO) A reimbursement model where hospitals, physicians, and other healthcare providers form partnerships whereby all are accountable for the quality of care, efficiency of medical services (to contain costs), and patient satisfaction; a pay-for-performance model of healthcare reimbursement.

Medicare Access and CHIP (Children's Health Insurance Program) Reauthorization Act (MACRA) Act that ended the Sustainable Growth Rate formula that had been used to determine payments to providers for healthcare services billed to Medicare beneficiaries. Also known as the Doc Fix Act.

Merit-based Incentive Payment System (MIPS) A new Medicare provider payment program based on quality of care, resource use, clinical practice improvement, and meaningful use of certified EHR technology.

for your information

Examples of Medicare Shared Services Accountable Care Organizations include Adena Healthcare Collaborative, LLC; Bassett Accountable Care Partners, LLC; Bluegrass Clinical Partners, LLC; and Carroll ACO, LLC. An Internet search of any of these will give you a better understanding of an Accountable Care Organization and its structure.

Master Patient Index (MPI)/Patient List A permanent listing of all patients who have received care in a hospital (inpatient or outpatient). In physicians' offices often referred to as a Master Patient List or Patient List. May also be known as a Master Person List or Master Person Index.

The **Master Patient Index (MPI)** contains the identifying, or administrative, data on each patient. The acronym MPI is used more in the hospital setting than in the outpatient setting, although the objective is the same: one file of all the patients seen in the facility, with each patient listed in the index only *once*. In a medical practice, this may be referred to as the Patient List or **Master Patient List**. Each patient then has a second level of information that reflects individual visits to the facility/practice. For instance, James Philips has been a patient at Memorial Hospital. He was admitted as an inpatient in January 2018 for appendicitis. He was then seen in the emergency department of the hospital in June 2019 for a fracture of his right radius. In September he underwent outpatient blood work ordered by his primary care physician. In this instance, James will have one entry in the MPI, but he will have three individual encounters attached to his record (one inpatient, two outpatient encounters).

The MPI must be kept permanently, since it is the master file of all patients seen at a particular facility. In the hospital setting, records are filed by **medical record number**, which is a unique number assigned to each patient. The medical record number for each patient is linked to the patient's name in the MPI. Thus, if the MPI were destroyed or unavailable for some reason, it would be difficult, if not impossible, to locate the patient's health record in a paper record system. Though physicians' offices typically file alphabetically by the patient's last name, best practice still dictates that a master index (list) of all patients be kept.

Medical record number A unique number assigned to each patient seen by a facility or an office.

In some facilities and offices, the MPI is still kept manually. Now that records are in electronic format, and registration of patients is electronic, the MPI is also in electronic rather than manual form. Since manual MPIs still exist from previous years, it is important to be familiar with "MPI cards," as seen in Figure 3.3. Figure 3.4 is an example of the equivalent of an MPI entry in EHRclinic (for a different patient). Notice that in the electronic version, much more demographic information is collected and stored in this patient's master file than for the patient with the manual MPI card.

MEMORIAL HOSPITAL 7652 HORIZON WAY ARCADIA, OH 44804			
Last Name, First Name, Middle Name Phillips, James Bernard		**DOB** 7/31/1990	**Gender** Male **Race** Caucasian **Medical Record Number** AA005
Home Address 34951 Hickory Lane, Arcadia, OH 44804			**Telephone Number** 567-555-4192
Previous Name N/A			**Social Security Number** 678-90-1234
ADM/ENCOUNTER DATE	**DISCHARGE DATE**	**TYPE OF SERVICE**	**PROVIDER**
1/15/2018	1/28/2018	IP	Howard Hinkins, MD
6/22/2019	6/22/2019	ED	Sylvia Crowell, MD
9/30/2019	9/30/2019	OP	Lloyd Wright, MD

Figure 3.3   **Master Patient Index (MPI) Card**

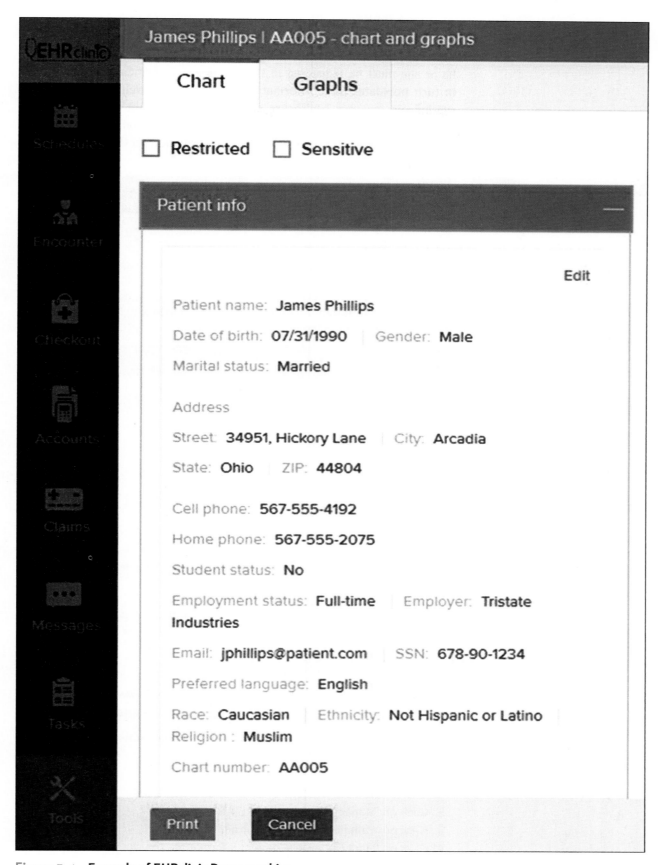

Figure 3.4   Example of EHRclinic Demographics

3.5 Registering a New Patient in EHRclinic

Before any information, administrative or clinical, is entered for a patient, he or she must be registered in the practice management software, which in turn populates basic information in the EHR as well. This function is carried out in every healthcare setting. It is important to have pertinent information about the patient available to the office staff. In Exercise 3.1, perform the steps necessary to view this information on the desktop.

EXERCISE 3.1 Go to https://connect.mheducation.com to complete this exercise. To see instructional notes with the steps, visit the eBook in Connect or download them from www.mhhe.com/iehr4.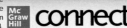

The Patient Information Screen

Using a computer to store data about all patients allows us to retrieve that data more quickly and is more efficient than using manual systems. There are certain data elements the healthcare professional needs to access often.

The Patient Information Settings screenshot in Figure 3.5 shows the screen used to change the information settings.

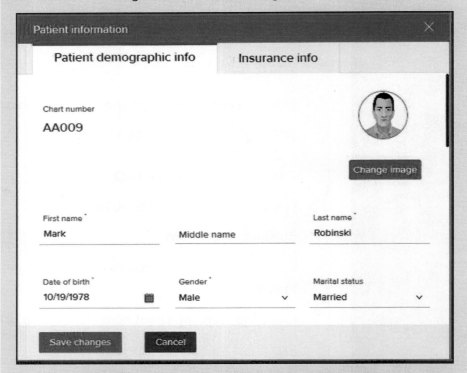

Figure 3.5 Patient Information Settings Screenshot in EHRclinic

In this exercise, you will select common data elements to display on the Desktop screen.

Follow these steps to complete this exercise:

1. Click on 'Tools' module.
2. Click on 'Manage practice data' button.
3. Click on 'Patient information' button.
4. Click on 'Mark Robinski's' patient information.
5. Click on 'Insurance info' tab.
6. Click on 'View chart' button.
7. Click on 'Collapse patient info' header.

8. Click on 'Collapse patient medical history' header.
9. Click on 'Collapse problem list' header.
10. Click on 'Collapse surgical history' header.
11. Click on 'Collapse family medical history' header.
12. Click on 'Collapse Social history' header.
13. Click on 'Collapse immunizations' header.
14. Click on 'Collapse medication list' header.
15. Click on 'Collapse allergies' header.
16. Click on 'Collapse list of lab reports' header.
17. Click on 'Collapse patient office visits' header.
18. Click on 'Collapse list of forms' header.
19. Click on 'Collapse messages' header.
20. Click on 'Collapse list of imaging reports' header.
21. Click on 'Collapse list of notes' header.
22. Click on 'Collapse list of letters' header.
23. Click on 'Collapse guarantor' header.
24. Click on 'Expand all' button.
25. Click on 'Add new note' button (in the Notes area).
26. Click on 'Note title' button and enter 'Review'.
27. Click on 'Note' button and enter 'Patient chart reviewed'.
28. Click on 'Done' button.

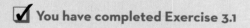 **You have completed Exercise 3.1**

In a physician's office, the registration process is completed by the reception staff at the time the patient arrives for care. In the hospital setting, the process takes place when the patient presents for care and is done by registration staff, often called Patient Access. Some hospitals have a centralized registration department, meaning that regardless of the type of patient (inpatient or outpatient), all registration is done from a central location. Other hospitals have decentralized registration, meaning that there is an admissions department that registers inpatients, an emergency department registration area for emergency patients, and an outpatient registration area for diagnostic testing such as radiology, laboratory, and physical therapy. It is important for the physician's office reception and scheduling staff to know what type of registration model is used by the local hospital(s), since communication with the registration staff is common. In Exercise 3.2 we will follow a patient through registration in a physician's office.

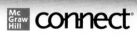 Go to https://connect.mheducation.com to complete this exercise. To see instructional notes with the steps, visit the eBook in Connect or download them from www.mhhe.com/iehr4. **EXERCISE** **3.2**

Register a New Patient

In this exercise, we will be registering a new patient, Alfredo J. Garza. He has called Summit Bay Health Center, asking if any of the providers are taking new patients. The healthcare professional tells him that Dr. Ingram, a family practice physician, is taking new patients and asks if he would like to

(continued)

establish care with Dr. Ingram. Since Mr. Garza does want to do so, the following steps are completed to register him in the practice management and EHR system of Summit Bay Health Center.

From the initial phone call, basic information such as full name, date of birth, address, and telephone number(s) is taken. He tells the healthcare professional that his name is Alfredo Jose Garza. He was born on 07/31/1958. His address is 117 Allenton Blvd., Bluffton, OH, 45817 and his phone number is 419-555-6179.

The healthcare professional will mail Mr. Garza some paperwork to complete before he arrives for his appointment. Typically, the paperwork includes a form to collect administrative information, a past medical history form, and authorization forms. The administrative information includes information such as address, telephone number, next of kin, insurance information, ethnicity, and race. The insurance information is entered as soon as it is available, so that verification of insurance can be done (more about insurance verification is in the financial management chapter).

For our purposes, we will assume that Mr. Garza completed the initial paperwork and brought it to the office before the day of his appointment with Dr. Ingram, as noted in Figure 3.6.

Follow these steps to complete the exercise on your own once you have watched the demonstration and tried the steps with helpful prompts. Use the registration form in Figure 3.6 to complete the following steps:

1. Click on 'Tools' module.
2. Click on 'Manage practice data' button.
3. Click on 'Patient information' button.
4. Click on 'Add new patient' button.
5. Click on 'First name' field and enter 'Alfredo'.
6. Click on 'Middle name' field and enter 'Jose'.
7. Click on 'Last name' field and enter 'Garza'.
8. Click on 'Date of birth' field and enter '07/31/1958'.
9. Click on 'Gender' drop-down and select 'Male'.
10. Click on 'Marital status' drop-down and select 'Single'.
11. Click on 'Street' field and enter '117 Allenton Blvd'.
12. Click on 'City' field and enter 'Bluffton'.
13. Click on 'Zip' field and enter '45817'.
14. Click on 'State' button and select 'Ohio'.
15. Click on 'Cell phone code' field and enter '419'.
16. Click on 'Cell phone' field and enter '555-6179'.
17. Click on 'Home phone code' field and enter '419'.
18. Click on 'Home phone' field and enter '555-6173'.
19. Click on 'Work phone code' field and enter '419'.
20. Click on 'Work phone' field and enter '555-0037'.
21. Click on 'Student status' drop-down and select 'No'.
22. Click on 'Employment status' drop-down and select 'Full-time'.
23. Click on 'Employer' field and enter 'Guardian Industries'.
24. Click on 'Email' field and enter 'agarza@guardianind.com'.
25. Click on 'SSN' field and enter '349-19-3741'.
26. Click on 'Preferred language' drop-down and select 'English'.
27. Click on 'Race' drop-down and select 'Declined to specify'.
28. Click on 'Ethnicity' drop-down and select 'Hispanic or Latino'.
29. Click on 'Religion' drop-down and select 'Catholic'.

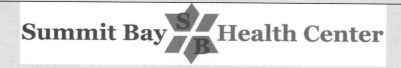

REGISTRATION FORM

(Please Print)

Today's date: March 17, 2022	Care Provider: Dr. Ingram

PATIENT INFORMATION

Patient's last name:	First:	Middle:	☒ Mr. ☐ Miss ☐ Mrs. ☐ Ms.	Marital status (circle one)
Garza	Alfredo	Jose		(Single) / Mar / Div / Sep / Wid

Is this your legal name?	If not, what is your legal name?	(Former name):	Birth date:	Age:	Sex:
☒ Yes ☐ No			07/31/1958	63	☒ M ☐ F

Street address:	Social Security no.:	Home phone:	Cell phone:
117 Allenton Blvd	349-19-3741	419-555-6173	419-555-6179

P. O. Box:	City:	State:	ZIP Code:
	Bluffton	OH	45817

Occupation:	Employer:	Employer phone no.:
Project Manager	Guardian Industries	419-555-0037

E-mail address: agarcia@guardianind.com

Race: declined	Ethnicity: Hispanic	Primary language: English	Religion: Catholic

Other family members seen here: none

INSURANCE INFORMATION

(Presentation of Insurance Card is required at time of each visit)

Person responsible for bill:	Date of birth:	Address:	Home phone:	Cell phone:
Alfredo Garza	07/31/1958			

Is this person a patient here?	☒ Yes ☐ No

Occupation:	Employer:	Employer address:	Employer phone no.:

Is this patient covered by insurance?	☒ Yes ☐ No

Please indicate primary insurance	☒ McGraw-Hill Healthmark Insurance	☐ BlueCross/ Blue Shield	☐ [Insurance]	☐ [Insurance]	☐ [Insurance]

☐ [Insurance]	☐ Workers' Compensation	☐ Medicare	☐ Medicaid *(Please provide card)*	☐ Other

Subscriber's name:	Subscriber's S.S. no.:	Date of birth:	Group no.:	Policy no.:	Co-payment:
Alfredo Jose Garza	349-19-3741	07/31/1958	6500	GAR5679009	$ 20.00

Patient's relationship to subscriber:	☒ Self ☐ Spouse ☐ Child ☐ Other	Effective Date: 01/01/2022

Name of secondary insurance (if applicable): None	Subscriber's name:	Group no.:	Policy no.:

Patient's relationship to subscriber:	☒ Self ☐ Spouse ☐ Child ☐ Other

IN CASE OF EMERGENCY

Name of local friend or relative (not living at same address):	Relationship to patient:	Home phone no.: ( )	Work phone no.: ( )

The above information is true to the best of my knowledge. I authorize my insurance benefits be paid directly to the physician. I understand that I am financially responsible for any balance. I also authorize [Name of Practice] or insurance company to release any information required to process my claims.

Alfredo Garza

03/17/2022

Patient/Guardian signature

Date

Figure 3.6 Alfredo Garza Registration Form

(continued)

30. Click on 'Search by insurance carrier name' search field and enter 'mcg'.
31. Click on 'McGraw-Hill Healthmark'.
32. Click on 'Patient insurance id' field and enter 'GAR5679009'.
33. Click on 'Add patient' button.
34. Click on 'Okay' button.

✔️ **You have completed Exercise 3.2**

 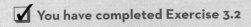
3.6 Scheduling an Appointment

In EHRclinic, the "Appointment Scheduling" function is used to make the appointment with the provider who has been assigned to that patient. In Alfredo Garza's example, he was a new patient and was assigned to Dr. Ingram.

In an office setting, the healthcare professional will need to know the reason for the visit in order to allot enough time for it. For example, a follow-up visit for hypertension is going to take less time than a physical exam. The scheduler or healthcare professional will also ask for convenient days and times before beginning the search for the appointment. In a hospital setting, outpatient procedures such as CT scans or MRIs are scheduled in advance, and the process is similar.

Each care provider is set up in the PM system to show his or her typical schedule. For instance, Dr. Ingram may prefer to start the day at 9:00 a.m., break for lunch from noon to 1 p.m., and end his day at 5:30 p.m. Dr. Pueblas, on the other hand, may prefer to start seeing patients at 8 a.m., break from seeing patients between 11 and 11:30 a.m. to return phone calls and perform administrative tasks, see patients from 11:30 a.m. until 1:00 p.m., and then break for lunch from 1:00 p.m. until 2:00 p.m. Her last appointment of the day is scheduled for 4:30 p.m. In addition, some care providers prefer to do complete physical exams only in the morning. Many offices leave open appointment times for urgent visits. Patients who do not show up for an appointment, or who cancel at the last minute, can wreak havoc on a schedule!

EXERCISE 3.3

Go to https://connect.mheducation.com to complete this exercise. To see instructional notes with the steps, visit the eBook in Connect or download them from www.mhhe.com/iehr4.

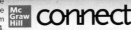

Schedule an Appointment

Recall that we registered Mr. Garza in Exercise 3.2, so his name is located in EHRclinic's Master Patient List. The healthcare professional asked Mr. Garza which days of the week work best for him. He does not have a preference of day, but he would like to be seen soon, so the healthcare professional starts the search beginning with March 28th. Since Mr. Garza is establishing care with this office, the type of visit he will have is a Routine Office Visit (ROV). He will be having a complete exam. When the correct type of visit is selected, the amount of time allotted for that visit is automatically assigned by the system. In this case, it will be a 30-minute appointment. He then states that a morning visit on a Wednesday is best for him, so 9:30 on March 30th is selected by the healthcare professional. Mr. Garza also states that he is having shortness of breath, so that will be entered as his **chief complaint**, which is the reason (in the patient's own words) that he has made the appointment.

Now we will perform the process of scheduling an appointment for Alfredo Garza.

Follow these steps to complete the exercise on your own once you have watched the demonstration and tried the steps with helpful prompts:

1. Click on 'New appointment' button.
2. Click on 'Search patient' field and enter 'gar'.
3. Click on 'Alfredo Garza' patient.
4. Click on 'Date & time' icon and select 'March 30, 2022 - 12:00 am'.
5. Click on 'Increase hour' button until 9:00 am.
6. Click on 'Increase minute' button until 9:30 am.
7. Click on 'Done' button.
8. Click on 'Duration' icon.
9. Click on 'Increase minute' button until 30 minutes.
10. Click on 'Done' button.
11. Click on 'Reason for visit' field and enter 'Shortness of breath'.
12. Click on 'Schedule' button.

✓ **You have completed Exercise 3.3**

> **Chief complaint** The reason for which a patient has made an appointment (usually in his or her own words, for instance, "I have a sore throat").
>
> **EHRclinic Tip** 〔EHRclinic〕
>
> In EHRclinic, the Search function is triggered once three characters are entered. Patients whose last names contain those three letters will appear in the list. The healthcare professional should then search for the correct patient carefully by matching the remainder of the patient's last name, first name, and middle name and finally verify by checking the patient's date of birth against the names listed in the Master Index.
>
> **EHRclinic Tip** 〔EHRclinic〕
>
> When choosing dates by using the EHRclinic datepicker icon (calendar icon in date fields), first select the month, then the year, and then the day.

3.7 Editing Demographic Data

People move, their last names change, their emergency contact information changes—just about anything except their first name and date of birth can change. It is important that an office always have up-to-date information on a patient.

At the time of check-in, many offices print out the identification page and have the patient review it, either on a yearly basis or even every time a patient is seen. If changes need to be made, the patient communicates them to the office staff, and the information is edited appropriately. To save paper, some offices have a computer terminal where the patient can view the information on the screen, or the healthcare professional may just swivel the screen around for the patient to view and either verify that no changes are necessary or state what information does need to be changed.

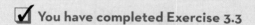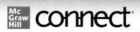

McGraw Hill **connect** Go to https://connect.mheducation.com to complete this exercise. To see instructional notes with the steps, visit the eBook in Connect or download them from www.mhhe.com/iehr4.

EHR PM EXERCISE 3.4

Edit Demographic Information

In this exercise, Mr. Garza realizes that he has moved since initially completing the registration paperwork; he calls in to the office to give his new address. He tells the healthcare professional that his street address is now 3729 Clearwater St. His other demographic information remains unchanged.

(continued)

Follow these steps to complete the exercise on your own once you've watched the demonstration and tried the steps with helpful prompts:

1. Click on 'Tools' module.
2. Click on 'Manage practice data' button.
3. Click on 'Patient information' button.
4. Click on 'Search patient' field.
5. Enter 'gar' in 'Search patient' field.
6. Click on 'Alfredo Garcia's' patient information.
7. Click on 'Street: 117 Allenton Blvd' field.
8. Enter '3729 Clearwater St' in 'Street' field.
9. Click on 'Add image' field.
10. Click on Alfredo Garza's image.
11. Click on 'Choose' button.
12. Click on 'Save changes' button.

☑ **You have completed Exercise 3.4**

Default value A value that automatically appears in a field each time it appears on a screen (e.g., the current date in a date field, the local area code in a home phone number field).

for your information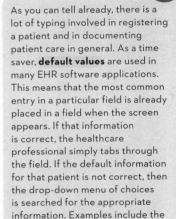

As you can tell already, there is a lot of typing involved in registering a patient and in documenting patient care in general. As a time saver, **default values** are used in many EHR software applications. This means that the most common entry in a particular field is already placed in a field when the screen appears. If that information is correct, the healthcare professional simply tabs through the field. If the default information for that patient is not correct, then the drop-down menu of choices is searched for the appropriate information. Examples include the Visit Type and Service Location fields.

3.8 Checking In a Patient

One of the advantages of using PM software is the ability to track a patient's flow through the office. The flow starts when the patient checks in. As a patient, you are aware of this part of the process—it is when you either sign your name on a log sheet or verbally inform the healthcare professional that you have arrived. This process is used in a physician's office setting but would not necessarily have a use in the hospital environment, other than in the outpatient registration area.

The typical flow is the following:

Patient checks in at front desk > patient is seen by the clinical support team (MA or nurse) > patient is seen by the care provider (physician or physician's assistant or nurse practitioner) > patient stops at the cashier or check-out desk > billing processes begin

EXERCISE 3.5 Go to https://connect.mheducation.com to complete this exercise. To see instructional notes with the steps, visit the eBook in Connect or download them from www.mhhe.com/iehr4.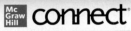

Check In a Patient Who Has Arrived

In the following exercise, Alfredo Garza has arrived and he has just signed the log, which alerts the healthcare professional to check him in for his appointment.

Follow these steps to complete the exercise on your own once you have watched the demonstration and tried the steps with helpful prompts:

1. Click on 'Schedules' module.
2. Double-click on 'Alfredo Garza's' appointment.
3. Click on 'Check-in' button.
4. Click on 'Check-in' button.
5. Click on 'Okay' button.

EHRclinic Tip EHRclinic

In some EHRclinic exercises, the Path window may obstruct areas you need to click. If this happens, you can collapse the path within the window or click to hide it in the upper left corner of the screen.

☑ **You have completed Exercise 3.5**

Although a medical practice or hospital is in business to care for patients, in the end, it is also just that—a business. In order to stay financially viable, there must be organized, effective policies and procedures in place to ensure cash flow and fiscal success.

You will learn about the intricacies of setting up fee schedules, billing insurance plans, and collection procedures in another course. In Exercise 3.6, though, you will learn about the information that must be collected for any patients who have a private or group insurance plan or who participate in a government health plan.

Figure 3.7 is a sample insurance card. The patient should present this card each time he or she arrives for an encounter. Office staff may scan the front and back of the card as an image that will reside in EHRclinic, or they may photocopy the front and back of the card and keep it in the patient's chart.

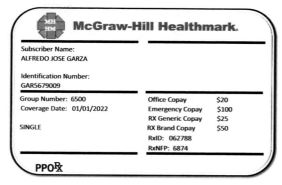

Figure 3.7   Sample Insurance Card

The information must be entered in EHRclinic exactly as it appears on the insurance card. For instance, say Alfredo Jose Garza does not use his first name; instead, he uses A. Jose Garza. But his insurance card reads Alfredo Jose Garza. In EHRclinic, or any other PM software, he should be entered as Alfredo Jose Garza.

Any typographical errors within EHRclinic will result in a delayed or denied claim. That will slow payment, which is not good business practice for the office!

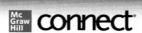 Go to https://connect.mheducation.com to complete this exercise. To see instructional notes with the steps, visit the eBook in Connect or download them from www.mhhe.com/iehr4.

 EXERCISE 3.6

Capture Insurance Information of a Patient

In this exercise, Mr. Garza has presented his insurance card to the health-care professional and has completed the insurance information on his registration form (Figure 3.6). Mr. Garza has coverage through only one insurance company, so that is the primary insurance (the first insurance that is billed).

Follow these steps to complete the exercise on your own once you have watched the demonstration and tried the steps with helpful prompts:

1. Click on 'Schedules' module.
2. Double-click on 'Alfredo Garza's' appointment.
3. Click on 'Insurance info' tab.
4. Click on 'Edit primary insurance' button.
5. Click on 'Is the plan active' drop-down and click 'Yes'.
6. Click on 'Patient responsibility' drop-down and click 'Copay'.
7. Click on 'Copay' field and enter '20'.
8. Click on 'Deductible' field and enter '0'.
9. Click on 'Deductible met' drop-down and click 'N/A'.
10. Click on 'Effective start date of coverage' field and select 'January 01 2022' date.

(continued)

11. Click on 'Effective end date of coverage' field and select 'December 31 2022' date.
12. Click on 'Group insurance ID' field and enter '6500'.
13. Click on 'Done' button.
14. Click on 'Save changes' button.

✓ **You have completed Exercise 3.6**

3.10 Guiding Staff Through the Use of an Electronic System

The use of electronic health records systems is not terribly difficult once one knows how to navigate through the various screens and has knowledge of the content of each section of the EHR. With practice, using an EHR becomes second nature. But a user's manual and a place to go for help is imperative in any computer system—healthcare or otherwise.

As mentioned in Chapter 1, typically, there is a User's Guide, which is lengthy, gives an overview of all the functionality of the system, and is then broken down by the individual functions of the system. It is usually accessible online from within the computer software itself. Any new employee and any employees who are using a new system, whether to input or access information (or both), should be familiar with the User's Guide.

However, on a daily basis, the Help feature is a staple of almost any computer software program. Remember that the User's Guide, tutorials, and any pop-up Help feature is there to be *used* when needed! For many of us, it is easier to ask someone how to perform a particular function than to search for the solution ourselves. The problem is that the person you are asking may give you the incorrect answer, or you may need an answer fast and there is no one around to ask. It shows initiative and will help you remember the steps more easily if you seek out answers on your own. Consider this analogy—you remember how to get to a particular destination when you have driven there yourself rather than as a passenger, correct? The same applies here. You will remember and *understand* the process if you look up the steps on your own.

Often, electronic systems also have on-demand Frequently Asked Questions (FAQs) and will post information about new upgrades in functionality. Readily available in EHRclinic Help is material that speaks to the newest upgrades in functionality, designed to help users maximize their EHR experience (Figure 3.8).

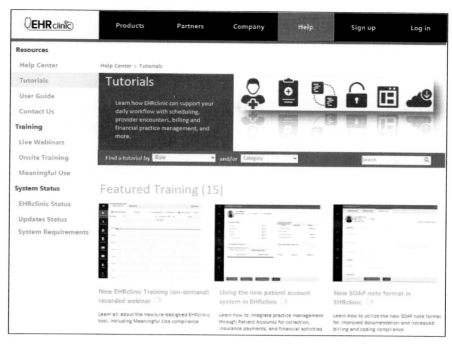

Figure 3.8   EHRclinic User Training and Help Options

APPLYING YOUR SKILLS

In this chapter we discussed how important accurate data is. Let's take a look at a situation that is not all that uncommon.

Cindy, at Dr. Clark's office, is in the midst of checking in a patient, Diana G. Pike, while also listening to her supervisor, Emily, give her instructions about something unrelated. Mrs. Pike has filled out the new patient registration form and mentioned to Cindy that she is a new patient. Mrs. Pike has a seat, and Cindy is completing her registration. She types in the last name of Pike and sees that there is a Diana Pike in the system. Diana G. Pike has a date of birth of 9/18/1957 and lives at 367 Georgetown Way, Bluffton, OH 45817. Diana Pike has a date of birth of 8/18/1957 and lives at 387 Warren Blvd, Bluffton, OH 45817. She assumes that someone inaccurately entered Diana Pike into the system, and she enters information about today's appointment under Diana Pike's record in the Master Patient Index.

Is there a problem? If so, what is it? How could it have been avoided? What impact could this have on other steps of the process?

chapter 3 summary

LEARNING OUTCOME	CONCEPTS FOR REVIEW
3.1 Identify administrative data elements.	– Demographic data are identifying data – Administrative data include demographic data as well as additional nonclinical data – A data dictionary is necessary to ensure consistency and reliability of data – CMS-1500, UB-04, and HIPAA regulations dictate much of the administrative data captured

3.2 Explain the administrative uses of data.	– Insurance purposes (file claims)
	– Satisfy regulatory requirements and Meaningful Use
	– Five sections of the claim form
	  • Provider
	  • Subscriber
	  • Payer
	  • Claim detail
	  • Services

3.3 Explain the use of EHR data in an Accountable Care Organization (ACO).	– Patient Protection and Affordable Care Act (ACA)
	– Definition of an ACO
	  • A new healthcare reimbursement model
	  • Partnership between healthcare providers to provide high-quality, coordinated care
	– Reimbursement based on quality measures, not fee for service
	– Need data from EHR to report results of each quality measure
	– ACO model used by Medicare and some commercial insurance plans
	– Medicare Access and CHIP Reauthorization Act (MACRA)
	  • Merit-based Incentive Payment System (MIPS)
	– Health information professionals as well as office administrators must ensure quality data collection and reporting

3.4 Explain the use of the Master Patient Index (MPI).	– Means of tracking that a patient was seen in a healthcare facility – Only one entry per patient • Each encounter has its own entry, filed under the patient's master entry – Medical record (chart) number unique to each patient—links the patient to his or her health record – Can be manual or electronic – Kept permanently

LEARNING OUTCOME	CONCEPTS FOR REVIEW
3.5 Apply procedures to register a new patient in EHRclinic.	– Patient must have an entry in the Master Patient Index or Patient List before any other functions can occur (scheduling, patient's chart, etc.) – Registration process occurs in every healthcare setting – Registration process ultimately results in the patient's being a part of the MPI – In a physician's office setting, this is done by a healthcare professional – In a hospital setting, this is done by the registration department
3.6 Apply procedures to schedule a patient's appointment in EHRclinic.	– Before scheduling an appointment, a provider has to be assigned, if a new patient, or select the patient's usual provider – Must know the reason for the visit in order to allot sufficient time for the visit – Select a date and time that works for the patient
3.7 Apply procedures to edit demographic information in EHRclinic.	– All information about a patient must be current and correct – Verification of demographic and administrative information is done by administrative personnel at the time a patient checks in – Information is edited, added, or deleted as appropriate

3.8 Identify the steps performed upon patient check-in.	– Knowing where the patient is in the flow through the office is important to maintain efficiency
	– Typical flow:
	  • Patient checks in at reception desk
	  • Patient is called back to the exam room by the healthcare professional
	  • Patient is seen and examined by the provider
	  • Patient checks out
	  • Claim process begins

3.9 Apply procedures to capture insurance information in EHRclinic.	– Capturing complete, correct insurance information is vital to cash flow and financial success – Require patients to present their insurance card on every visit – Information in the practice management system must match what is on the insurance card
3.10 Locate the User's Guide and Help feature in EHRclinic.	• User's Guide available on demand in most software systems • Frequently Asked Questions (FAQs) also may be available • Specific Help features by function in most software

chapter review

MATCHING QUESTIONS

Match the terms on the left with the definitions on the right.

_____ 1. **[LO 3.6]** chief complaint

_____ 2. **[LO 3.1]** account (billing) number

_____ 3. **[LO 3.1]** CMS-1500

_____ 4. **[LO 3.1]** administrative data

_____ 5. **[LO 3.1]** Clinical Documentation Architecture (CDA)

_____ 6. **[LO 3.4]** Master Patient Index (MPI)

_____ 7. **[LO 3.1]** UB-04

_____ 8. **[LO 3.1]** Continuity of Care Document (CCD)

_____ 9. **[LO 3.1]** library

_____ 10. **[LO 3.1]** data dictionary

a. information, such as a patient's insurance information, marital status, employer

b. list of correct definitions for a facility's unique terms and jargon

c. form used to submit insurance claims in an outpatient setting such as physician's office

d. in terms of computer software, a comprehensive listing of related entities to choose from, such as ICD-10 codes

e. form used to submit insurance claims in a hospital setting

f. permanent roster of all patients ever seen in a healthcare setting

g. reason for a patient's appointment; may determine the length of an exam visit

h. HL7 standard that outlines the format of clinical documentation, such as reports and discharge summaries

i. document exchange standard that guides how patient information is shared among providers and healthcare settings

j. a unique number assigned to every new encounter

MULTIPLE-CHOICE QUESTIONS

Select the letter that best completes the statement or answers the question:

1. **[LO 3.1]** _____ data include demographic data.
   a. Clinical
   b. HIPAA
   c. Administrative
   d. Financial

2. **[LO 3.4]** Anna Jacobs presented to the ER of County Hospital three times in the past year. She will appear in County's MPI
   a. once.
   b. twice.
   c. three times.
   d. four times.

3. **[LO 3.1]** Which of the following is NOT an example of demographic data?
   a. full name
   b. primary physician
   c. Social Security number
   d. date of birth

4. **[LO 3.2]** Administrative data are used to satisfy _____ requirements.
   a. CCHIP
   b. HITECH
   c. HIPAA
   d. ONC

5. **[LO 3.5]** Before a patient can be treated at a healthcare setting, she must be
   a. prepped.
   b. registered.
   c. logged.
   d. admitted.

6. **[LO 3.4]** How long should a facility's Master Patient Index be kept?
   a. three years
   b. five years
   c. seven years
   d. permanently

7. **[LO 3.1]** Recording a patient's previous or married name might help with
   a. cross-referencing data.
   b. compiling family history.
   c. legal proceedings.
   d. Privacy Rule compliance.

8. **[LO 3.10]** Where should staff go for help if they need it in EHRclinic?
   a. Work Flow Help
   b. User's Guide
   c. Frequently Asked Questions
   d. Any of the above

9. **[LO 3.5]** _____ is part of a patient's administrative information found on a registration form.
   a. Occupation
   b. Chief complaint
   c. Provider number
   d. Co-pay amount

10. **[LO 3.1]** Patient demographic information should be verified
    a. at the initial visit.
    b. at each visit.
    c. once a year.
    d. when the patient initiates a change.

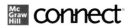

Enhance your learning by completing these exercises and more at https://connect.mheducation.com!

11. **[LO 3.9]** An insurance claim may be denied if the receptionist fails to
    a. collect a patient's co-pay.
    b. make a copy of the patient's insurance card.
    c. enter all data correctly.
    d. have the patient sign the front-desk log.

12. **[LO 3.6]** _____ is part of the Appointment scheduling feature of EHRclinic.
    a. Occupation
    b. Chief complaint
    c. Provider number
    d. Co-pay amount

13. **[LO 3.3]** Accountable Care Organizations rely on EHR
    a. data.
    b. functionality.
    c. compliance.
    d. format.

14. **[LO 3.2]** A facility's collection of patient data might be used to satisfy _____ requirements.
    a. data dictionary
    b. Meaningful Use
    c. incentive
    d. interoperability

15. **[LO 3.7]** Editing a patient's mailing address is accomplished by using
    a. drop-down menus.
    b. free-text fields.
    c. Help topics.
    d. patient flags.

16. **[LO 3.4]** In a hospital's health information department, patient records are most often filed by
    a. patient's last name.
    b. number of patient encounters.
    c. provider identification number.
    d. medical record number.

17. **[LO 3.8]** Patient check-in is
    a. essential for claims processing.
    b. important for efficient patient tracking.
    c. done in the patient chart.
    d. an optional function in EHRclinic.

18. **[LO 3.2]** Information such as a policyholder name and insurance plan name appears in the _____ section of a claim form.
    a. payer
    b. provider
    c. services
    d. subscriber

SHORT-ANSWER QUESTIONS

1. **[LO 3.3]** What is the role of an Accountable Care Organization?

2. **[LO 3.5]** What is the difference between centralized and decentralized registration centers in a hospital setting?

3. **[LO 3.9]** Explain why it is important to enter insurance information into EHRclinic exactly as it appears on a patient's insurance card.

4. **[LO 3.7]** List at least three ways that an office can obtain updated patient information.

5. **[LO 3.1]** Why is it important that every staff member in a facility use terminology consistently?

6. **[LO 3.10]** Carolyn is a new employee at a cardiology practice. She will be registering patients as well as doing some coding and billing. She has never used EHRclinic, though she has had experience with other EHR software. She is having trouble catching on. What might her supervisor have her do, so that she is more comfortable with the use of EHRclinic and so that she knows where to go for answers?

7. **[LO 3.6]** Explain why the receptionist needs to ask the reason for a patient visit when scheduling an appointment.

8. **[LO 3.2]** The CMS-1500 form is used to submit claims for _____ encounters, whereas the UB-04 form is used to submit _____ claims.

9. **[LO 3.7]** Discuss the importance of reliable, up-to-date patient information.

10. **[LO 3.1]** List at least five required pieces of demographic information collected for each patient.

11. **[LO 3.8]** Fields, such as Visit Type, that contain a list of options to choose from are known as what type of menus?

12. **[LO 3.4]** Explain the use of a medical record number.

13. **[LO 3.2]** List the five major sections on a standard claim form.

14. **[LO 3.9]** A patient may _____ to provide certain optional pieces of information if he or she feels uncomfortable.

15. **[LO 3.9]** List at least three pieces of information typically found on a patient's insurance card.

16. **[LO 3.3]** Define and explain the purpose of MACRA.

APPLYING YOUR KNOWLEDGE

1. **[LOs 3.5, 3.6, 3.7, 3.8, 3.9, 3.10]** Which of the EHRclinic exercises completed in this chapter do you think will be used most often in the office setting? Explain your answer.

2. **[LOs 3.1, 3.2, 3.7]** As the receptionist for Summit Bay Health Center, you recently mailed an informational letter to all patients listed in your MPI. One morning you come into work and see Alfredo Garza's letter marked "Return to Sender, Address Unknown" sitting on your desk. What do you do?

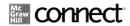

Enhance your learning by completing these exercises and more at https://**connect.mheducation.com**!

3. **[LOs 3.1, 3.2]** Discuss why administrative data such as race, ethnicity, and preferred language might need to be reported to satisfy Promoting Interoperability (Meaningful Use) requirements.

4. **[LO 3.4]** The text mentions that if an MPI were inaccessible or unavailable for any reason, it would be nearly impossible to locate a patient's record. Is that true for paper and electronic health records alike? Explain that statement.

5. **[LOs 3.1, 3.2, 3.4]** One of your colleagues has been asked to update the office's data dictionary. She remarks that she does not see why having the data dictionary is so important, because most terms are easily understood by most people in the office. How would you explain to her, with examples, the importance of a solid data dictionary for your practice?

6. **[LOs 3.5, 3.6, 3.7, 3.8]** Discuss the advantages of using a practice management tool such as EHRclinic to complete tasks such as patient registration and appointment scheduling.

7. **[LOs 3.4, 3.5, 3.7]** Why is it important to search for a patient in the MPI before adding the person as a new patient? Explain the consequences of having a patient entered more than once.

8. **[LO 3.3]** Discuss the potential benefits and risks associated with the use of Accountable Care Organizations.

9. **[LO 3.1]** Visit the Commonwell Health Alliance website, at https://www.commonwellalliance.org. Discuss how they intend to increase the interoperability of EHR systems. Additionally, explain why interoperability is so important when using EHRs.

10. **[LO 3.3]** The Merit-based Incentive Payment System, or MIPS, is part of the Medicare Access and CHIP Reauthorization Act (MACRA). Explain how MIPS is linked to incentives.

chapter references

Centers for Medicare & Medicaid Services (CMS). *MACRA Delivery System Reform, Medicare Payment Reform.* Retrieved from https://www.cms.gov/Medicare/Quality-Initiatives-Patient-Assessment -Instruments/Value-Based-Programs/MACRA-MIPS-and-APMs/MACRA-MIPS-and-APMs.html.

Commonwell Health Alliance. Retrieved from https://www.commonwellalliance.org/.

Dimick, Chris. "Exposing Double Identity at Patient Registration" *Journal of AHIMA, 80*(11). (2009, November).

Dolin, R.H., Alschuler, L., Beebe, C., et al. (2001, November-December). The HL7 Clinical Document Architecture. *Journal of the American Medical Informatics Association, 8*(6): 552–569.

EHR Incentive Program. *Eligible Professional Meaningful Use Table of Contents Core and Menu Set Measures.* Retrieved from https://www.cms.gov/Regulations-and-Guidance/Legislation/EHRIncentivePrograms /downloads/EP-MU-TOC.pdf.

Mertz, Jon. (2010). HL7 Standards. HL7 Quality Reporting Document Architecture (QRDA) Defined. Retrieved from http://healthstandards.com/blog/2010/01/28/hl7-quality-reporting-document -architecture-qrda-defined/.

National Committee on Vital and Health Statistics. (1996). *Core Health Data Elements: Report of the National Committee on Vital and Health Statistics.* Retrieved from http://www.cdc.gov/nchs/data/ncvhs /nchvs94.pdf.

Newby, Cynthia. (2010). *From Patient to Payment: Insurance Procedures for the Medical Office* (6th ed.). New York: McGraw-Hill Companies.

SearchHealthIT. Continuity of Care Document (CCD). Retrieved from http://searchhealthit.techtarget.com /definition/Continuity-of-Care-Document-CCD.

Washington, Lydia. (2013, March 1). ACO Summit Highlights. *Journal of AHIMA.* Retrieved from http:// journal.ahima.org/2013/03/01/aco-summit-highlights/.

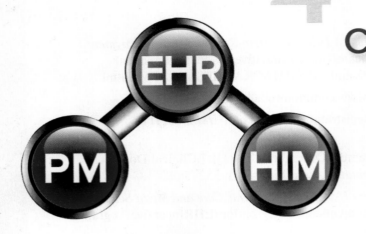

chapter **four**

Content of the Health Record—The Past Medical, Surgical, Family, and Social Histories

What You Need to Know and Why You Need to Know It

Before patients are seen by the care provider, they first meet with the healthcare professional, such as a medical assistant or nurse, to go over the reason for the visit and to capture historical information about their health status. In this chapter we will cover the types of history collected. We will also cover *why* knowing this information is so important in the care of the patient. As with all documentation in a health record, the history must be accurate because often the past history plays a part in the diagnosis and treatment of the current condition. The history generally begins with the chief complaint, which is documented in the patient's (or legal representative's) own words.

4.1 Forms as Data Collection Tools

Take a moment to think of forms that you have completed recently. Most likely they were on paper, and you can probably think immediately of one that was long and cumbersome and took quite a bit of thought to complete. You can also think of one or two that seemed rather logical, well organized, and easy to complete. The same goes for forms that are on-screen rather than on paper. When we speak of paper forms, we refer to "boxes" that we are filling out. On-screen, these boxes are called *fields*. In most healthcare settings, at this point in time, much of the information gathered from a patient will continue to be collected through the use of a paper form, and then that information will be transferred to the patient's EHR. Thus, it is important that the design of paper forms be logical to minimize the amount of time it takes to transfer the information and to minimize the likelihood of having missing or incorrect information end up in the EHR. More offices are coming into the digital age, however, and have placed computer terminals in waiting areas, so that patients can sign in from the terminals as well as update demographic information rather than "signing in" on a paper log. Even driver's licenses and insurance cards can be scanned from these terminals, thus capturing accurate (and valid) identification as well as accurate billing information. As the transition to an electronic record progresses, patients will increasingly complete other forms electronically, though paper forms will not disappear completely, since there will be patients who do not want to complete the forms electronically due to lack of a computer, lack of computer literacy, or privacy concerns, and when the computer system "goes down" we will still need to revert to paper and then enter the data manually into the EHR.

When designing a form, keep in mind the following:

- The form should have a name—a title that correlates to the information gathered on the form.
- The name of the office or facility should be added to the form.
- Each page of a multipage form should include the patient's name, the patient's date of birth (DOB), and the medical record number or chart number to guard against intermingling the records of patients with the same or similar names and to guard against documentation errors in general.
- The information collected should be relevant to the purpose of the form. Only data that are necessary should be collected—a medical history

Page 1

SUMMIT BAY HEALTH CENTER MEDICAL HISTORY FORM

PATIENT NAME	DOB	MEDICAL RECORD NUMBER

PLEASE ANSWER THE FOLLOWING QUESTIONS THOROUGHLY. IF A QUESTION DOESN'T APPLY, PLEASE ENTER N/A OR PLACE A LINE IN THAT AREA.

PRESENT MEDICAL CONDITION (why are you being seen today)

_____

_____

_____

ALLERGIES/REACTIONS TO MEDICINES/FOODS:

NAME OF MEDICATION/AGENT	TYPE OF REACTION

MEDICATIONS: Enter all prescription and non-prescription medicines, herbal remedies, vitamins, or birth control medications here:

MEDICATION	DOSE	HOW OFTEN?	TAKEN FOR?

PERSONAL MEDICAL HISTORY: Please check all conditions you have had (with approximate date or year)

Heart Disease ____ _____ Cancer ____ _____ Type _____

Heart attack ____ _____ Diabetes ____ _____ Type _____

Hypertension ____ _____ Thyroid ____ _____ Type _____

Stroke ____ _____ Bleeding Disorder ____ _____ Type _____

High cholesterol ____ _____ Other ____ _____

Depression/Suicide Attempt ____ _____ Other ____ _____

Alcoholism _____ Other ____ _____

1

Page 2

Patient Name _____ DOB _____ Med. Record Number _____

SURGICAL HISTORY: Please indicate all procedures or surgeries you have had (with approximate date or year)

Type of surgery	Date (year)	Name of surgeon

FAMILY HISTORY: Please place a check under the family member who has had any of the conditions:

CONDITION	Mom	Dad	Sib.	Child	Other	CONDITION	Mom	Dad	Sibling	Child	Other
Alcoholism						Environmental allergies					
Anemia						Loss of hearing					
Anesthesia problem						Heart problems (heart attack, coronary artery disease, congestive heart failure)					
Arthritis						Hypertension					
Asthma						High cholesterol					
Bleeding problem						Mitral valve disorders					
Cancer, breast						Lupus					
Cancer, colon						HIV/AIDS					
Cancer, melanoma/basal cell						Kidney disease					
Cancer, ovarian						Mental health disorders					
Cancer, prostate						Migraine headaches					
Cancer, other						Osteoarthritis					
Depression						Rheumatoid arthritis					
Type I Diabetes						CVA (stroke)					
Type II Diabetes						Cerebral hemorrhage					
Eczema						Thyroid disorder					
Seizure disorder or epilepsy						Other					
Glaucoma						Other					

IMMUNIZATION HISTORY: Please indicate date (or best guess) of last immunization for:

Hepatitis A _____ Hepatitis B ____ Measles ___ Mumps ____ Rubella ____ Pneumovax (pneumonia) ____

Tetanus (Td) _____ MMR ____ Chicken pox _____ Flu ____Other _____

SOCIAL HISTORY

Tobacco Use

Cigarettes (current use) ☐ yes ☐ no If yes, packs per day _____ for _____ years

Cigarettes (past use) ☐ yes ☐ no If yes, no. of years _____; quit when? _____

2

Page 3

Patient Name _____ DOB _____ Med. Record Number _____

____ Other current tobacco use: ☐ snuff/chew ☐ pipe ☐ cigar

____ Other past tobacco use: ☐ snuff/chew ☐ pipe ☐ cigar

Alcohol Use

Do you drink alcohol? ☐ yes ☐ no If yes, no. of drinks per week _____

Recreational Drug Use

Do you use any recreational drugs? ☐ yes ☐ no If yes, what and how often? _____

_____

Physical Activity

How often do you exercise? _____ times/week

Are you relatively active (engage in recreational sports, take stairs daily, job involves standing, walking often, etc). ☐ yes ☐ no

SOCIOECONOMIC HISTORY

Occupation _____ Student status ☐ Full time ☐ Part time

Education Completed : ☐ High School graduate ☐ College graduate ☐ Graduate School

Marital Status ☐ Single ☐ Married ☐ Separated ☐ Divorced ☐ Widowed

REVIEW OF SYSTEMS Answer the following questions for any current problems you are experiencing:

Constitutional: Are you experiencing?

____ Fever/chills/nigh-sweats   ____ Tiredness/weakness

____ Unexpected weight gain/loss   ____ Excessive thirst or urination

____ Tiredness/weakness   ____ Difficulty falling or staying asleep

Eyes, Ears, Nose, Throat and Mouth   *Skin*

____ Change in vision   ____ Rash

____ Difficulty hearing/ringing in ears ____ Change in moles

____ Teeth/gum problems

____ Hay fever or allergies

Cardiovascular   *Respiratory*

____ Chest pain or discomfort   ____ Cough/wheeze

3

Page 4

Patient Name _____ DOB _____ Med. Record Number _____

____ Leg pain during exercise   ____ Difficulty breathing/shortness of breath

____ Palpitations (racing heart)

Gastrointestinal   *Genitourinary*

____ Abdominal pain   ____ Frequent urination during night

____ Blood in stool   ____ Leaking urine

____ Nausea/vomiting/diarrhea   ____ Vaginal bleeding (not related to period)

Musculoskeletal   ____ Discharge from penis

____ Muscle/joint pain   *Breasts*

Neurological   ____ Lump or discharge

____ Headaches   *Psychiatric*

____ Dizziness/light-headed   ____ Anxiety/stress

____ Numbness   ____ Depression

____ Memory Loss   *Blood/Lymphatic*

                                       ____ Lumps

                                       ____ Easily bruises/bleeding

Is there anything you want the doctor to address with you today? _____

_____

WOMEN'S HEALTH HISTORY

No. pregnancies ____ No. deliveries _____ No. abortions ____ No. miscarriages _____

Date of last menstrual period _____ Frequency of periods _____ Length _____

_____   _____
Patient's Signature   Date

FOR INTERNAL USE ONLY (ENTER DATE REVIEWED AND INITIALS) ANY CHANGES, ADDITIONS, DELETIONS SHOULD BE DOCUMENTED ABOVE, DATED AND INITIALED.

4

Figure 4.1 Medical History Form

form in a dermatologist's office will probably not include the patient's menstrual history, for example. If that information were needed for some reason, it could still be added elsewhere in the patient's record.

- Related pieces of data should be adjacent—for instance, the street address, city, and ZIP code of a patient's address should be adjacent to one another on the form.
- The field names (also called labels) should be clearly marked by the use of bolding, colored font, or italics.
- If the form is lengthy, it should be separated into sections.
- The form should be easy to complete; in other words, it should be obvious whether the answer to each field is to be written on the same line as the field heading or needs to go in the line below.
- Each piece of data should be requested only once on a given form.
- Sufficient space should be provided for the answer to each field.
- Typically, a form should not duplicate questions that are answered on other forms; an exception to this is a question about medication allergies, which is often asked on more than one form due to the importance of the information. An allergy may slip a patient's mind when completing a form at home, but he or she will recall the allergy later in the interview process.

Paper forms are often the source documents used to enter data into the EMR. If that is the case, office policy must reflect what is considered the primary record—paper or EMR—and what will be done with the paper once the data are entered into the EMR. Will it be kept for a period of time and then destroyed, or will the paper be destroyed as soon the data are entered? And, of course, how will the paper be destroyed? Some paper forms may be ordered from an outside company and an inventory of each form kept on hand in the office; in other offices, each form is developed internally and the forms are printed as needed. That decision is often based on available storage space.

Following these guidelines will make it easy for the patient to complete a form. A thoroughly completed form will benefit the care provider as well. Care providers need complete, accurate information quickly, so proper development of data collection tools—whether on paper or on-screen—should be an important task in any healthcare setting.

The registration form used in the administrative data chapter is an example of a form that has individual fields in block format. The medical history form in Figure 4.1 is an example of one that has a more free-form format rather than individual fields.

Many "paperless" offices ask their patients to complete history forms online. Think of the last time you applied for a job or when you applied to the college you are attending. Most likely you did so online rather than with a paper application. The rules noted in this section about ease of completion apply to online forms as well as paper forms.

4.2 The Past Medical, Surgical, Family, and Social Histories

A patient's **past medical history (PMH)** often contains information that is pertinent to his or her current health status. It is important that the care provider be aware of the patient's past medical history, which includes

Past medical history (PMH)
Previous medical condition(s) for which the patient has been treated.

- Medical conditions (past and current) for which the patient has been treated or that the patient is experiencing
- Date of onset and date resolved for each medical condition
- Known allergies (particularly to medications) as well as the actual reaction
- Immunization status, particularly in children
- Current list of medications, including name, dosage, frequency, and reason it is being taken
- **Review of systems (ROS)**, that is, a body-system inventory of symptoms he or she is having

Review of systems (ROS) A body-system-by-body-system inventory of any symptoms the patient is having or has had based on a series of questions asked by the care provider.

Many offices include the patient's current condition on the history form, or the particulars of the current condition may be documented in the progress note for the visit. The information about the current condition includes

- Chief complaint (the reason the patient is being seen that day—generally speaking, the reason for the appointment)
- History of present illness: the location of the condition (for example, pain in the right shoulder); the type of pain (ache, sharp pain, etc.); its severity (mild, severe); the duration (how long the complaint has been present); and any associated signs and symptoms (for example, difficulty raising the arm above the head when pain is present)

Surgical history Previous surgical procedure(s) the patient has undergone, the approximate date(s), the name of the surgeon(s), the reason(s) for the procedure(s), and complications, if any.

The **surgical history** includes information about procedures the patient has undergone. If a patient, Carolyn Wright, is experiencing right lower quadrant pain, yet her history shows she had an appendectomy 14 years ago, the care provider will concentrate diagnostic testing on other possibilities. Surgical history includes

- Name of the operation or procedure
- Reason for the procedure
- Date the procedure was performed (may be approximate)
- Name of the surgeon who performed the procedure
- Anesthesia reactions or complications, if any

Family history (FH) Documentation of conditions and diseases found in immediate family members (e.g., diabetes mellitus, cancer, or heart disease).

The **family history (FH)** includes information that will alert the care provider to any conditions that may affect the patient's overall health now or in the future. For example, Neil Alexander is a 45-year-old patient who has been experiencing chest pains and shortness of breath. He notes that both his father and paternal grandfather had a myocardial infarction (heart attack) before the age of 50. In this case, that information is important to the care provider in order to make diagnostic and treatment decisions for the patient. Family history includes

- Name(s) of the condition(s)
- Family member(s) who had the condition(s)
- Sometimes, whether immediate family members (parent, sibling) are still alive and, if not, the date/cause of death

Social history (SH) Lifestyle or social habits of the patient. Examples include smoking history or current use, use of alcoholic beverages and frequency, and patient's profession.

The **social history (SH)** is important because the care provider needs to know the patient's habits in order to assess possible causes of conditions or potential health concerns that could arise as a result of the patient's habits or lifestyle. An example is a patient who is overweight, works in a sedentary job, and has noted that she does not exercise or participate in any type of strenuous activity. That patient would be at risk for heart disease, stroke, and other serious medical conditions. Elements of a social history include

- Smoking history—past or current use
- Other tobacco use (snuff, pipe, or cigar, for example)
- Alcohol use—current or past
- Recreational drug use
- Socioeconomic data—occupation, education, marital status
- Sexual activity and use of protection
- Exercise and physical activity

Unlike a written record, an EMR lends itself to being copied from one encounter to the next relatively easily, particularly the past medical, surgical, family, and social histories. This is known as **cloning**, or more commonly as **copy and paste**. The reason providers and practitioners clone parts of a record is speed and efficiency. Let's say Dr. Ingram is reviewing the social history of a 58-year-old established patient, Mary Cay Gregory. Dr. Ingram goes over the social history that is already in the previous record with Mrs. Gregory, and she says that nothing has changed and she has nothing to add. Rather than type those notes again, the physician simply copies them from the previous record and pastes them into the current record. A patient's social history may contain sensitive information, and care should be taken to ensure that the copied information is verified. In Mrs. Gregory's case, for example, the information is copied from and to the same patient's health record. Although the practice of copying information between different patients' records is discouraged, some medical offices choose to do so; in these instances, it is imperative to pay attention to detail and to ensure the accuracy and completeness of the documentation.

Cloning (copy and paste) Used in an electronic environment, copying similar or identical information from a previous encounter of the same or a different patient.

Even copying from encounters belonging to the same patient has its dangers. Let's say that Dr. Ingram copies and pastes the diagnosis of pneumococcal pneumonia from Mrs. Gregory's last visit into the current problem list. Mrs. Gregory's last visit was two years ago, and she no longer has pneumococcal pneumonia. Including pneumococcal pneumonia as an active condition on this visit is not accurate; it is not an acute condition and therefore should not appear as such on this current record. Doing so brings into question the validity of the record in general.

Thus, although it may seem efficient, cloning entries can be dangerous, particularly if incorrect medications, prior or current treatments, or past histories are incorrectly carried over to a patient's record. Before the cloning feature of an EMR is used, it is imperative that the providers, practitioners, and staff understand the serious nature of incorrect information within the record. They must remember the importance of the health record; it serves as a basis for medical decision making, and it is a record upon which legal decisions are based in cases of medical malpractice, liability (such as in the case of a car accident), and Workers' Compensation. Additionally, reimbursement is tied to the documentation found in the health record—as proof of what is wrong with the patient, what was done to or for the patient, and the quality of care provided to the patient (Haugen).

Past medical and surgical histories, family and social histories, and the findings of the physical examination and the patient's signs and symptoms, which we will discuss in more detail in the next section, are all pieces of the puzzle that allow the care provider to accurately diagnose and treat the patient.

Enter a Patient's Past Medical History

In this exercise, we will be following the past medical history of a patient, Amy Peterson. She has arrived and checked in for her appointment with Dr. Rodriguez at Summit Bay Health Center. The healthcare professional has called Mrs. Peterson back to the exam room for the initial portion of the visit. Mr. Peterson has accompanied the patient to the appointment and is in the exam room as well. The healthcare professional begins by accessing Mrs. Peterson's Facesheet screen in EHRclinic, as noted in Figure 4.2.

The healthcare professional will verify Mrs. Peterson's information and change it, if necessary, before going on to the past medical history. The healthcare professional clicks on the Past Medical History screen from the facesheet.

Though some information may be entered previously, the healthcare professional should ask about any other conditions. Mrs. Peterson's husband confirms she has osteoporosis and osteoarthritis, but no other medical conditions. The healthcare professional asks about any previous surgeries. In addition to the hysterectomy that has been previously recorded, Mr. Peterson responds that she had an appendectomy back in 1991 and she had a cataract removed from her right eye in 2013. They are the only surgical procedures Mrs. Peterson has had, but she does have one child, so the healthcare professional asks Mrs. Peterson about her reproductive history. Mrs. Peterson says she was pregnant once and has one child. The pregnancy was a full-term pregnancy.

Follow these steps to complete the exercise on your own once you have watched the demonstration and tried the steps with helpful prompts. Use the information provided in the scenario to complete the information.

1. Click on 'Tools' module.
2. Click on 'Manage reports' button.

EHRclinic Tip [EHRclinic]

Often, patients will not know the exact dates of their past medical history diagnoses or surgical procedures. If they can recall the month and year, or just the year, the healthcare provider can use the closest estimated date in EHRclinic.

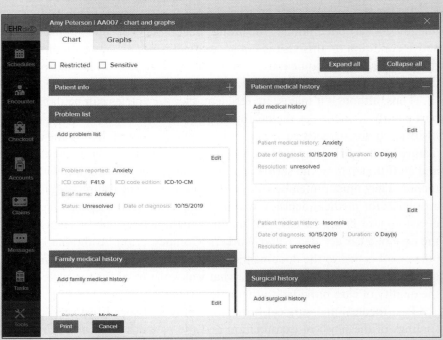

Figure 4.2 Amy Peterson's Facesheet

3. Click on 'Patient charts and graphs' button.
4. Click on 'Search by patient first name/last name/chart number/SSN' field and enter 'pet'.
5. Click on 'Amy Peterson's' info.
6. Click on 'Add medical history' button.
7. Click on 'Patient medical history' input field and enter 'Osteoporosis'.
8. Click on 'Resolution' drop-down and click on 'Unresolved'.
9. Click on 'Done' button.
10. Click on 'Add medical history' button.
11. Click on 'Patient medical history' input field and enter 'Osteoarthritis'.
12. Click on 'Resolution' drop-down and click on 'Unresolved'.
13. Click on 'Done' button.
14. Click on 'Add surgical history' button.
15. Click on 'Past surgery' input field and enter 'Appendectomy'.
16. Click on 'Date of surgery' field and enter '01/01/1991' in 'Date of surgery' field.
17. Click on 'Done' button.
18. Click on 'Add surgical history' button.
19. Click on 'Past surgery' input field and enter 'Cataract removal right eye'.
20. Click on 'Date of surgery' field and enter '01/01/2013' in 'Date of surgery' field.
21. Click on 'Done' button.
22. Click on 'Add new note' button.
23. Click on 'Note title' button and enter 'Reproductive history'.
24. Click on 'Note' button and enter 'One full-term pregnancy with one living child'.
25. Click on 'Done' button.

☑ You have completed Exercise 4.1

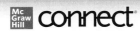 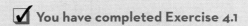 Go to https://connect.mheducation.com to complete this exercise. To see instructional notes with the steps, visit the eBook in Connect or download them from www.mhhe.com/iehr4. **EXERCISE 4.2**

Enter a Patient's List of Current Medications

In this exercise, the patient's current medications are entered. Part of the functionality of EHRclinic is the differentiation between those medications prescribed by Summit Bay Health Center and those prescribed by another provider or bought over the counter.

This process begins by accessing Mrs. Peterson's facesheet in EHRclinic and then selecting Medications to access the medication list (Figure 4.2). Mrs. Peterson shares with the healthcare professional that she takes ibuprofen for her osteoarthritis. She takes 800 mg tablets three times a day. She also takes glucosamine chondroitin every day. These are tablets as well, and she takes the 750-600 mg tablets. She is also taking alendronate, which is a drug for post-menopausal osteoporosis prevention. These are taken in tablet form as well, 35 mg one time a week.

Follow these steps to complete the exercise on your own once you have watched the demonstration and tried the steps with helpful prompts. Use the information provided in the scenario to complete the information.

(continued)

1. Click on 'Search by patient first name/last name/chart number/SSN' field and enter 'pet'.
2. Click on 'Amy Peterson's' info.
3. Click on 'Add medication list' button.
4. Click on 'Status' button and select 'Active'.
5. Click on 'Drug type' button and select 'Rx'.
6. Click on 'Drug name' input field and enter 'Ibuprofen'.
7. Click on 'Dosage' input field and enter '800 mg'.
8. Click on 'Drug form' drop-down and select 'Tablet'.
9. Click on 'Route' drop-down and select 'Oral'.
10. Click on 'Frequency' input field and enter 'three times a day'.
11. Click on 'Done' button.
12. Click on 'Add medication list' button.
13. Click on 'Status' button and select 'Active'.
14. Click on 'Drug type' button and select 'OTC'.
15. Click on 'Drug name' input field and enter 'Glucosamine chondroitin'.
16. Click on 'Dosage' input field and enter '750-600 mg'.
17. Click on 'Drug form' drop-down and select 'Tablet'.
18. Click on 'Route' drop-down and select 'Oral'.
19. Click on 'Frequency' input field and enter 'one daily'.
20. Click on 'Done' button.
21. Click on 'Add medication list' button.
22. Click on 'Status' button and select 'Active'.
23. Click on 'Drug type' button and select 'Rx'.
24. Click on 'Drug name' input field and enter 'Alendronate'.
25. Click on 'Dosage' input field and enter '35 mg'.
26. Click on 'Drug form' drop-down and select 'Tablet'.
27. Click on 'Route' drop-down and select 'Oral'.
28. Click on 'Frequency' input field and enter 'once a week'.
29. Click on 'Done' button.

☑ **You have completed Exercise 4.2**

EXERCISE 4.3

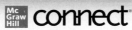

Go to https://connect.mheducation.com to complete this exercise. To see instructional notes with the steps, visit the eBook in Connect or download them from www.mhhe.com/iehr4.

Enter a Patient's Known Drug Allergies

Mrs. Peterson has a severe allergy to Reglan, identified in adulthood. Knowing the patient's medication allergies is a very important piece of information. Not knowing her allergies, and prescribing a drug that she is allergic to, could cause a very serious reaction. Her allergy to Reglan will be documented in the Allergies List section of the facesheet (Figure 4.2).

Follow these steps to complete the exercise on your own once you have watched the demonstration and tried the steps with helpful prompts. Use the information provided in the scenario to complete the information.

1. Click on 'Search by patient first name/last name/chart number/SSN' field and enter 'pet'.
2. Click on 'Amy Peterson's' info.

3. Click on 'Add allergies' button.
4. Click on 'Allergy type' button and select 'Drug allergy'.
5. Click on 'Allergy details' input field and enter 'Reglan'.
6. Click on 'Onset' button and select 'Adulthood'.
7. Click on 'Severity' button and select 'Severe'.
8. Click on 'Status' drop-down and select 'Active'.
9. Click on 'Allergies done' button.

☑ **You have completed Exercise 4.3**

EHRclinic Tip [EHRclinic]

In some EHRclinic exercises, the Path window may obstruct areas you need to click. If this happens, you can collapse the path within the window or click to hide it in the upper left corner of the screen.

4.3 Handling Inconsistent or Unclear Information

As we discussed earlier, a patient's history is gathered by use of a form, as well as through an interview with the patient. Sometimes, what a patient has documented on the history form contradicts what comes out during the interview. When entering any information about a patient—for instance, if you are reviewing a past medical history with the patient and you see on the past medical history form that the patient had an appendectomy in 2016, yet she tells you verbally that she has never had any surgeries—you need to question the patient to determine the correct answer. Though the patient completed the form, she could have checked the wrong box on the form, or she may have forgotten that she had had the surgery. Sometimes, patients choose not to tell the healthcare professional or care provider all the facts. Often, the healthcare professional senses that the patient is being evasive or is only partly answering questions. It is part of the healthcare professional's role to act in such a way that instills trust; communicating *why* these questions are being asked is often all that is needed for a patient to become more comfortable. The fact that there is a discrepancy (or that information is missing) should never be ignored and should be documented. The medical practice or hospital must have written policies on how to handle such situations.

Following is an example of a policy statement regarding inconsistent information: *In the event that an error or inconsistency is found in a health record or in the information given verbally by a patient/legal representative, an attempt should be made to verify the information and document the same. The circumstances surrounding the discrepancy should be documented sufficiently in the health record to explain the situation thoroughly.*

Documentation in a health record must be accurate, precise, reliable, and consistent, not only because it is a legal document but also to ensure quality medical care. EHRclinic, like other EHR software, has built-in mechanisms to amend, delete, or add documentation without compromising the integrity of the record. Though a change to documentation may occur, the original version of the documentation is always retrievable. Remember, the health record is a *legal document*, so any written information upon which care may have been based or that may have been released to other care providers, insurance companies, or other third parties must remain retrievable. In the previous example regarding the discrepancy about the patient's surgery, the explanation of the discrepancy can be documented in a details box, found in the past surgical history section of the record. Later in this worktext, when covering data integrity, we will further examine correcting and amending entries and will test your knowledge through EHRclinic exercises.

4.4 Documenting Vital Signs

Vital signs Measurements taken (temperature, heart rate, respiratory rate, blood pressure, height and weight, and sometimes Body Mass Index) to determine the status of basic body-system functions.

The patient's **vital signs** are taken by the healthcare professional—some offices take them before completing the history, and others take them after. EHRclinic software includes a very helpful feature: the ability to see a patient's vital signs over time. The tracking of the vital signs can be seen graphically or chronologically. This helps the provider assess such conditions as hypertension or significant weight gain or loss.

Like the documentation of the patient's history, entering the vital signs is done from the vital signs section of the facesheet.

The vital signs include the patient's blood pressure, heart rate, respiratory rate, temperature, height, weight, Body Mass Index (BMI), and oxygen saturation. Technically, height and weight and BMI are not vital signs, but all are taken or calculated about the same time as the vital signs and therefore are included in that section of the record.

EXERCISE 4.4

Go to https://connect.mheducation.com to complete this exercise. To see instructional notes with the steps, visit the eBook in Connect or download them from www.mhhe.com/iehr4.

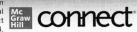

Enter a Patient's Vital Signs

EHRclinic allows documentation of the position the patient is in when the blood pressure is taken: sitting, standing, or lying down.

In our example, the healthcare professional is in the process of taking Amy Peterson's vital signs. She asks Mrs. Peterson to sit on the exam table and takes her blood pressure. The reading is 110/65, examined on the right arm. Her heart rate is 68 beats per minute (bpm) and regular, with a respiratory rate of 22. Mrs. Peterson's temperature is 97.6 F (oral). She reports no pain during this visit. Her weight was taken before coming into the exam room, and she weighed 135 pounds. She is 5 feet 2 inches (62 inches) tall. Her oxygen saturation today is 99%.

Follow these steps to complete the exercise on your own once you have watched the demonstration and tried the steps with helpful prompts. Use the information provided in the scenario to complete the information.

1. Click on 'Encounter' module.
2. Click on 'Provider: Selected All providers' field and select 'Dr. Maria Rodriguez'.
3. Click on 'Amy Peterson's' check-in.
4. Click on 'Height' input field and enter '62' (inches).
5. Click on 'Weight' input field and enter '135' (pounds).
6. Click on 'Blood pressure systolic' input field and enter '110'.
7. Click on 'Blood pressure diastolic' input field and enter '65'.
8. Click on 'Arm examined' drop-down and click 'Right'.
9. Click on 'Patient position' drop-down and click 'Sitting'.
10. Click on 'Pulse' input field and enter '68'.
11. Click on 'Respiratory rate' input field and enter '22'.

12. Click on 'Pain scale' input field and enter '0'.
13. Click on 'Temperature' input field and enter '97.6'.
14. Click on 'Temperature type' drop-down and enter 'Oral'.
15. Click on 'SpO2' input field and '99'.
16. Click on 'Ready for provider' button.
17. Click on 'Okay' button.

☑ **You have completed Exercise 4.4**

for your information **fyi**

The Body Mass Index (BMI) is now a standard entry in most health records. BMI is a formula showing body weight adjusted for a patient's height. A healthy BMI is between 18.5 and 24.9. EHR software will automatically compute the BMI once the patient's height and weight are entered in the Vital Signs field.

At this point in the process, the patient has been taken to the exam room, vital signs have been taken, and she is ready to be seen by the care provider.

APPLYING YOUR SKILLS

1. What is meant by using a paper form as a "source document"?
2. Why is a social history important in the care of a patient?
3. Would a patient's vital signs ever be cloned from one record to another? Explain your answer.

chapter 4 **summary**

LEARNING OUTCOME	CONCEPTS FOR REVIEW

4.1 Outline the use of forms as data collection tools.	– Paper form versus computer screen
	– When designing a form, keep the following in mind:
	  • Name of the form
	  • Name of the office or facility
	  • Patient's name on every page
	  • Purpose of the form
	– Keep related information close together on the form
	– Clearly mark field headings
	– Lengthy forms should be separated into sections
	– Ease of completion and of reading
	– Don't duplicate information on the form
	– Sufficient space for answers on paper forms

4.2 Execute a step-by-step procedure to document past medical, surgical, family, and social histories in EHRclinic.	– All histories are important in the assessment of patients – Past medical history includes current and past medical conditions; allergies; medications; immunization status; chief complaint; history of present illness; review of systems – Surgical history includes all surgeries or procedures the patient has had and the dates (even if approximate) – Family history is collected to assess whether the patient is predisposed to certain conditions – Social history is collected to determine if the patient may be at a greater risk for certain conditions – The use of cloning (copy and paste) in an EMR/EHR
4.3 Examine the necessity of properly documenting and correcting inconsistent or unclear information.	– Office or facility must have clear policies to deal with inconsistent information – When a discrepancy is found and the patient is present, ask which is correct; amend the record according to policy – If the correct information is not certain, document that as well

4.4 Apply procedures to document vital signs in EHRclinic.	– Vital signs include
	  • Blood pressure
	  • Temperature
	  • Heart rate
	  • Respiratory rate
	  • Height
	  • Weight
	  • Body Mass Index
	  • Blood oxygen saturation
	– EHRclinic will show vital signs over time, which may alert the provider to certain risk factors such as high blood pressure or significant weight loss or gain

chapter review

MATCHING QUESTIONS

Match the terms on the left with the definitions on the right.

_____ 1. **[LO 4.2]** review of systems (ROS)

_____ 2. **[LO 4.2]** surgical history

_____ 3. **[LO 4.2]** past medical history (PMH)

_____ 4. **[LO 4.2]** social history (SH)

_____ 5. **[LO 4.2]** family history (FH)

_____ 6. **[LO 4.4]** vital signs

a. patient information such as blood pressure and respiratory rate

b. patient information that includes immunizations and allergies

c. patient information that includes information such as frequency of drinking and smoking

d. comprehensive inventory of patient symptoms such as headaches, vision, heart palpitations, and swelling of joints

e. patient information that includes past procedures and who performed the procedures

f. patient information that includes possibly inherited conditions

MULTIPLE-CHOICE QUESTIONS

Select the letter that best completes the statement or answers the question:

1. **[LO 4.1]** An on-screen item of data is known as a
   a. box.
   b. crate.
   c. carton.
   d. field.

2. **[LO 4.3]** EHRclinic allows you to note discrepancies in the_____field.
   a. Details
   b. Discrepancies
   c. Information
   d. Registration

3. **[LO 4.1]** It is important to keep the design of paper forms
   a. cumbersome.
   b. detailed.
   c. logical.
   d. short.

4. **[LO 4.2]** Which of the following is NOT a required patient history?
   a. family
   b. birth
   c. social
   d. surgical

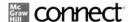

Enhance your learning by completing these exercises and more at **https://connect.mheducation.com!**

5. **[LO 4.1]** Of the following, who will benefit from thoroughly completed paper forms?
   a. care providers
   b. patients
   c. receptionists
   d. all of these

6. **[LO 4.2]** The patient's _____ history can help predict a future health condition.
   a. family
   b. medical
   c. social
   d. surgical

7. **[LO 4.4]** A patient's vital signs can be easily viewed via EHRclinic's _____ screen.
   a. Facesheet
   b. Help
   c. Patient Vitals
   d. Registration

8. **[LO 4.3]** Which of the following is NOT a method of gathering a patient's history?
   a. patient/guardian completes the history form
   b. provider interviews patient/guardian
   c. HIM professional interviews patient/guardian
   d. review of past health (medical) records by the provider, if available

9. **[LO 4.1]** Which piece of information might be included multiple times on a form?
   a. address
   b. drug allergies
   c. marital status
   d. patient history

10. **[LO 4.1]** What information should you see on all forms in a patient chart?
    a. name
    b. DOB
    c. medical record number
    d. all of these

11. **[LO 4.2]** A patient's surgical history includes the
    a. approximate date of the procedure.
    b. name of the attending physician.
    c. patient's recovery time.
    d. type of sutures used.

12. **[LO 4.1]** For ease of completion, related information should be _____ on a form.
    a. adjacent
    b. duplicated
    c. labeled
    d. separate

13. **[LO 4.4]** What does BMI stand for?
    a. Basic Medical Information
    b. Body Mass Index
    c. Body Matter Indicator
    d. Base Measurement Index

14. **[LO 4.2]** Which of the following includes the patient's frequency of alcohol consumption?
    a. family history
    b. medical history
    c. social history
    d. surgical history

15. **[LO 4.3]** Any discrepancies in patient information need to be
    a. detailed.
    b. documented.
    c. filed.
    d. transcribed.

SHORT-ANSWER QUESTIONS

1. **[LO 4.1]** Explain why it is important to keep the design of paper forms logical and orderly.

2. **[LO 4.2]** Explain why a patient's social history is important.

3. **[LO 4.1]** Why is it recommended that a patient's name, DOB, and chart number/medical record number appear on each page of a multipage form?

4. **[LO 4.4]** List the vital signs that are typically taken at each patient visit.

5. **[LO 4.1]** Why, in the age of EHRs, is patient information still gathered mainly through the use of paper forms?

6. **[LO 4.2]** Differentiate between social and family histories.

7. **[LO 4.3]** Why does a medical office need to have clear policies in place for dealing with discrepancies in patient information?

8. **[LO 4.4]** EHRclinic includes a feature to allow the provider to view the patient's vital signs in different ways. Explain the benefit of this feature.

9. **[LO 4.2]** Why might so many patient histories need to be taken?

10. **[LO 4.2]** Dr. Stephens copied and pasted the physical exam from Jeanie Lopez's visit for strep pharyngitis to the physical exam of Shelly Lopez's visit for strep pharyngitis. Could that cause any problems with the care rendered to Shelly Lopez? Explain your answer.

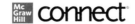

Enhance your learning by completing these exercises and more at https://connect.mheducation.com!

APPLYING YOUR KNOWLEDGE

1. **[LO 4.2]** Stephanie Lewis comes to your office for her annual wellness checkup. As the health-care professional who will be doing her initial interview, create a list of questions you might ask Stephanie to obtain her social history.

2. **[LO 4.4]** How can the EHRclinic Tracking feature assist you in analyzing a patient's vital signs over time? Give a specific example.

3. **[LO 4.1]** As an office manager for a large healthcare practice, you have been asked to design a new patient intake form. Sketch out your form's layout, keeping in mind the best practices discussed in the chapter.

4. **[LO 4.3]** Bob Larks is a new patient in your practice, and he brought his informational form with him on his first visit. During the patient history portion of his exam, he says that he does not drink, but while entering that information in Bob's chart you notice that his initial history stated that he was a "social drinker." What should you do?

5. **[LOs 4.2, 4.3]** As a healthcare professional, you are attempting to obtain the medical history of your patient, Lisa Sanchez. However, you are having difficulty because Lisa is evading your questions and is refusing to respond. What can you do?

chapter references

Booth, K.A., Whicker, L.G., Wyman, Terri D., and Moany Wright, Sandra. (2011). *Administrative Procedures for Medical Assisting* (4th ed.). New York: McGraw-Hill Companies.

Green, M.A., and Bowie, M.J. (2016). *Essentials of Health Information Management: Principles and Practices* (3rd ed.). Clifton Park, NY: Delmar, Cengage Learning.

Haugen, Heather. (2014, June). Overcoming the Risks of Copy and Paste in EHRs. *Journal of AHIMA, 85*(6): 54–55.

Newby, C. (2010). *From Patient to Payment: Insurance Procedures for the Medical Office* (6th ed.). New York: McGraw-Hill Companies.

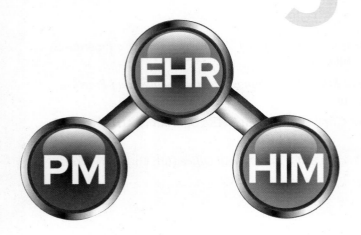

Content of the Health Record— the Care Provider's Responsibility

Key Terms

Computerized physician order entry (CPOE)

Discharge summary

ePrescribing

History & physical (H&P)

History of present illness (HPI)

Interface

Physical exam (PE)

Point of care (POC)

Problem list

Review of systems (ROS)

Scribe

SOAP note

Speech recognition technology

Voice recognition technology

What You Need to Know and Why You Need to Know It

In this chapter the EHR is assessed from the care provider's perspective. In the EHRclinic demonstrations, we will illustrate how a care provider captures clinical information.

Knowing where in a record certain information resides is important because it is often necessary for the medical assistant, coder, biller, or other healthcare professional to access a care provider's documentation to answer a question for another care provider or for an insurance company, or to complete forms.

5.1 The SOAP Note

SOAP stands for **S**ubjective, **O**bjective, **A**ssessment, and **P**lan. It is a format for documentation that reflects a patient's visit (typically an office visit) in an orderly fashion—from the time the visit begins to the time it ends. A SOAP note consists of four distinct areas of documentation. They are

Subjective (S): This is the information the care provider learns from the patient. The subjective findings are the patient's description of his or her symptoms. For instance, Henry Stewart is seen in Dr. Connors' office today; he tells the doctor that he has had a "cold and terrible headache" for three days. He also states that he "has been achy and has pressure over both eyes." These are all sensations that only the patient can feel and therefore are subjective. They are not measurable.

Objective (O): Objective findings include information the care provider gathers from performing a physical exam. These are measurable findings. For example, upon conducting a physical exam on Henry Stewart, the physician notes that the patient flinches when he palpates the area above the patient's eyebrows and his cheekbones; because the patient flinches, the physician knows that the patient is experiencing discomfort. The patient also has a green nasal discharge. Mr. Stewart is an established patient of Dr. Connors' and he has had three sinus infections in the past two years, as noted in the patient's past medical history, which is based on the documentation from his prior encounters. Objective findings also include measurable test results such as an x-ray finding or lab results.

Assessment (A): At the assessment stage, the care provider *assesses* the patient's signs and symptoms and the results of the physical exam in order to make a diagnosis or diagnoses. In many cases, it is necessary to await test results to determine a diagnosis; in the meantime, a diagnosis may be considered "probable," "possible," or "suspected." In the case of Henry Stewart, the physician has documented the diagnosis as acute sinusitis.

Plan (P): The plan is also known as the *plan of care*. The care provider will order any tests he or she feels are medically necessary, prescribe medications or recommend over-the-counter medications, order consultations with other care providers if necessary, educate the patient about his or her condition, and advise the patient of follow-up instructions. In Mr. Stewart's case, Dr. Connors wrote an order for a CT scan of the

SOAP note An acronym for the documentation used in a care provider's office to record the patient's symptoms, signs, assessment (diagnosis), and plan of care. SOAP stands for Subjective, Objective, Assessment, and Plan.

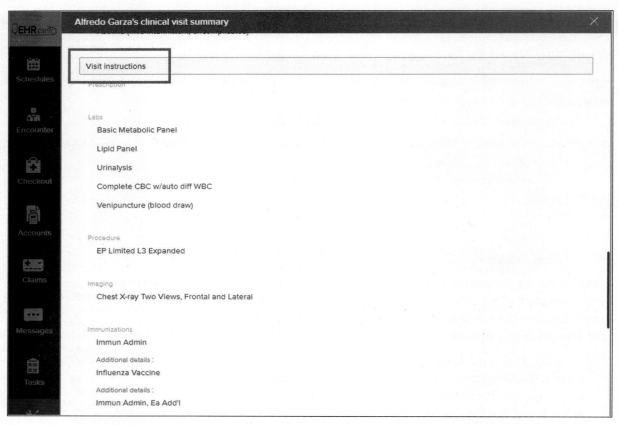

Figure 5.1   Example of Patient Visit Instructions (Plan) from EHRclinic

sinuses. His instructions to Mr. Stewart included drinking plenty of fluids and taking the next two days off from work. A prescription for a Z-Pak was ordered and he was given printed educational material about sinusitis (from the EHR software). He was told to schedule a follow-up appointment for 10 days from now.

An example of an instruction screen for a patient is found in Figure 5.1. In a paper record, the physician would hand-write the instructions under the 'Plan' in the patient's record, as seen in Figure 5.2.

EXERCISE   5.1

Go to https://connect.mheducation.com to complete this exercise. To see instructional notes with the steps, visit the eBook in Connect or download them from www.mhhe.com/iehr4.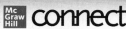

Look Up the Patient's Plan of Care

In this exercise, it is necessary to access the plan of care Dr. Ingram ordered for Alfredo Garza. Dr. Ingram is on the phone and has asked you to look up the treatment plan for Alfredo Garza because he has to return a call to Mr. Garza quickly and is not at a computer. This information can be found within the patient's last office visit notes. Once the information is accessed, you can print it and give it to Dr. Ingram to review.

Follow these steps to complete the exercise on your own once you have watched the demonstration and tried the steps with helpful prompts. Use the information provided in the scenario to complete the information.

1. Click on 'Tools' module.
2. Click on 'Manage reports' button.

3. Click on 'Patient charts and graphs' button.
4. Click on 'Search by patient first name/last name/chart number/SSN' field and enter 'gar'.
5. Click on 'Alfredo Garza's' info.
6. Click on 'Patient office visits 1' view button.
7. Click on 'Patient office visits' print button.
8. Click on 'Okay' button.
9. Click on 'Patient office visits' cancel button.
10. Click on 'Add new note' button.
11. Click on 'Note title' button and enter 'Review'.
12. Click on 'Note' button and enter 'Patient OV reviewed and printed'.
13. Click on 'Done' button.
14. Click on 'Chart and graphs' cancel button.

✓ **You have completed Exercise 5.1**

EHRclinic Tip ⓔEHRclinic

Unstructured data are not taken into consideration when EHRclinic calculates the charges for an office visit; structured data are included in the calculation of charges for the office visit. For example, procedure codes are forms of structured data that are used to calculate charges.

In an electronic health record, these elements are documented, but rather than being handwritten, a combination of free-text writing and use of drop-down menus and standard text makes documentation more thorough, consistent, easily retrievable, and legible. As you complete the exercises later in this chapter, you will see that the SOAP elements just described are present in the EHR.

When a patient is admitted to a hospital, the care provider documents the subjective and objective findings, along with the results of a physical exam, in the **History & physical** report, otherwise known as an **H&P**. The assessment and plan, as well as a recap of the patient's course in the hospital, are documented in a **discharge summary** (or note). Throughout the stay, nurses document in the nursing notes section of the record, and care providers document in the physician's progress notes. When handwritten or typed, these are *unstructured data*; when an electronic health record is used and the responses are chosen from a pre-formatted field, such as from a drop-down menu, the data are *structured*.

History & physical (H&P) A report completed by a care provider that includes the reason(s) the patient is being seen or admitted; the history of present illness; the pertinent past medical, surgical, social, and family histories; other current conditions/diseases the patient is being treated for; the report of a physical examination; working diagnoses; and plan of care.

Discharge summary A report completed by a care provider that summarizes a patient's stay in the hospital. It generally includes the final diagnoses, a summary of the patient's course in the hospital, any procedures performed, a recap of diagnostic results, and discharge instructions.

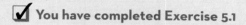

5.2   The History of Present Illness (HPI)

The **history of present illness**, or **HPI**, is the patient's depiction of his or her current illness as told to the healthcare professional or care provider. The typical elements of an HPI are

- Location of the condition (abdomen, arm, leg, head, etc.)
- Quality: pain is sharp, dull, or an ache, for example
- Severity: rating of pain/itch/cough/nausea and so on. Often, patients are asked to rate their symptoms on a scale of 1 to 10, with 1 being barely noticeable and 10 being intolerable. This may also mean the severity in terms of bleeding, vomiting, or diarrhea—for instance, profuse bleeding from a laceration versus a small amount of bleeding.
- Timing/duration: how long the condition has been present—hours, days, weeks, months, for example

EHRclinic Tip ⓔEHRclinic

In some EHRclinic exercises, the Path window may obstruct areas you need to click. If this happens, you can collapse the Path within the window or click to hide it in the upper left corner of the screen.

History of present illness (HPI) The patient's description of current complaints such as when the symptoms started, the location of the condition, the quality of the symptoms, the severity of the symptoms, anything that makes the symptoms better or worse, and additional symptoms the patient is experiencing.

Patient: Henry Stewart	DOB: July 31, 1991 **Date of Service:** 05/03/2022
S	Mr. Stewart presented today because he has had a headache for the past three days. He has not received any relief from OTC decongestants or antihistamines. He describes the pain as more of an ache, though when he pushes on his forehead, it is painful. He has had cold symptoms for about a week, but his symptoms are getting worse, and on a scale of 1 to 10, he says that his pain is an 8. He has also noted that he has had two minor nose bleeds in the past two days.
O	Vital signs noted in his chart. All within normal limits. Head and face: physical exam of nasal passages reveals a moderate amount of green discharge from both nares. The patient is tender to the touch above each eyebrow and cheek bone. Chest is clear to percussion and auscultation. Heart: Regular rate and rhythm. Abdomen: Non-tender. This is the third time Mr. Stewart has been diagnosed with a sinus infection in the past 18 months.
A	Acute sinusitis.
P	CT scan of sinuses to be done today or tomorrow at Memorial Hospital (order given to patient). Instructed to drink plenty of fluids and bedrest for two days. To return to office in 10 days for follow-up. Z-Pak single-dose pack was sent to The Corner Pharmacy via ePrescribe. Patient was given sinusitis literature.
	Jared Connors, MD 05/03/2022

Figure 5.2 **Written SOAP Note**

- Modifying factors: alternating ice and heat on a painful area, effect of pain medication, and so on
- Associated signs and symptoms: for instance, the cold symptoms described by Henry Stewart in Figure 5.2

Read Henry Stewart SOAP note in Figure 5.2 again. Match the information listed in the subjective portion of the note to the typical elements of an HPI. Not all elements are collected on all visits—only those that are necessary based on the patient's chief complaint would be documented.

Review of systems (ROS) A body-system-by-body-system inventory of any symptoms the patient is having or has had based on a series of questions asked by the care provider.

5.3 The Review of Systems (ROS)

The **review of systems (ROS)** is a body-system-by-body-system assessment of any signs or symptoms the patient is experiencing that may or may not be related to the reason for the visit. An ROS is not the same as a physical exam, because the ROS documents the patient's own responses, not an objective assessment by the care provider. Thus, the patient's responses constitute subjective content in the health record. Often, the ROS is accomplished by the completion of a medical history form by the patient, which was covered earlier. Or the care provider may use that as a starting point and ask questions based on the patient's responses on the form. The completion (or review) of the ROS is an integral component in assessing the patient's overall health as well as gaining a better picture of any additional signs or symptoms that may be related to the patient's chief complaint. In addition, the ROS plays a role in how much the patient will be charged for the visit, since it takes into account the care provider's time and medical expertise during an office visit. Regardless of whether (1) the history form is already completed and the care provider reviews it or (2) the care provider completes the form during an office

for your information fyi

Below are common questions asked during the Review of Systems (ROS) though the questions asked by the care provider may be governed by the patient's chief complaint.
Have you been having any unusual headaches?
Have you been having any blurry or double vision?
Have you had any change in bowel habits?
Have you had any swelling of your joints?

visit, there must be some form of documentation to show that the ROS was done or reviewed in order to receive reimbursement for it. The particulars of procedure coding, charging, and reimbursement will be covered briefly in the financial management chapter.

Usually, a care provider will start at the head and work down through the body to the lower extremities. Following are examples of questions that may be asked of the patient regarding his/her general health or issues with particular body systems:

- General, also referred to as constitutional (how the patient is feeling in general, any complaints or concerns, and a recap of vital signs)
- Skin (any rashes or wounds that will not heal, any unusual moles or markings that have appeared, and so on)
- Head, eyes, ears, nose, and mouth (headaches, double vision, blurring of vision, ringing of ears, earache, nosebleeds, dry mouth,dental issues)
- Throat (persistent sore throat, difficulty swallowing)
- Breasts (whether monthly self-exams are done; any changes, lumps, nipple discharge)
- Respiratory (difficulty breathing, shortness of breath)
- Cardiovascular (any chest pain, palpitations, or fluttering)
- Gastrointestinal (problems with stomach pain, constipation, diarrhea; changes in stool, signs of blood in stool)
- Genitourinary (problems voiding, cloudiness of urine, changes in color or odor of urine, difficulty starting to urinate, nighttime urination, signs of blood in urine)
- Musculoskeletal (pain in joints or extremities, difficulty walking)
- Neurologic (dizziness; light-headedness; difficulty with memory, cognition, coordination; severe headaches)
- Endocrine (if female, problems with menses; swelling of the thyroid)
- Psychological (depression, changes in mood)
- Hematologic/lymphatic (unexplained or profuse bleeding, swelling of lymph glands)
- Allergies (problems with environmental allergies, known allergies or reactions to medications)

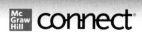 Go to https://connect.mheducation.com to complete this exercise. To see instructional notes with the steps, visit the eBook in Connect or download them from www.mhhe.com/iehr4. **EXERCISE 5.2**

Locate Alfredo Garza's Blood Pressure

In this exercise, Alfredo J. Garza stopped by the office and wants a graph to document what his blood pressure was on his last visit. He is also asking for a printout of his clinical visit summary to take to another provider. To look this up, you will access Alfredo Garza's health record.

(continued)

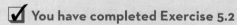
You will start by going to Alfredo J. Garza's facesheet. The vital signs graph area is found there, and you do not need to leave the facesheet to obtain his blood pressure readings and the clinical visit summary.

Follow these steps to complete the exercise on your own once you have watched the demonstration and tried the steps with helpful prompts.

From the EHRclinic Tools, access the patient's facesheet through the Charts, graphs, and reports area and then follow these steps:

1. Click on 'Patient charts and graphs' button.
2. Click on 'Search by patient first name/last name/chart number/SSN' field and 'gar'.
3. Click on 'Alfredo Garza's' info.
4. Click on 'Graphs' tab.
5. Click on 'Chart and graphs' print button.
6. Click on 'Okay' button.
7. Click on 'Chart' tab.
8. Click on 'Patient office visits 1' view button.
9. Click on 'Patient office visits' print button.
10. Click on 'Okay' button.
11. Click on 'Patient office visits' cancel button.
12. Click on 'Add new note' button.
13. Click on 'Note title' and enter 'Print'.
14. Click on 'Note' button and enter 'Patient's graph printed'.
15. Click on 'Done' button.
16. Click on 'Chart and graphs' cancel button.

Once you locate the vital signs, you will provide Mr. Garza with his print-outs and tell him that on his visit of April 4, 2022 his blood pressure reading was 136/88.

☑ **You have completed Exercise 5.2**

In EHRclinic and most other EHR software, the ROS choices are determined by the patient's chief complaint or the corresponding body system. Not every ailment requires a thorough ROS. For instance, for a patient being seen with cold symptoms, the care provider may review just the head, eyes, ears, nose, and throat (HEENT) and the chest (which essentially makes up the respiratory system). The care provider typically has no need to review the breasts or the neurologic, psychological, or reproductive systems.

Figure 5.3 shows the master ROS file in EHRclinic, and Figure 5.4 shows the full ROS.

Each office must construct a master ROS file; however, each care provider chooses the content of each ROS screen and how it displays. Thus, in EHRclinic the ROS screens are user based and can be customized to each user's needs or preferences. (Figure 5.4 shows a completed ROS in narrative form.)

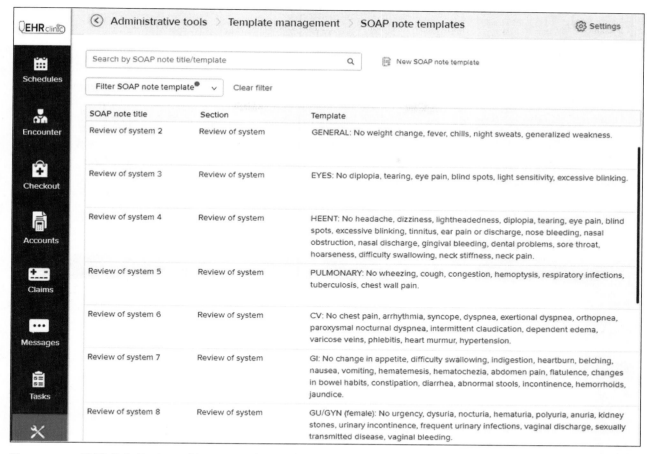

Figure 5.3 EHRclinic Review of Systems Admin Screen

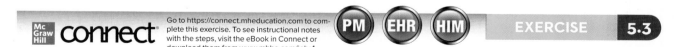

Go to https://connect.mheducation.com to complete this exercise. To see instructional notes with the steps, visit the eBook in Connect or download them from www.mhhe.com/iehr4.

PM   EHR   HIM   **EXERCISE**   5.3

Add New Options to the ROS

Even though the EHRclinic ROS Admin function is comprehensive, your practice may want to customize specific sections by adding new choices or adjusting existing ones. This is done through the Tools Template Management screen in EHRclinic.

Follow these steps to complete the exercise on your own once you have watched the demonstration and tried the steps with helpful prompts.

From the EHRclinic Tools, access the Review of Systems administration page through the Template Management area and then follow these steps:

1. Click on 'Manage templates' button.
2. Click on 'SOAP note templates' button.
3. Click on 'Filter SOAP note template' drop-down.
4. Select 'Review of system' option.

(continued)

5. Click on 'Close' button.

6. Click on 'New SOAP notes template' button.

7. Click on 'SOAP note field' drop-down and select 'Review of system'.

8. Click on 'Title' field and enter 'Review of system 18'.

9. Click on 'Template' field and enter '+ headache upon wakening'.

10. Click on 'Add template' button.

You have now customized your ROS Admin screen. If you are the office manager in charge of customizing the practice's screens, you may be responsible for updating the SOAP notes templates frequently.

☑️ **You have completed Exercise 5.3**

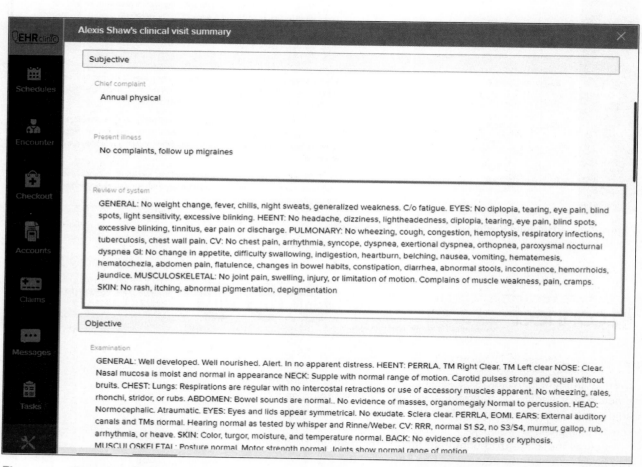

Figure 5.4   Completed ROS

5.4   The Physical Exam

Physical exam (PE) An examination of the patient's body for signs of disease.

The **physical exam (PE)** is performed by the care provider. As we discussed earlier, in a physician's office, the care provider is the physician, a physician's assistant, a nurse practitioner, or a nurse midwife. The extent of the physical exam is typically driven by the patient's chief complaint, the reason the patient is being seen that day. For instance, if a patient is being seen for an annual physical exam, the PE will be more extensive than the PE performed for a patient being seen with a chief complaint of a splinter in the right ring finger.

The care provider will also determine the extent of the PE based on the patient's responses to the ROS questions. If the patient with a splinter in the right ring finger has also been falling more than usual, then the PE will be more extensive and may include the musculoskeletal and neurologic systems.

Figure 5.5 depicts a written physical exam similar to one found in a paper health record. Figure 5.6 shows a physical exam as documented using EHRclinic.

The healthcare professional who needs to know the results of a patient's physical exam on a future visit or to answer questions, complete forms, or handle insurance issues will need to access the patient's physical exam.

PHYSICAL EXAM

Alexis Shaw is a 25-year-old African American female being seen today for her annual physical. Her ROS has been reviewed; and is unremarkable.

HEENT: Scalp clear; eyes and ears within normal limits. Nose: Some congestion noted. Throat: post-nasal drip noted.

Chest: Lungs clear to auscultation, no wheezes or rales.

Cardio: Heart rate and rhythm normal; no murmurs.

Abdomen: Soft, non-tender, no guarding or rebound noted.

Skin: No rashes, broken skin, or open wounds. Nails: bites her nails, but otherwise unremarkable.

Breasts & Genitalia: Deferred - she has an appointment with her GYN in two months. Her LMP was April 15 of this year. Periods are normal.

Extremities: Range of motion intact; no swelling.

Neuro: Within normal limits.

Figure 5.5   Written PE

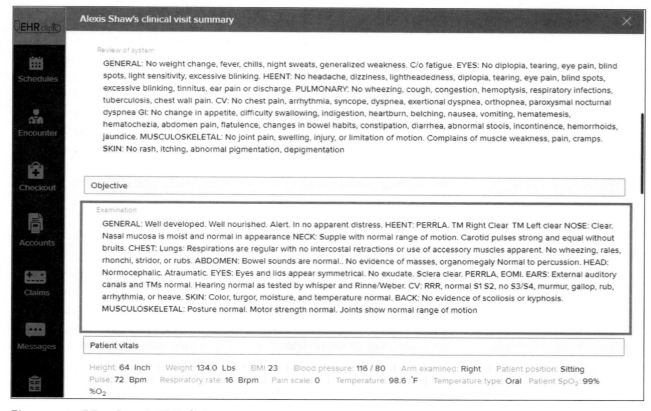

Figure 5.6   PE as Seen in EHRclinic

Though an EHR results in more detailed, timely documentation, it is still labor intensive for the care provider, and patients might leave with the perception that the physician was more interested in the computer than in them. To counter this, many physicians, hospitals, emergency departments, and clinics are utilizing **scribes** to enter data into the EHR. A scribe is not a clinician and does not have to have any clinical education. The qualifications differ by setting (hospital, physician's practice, urgent care, long-term care facility, etc.) and individual facility. For all scribes, however, excellent keyboarding skills, including speed and, most importantly, accuracy, are a must. In addition, the scribe works only under the supervision of the care provider and must have knowledge of medical terminology, human disease, and pharmacology. The care provider is ultimately responsible for the information entered into the EHR. The entries made by the scribe are electronically signed or attributed to the scribe, but the care provider must countersign the documentation. Best practice dictates that the care provider not countersign any notes until he or she has read and verified their accuracy.

Scribes may have other duties in addition to entering information into the health record as the physician or other healthcare provider is examining the patient. Scribes may locate information in the EHR that the physician asks for while seeing the patient. For instance, the physician may need to know when a patient was started on a particular medication or how long the patient has been seen for a particular condition.

Regulations covering the use and responsibilities of scribes vary from state to state and by accrediting agency; thus, it is important to do a thorough search of regulations and standards prior to implementing the use of scribes in your organization (AHIMA).

The use of scribes is not an entirely new practice. Many care providers have long used scribes to document in their paper or electronic records. Dermatologists, for example, not only are examining skin with their eyes but also must hold measuring tools and a magnifier and therefore cannot stop to document each lesion. A scribe is needed to document as the dermatologist verbally describes each lesion. The same applies to an ophthalmologist, who uses instruments to examine a patient's eyes and therefore cannot stop to write or type in findings. However, the general use of scribes is a relatively new practice. Even so, a good deal of research has been done on the effectiveness of the use of scribes on productivity, reimbursement, quality of documentation, and patient (and provider) satisfaction. So far, results are showing positive outcomes in all areas (Shultz and Holmstrom).

Scribe An assistant who enters data, either in writing or electronically, into the health record as the care provider verbally dictates recent findings.

5.5 Medical Dictation and Transcription

With a manual record system, care providers may choose to handwrite their charts. That has often been problematic because handwriting is often illegible. A record that is not legible can cause safety concerns and negative patient outcomes, and it wastes time for the healthcare professional who cannot read the writing and has to track down the care provider for clarification. You have no doubt read or heard horror stories of wrong medications or wrong dosages being given to patients because of illegible handwriting. Health insurance companies may also deny payment based on illegible handwriting.

One solution many physicians used in the past was to dictate their notes into a dictation system, and a transcriptionist then transcribed the physician's words into a typed document. Dictation used as a business tool dates back to the early 20th century when Thomas Edison, Inc., and Columbia Graphophone Company distributed their first versions of voice recorders, known as the Ediphone and Dictaphone, respectively. Dictation has evolved considerably—from handheld machines to less cumbersome systems that require the use of only a telephone.

The use of dictation and transcription software resulted in greater accuracy (because of better recording quality), faster turnaround time than the original dictation systems, and more advanced reporting capabilities, which allowed physicians' offices and hospitals to analyze the cost of dictation and transcription as a means of documentation.

The cost of dictation, and the required transcriptionists who translate the spoken word into the written word, is not negligible. As technology progressed, so did the price of dictation systems. As the requirements of government agencies and insurance companies rose, as well as escalating malpractice and negligence cases, the need for better, faster documentation grew. But recording a physician's words on paper also needed to be done in a timely manner. The need for qualified transcriptionists grew, but they were often in short supply.

5.6 Speech Recognition Technology

Over the past 30 years or so, speech recognition technology has replaced traditional dictation to a great degree. You will hear this referred to as voice recognition technology as well. In healthcare, **speech recognition technology** is software that converts the care provider's speech (dictation) into digital data, resulting in a transcribed report or, in the case of an electronic record, the data appearing within the EHR. **Voice recognition technology** is technically the process of identifying the person who is speaking. Chances are you are already using speech recognition technology and do not even realize it. For instance, your cell phone has a feature that allows you to voice dial, or you call your local cable company and go through a series of questions to which you respond by "saying or pushing 3." Both are forms of speech recognition. In these two examples, a command is carried out based on your response. With speech recognition used in the medical environment, as the care provider dictates, the words appear on the computer screen and as a printed report, when needed. The software "learns" the dictator's voice. However, the words that end up on the screen may not be perfect; for instance, "there" may be typed rather than "their" or "Xanax" may be heard as "Zantac." But, because medicine requires accurate information, the medical transcriptionist's role has become more that of an editor than that of a transcriptionist. The transcriptionist may listen to the entire piece of dictation and compare it against what appears on the screen, or, once the system learns a particular physician's voice and becomes more accurate, the transcriptionist may only read what is on the screen to look for obvious errors. The decision is dependent on the particular facility or department and is based on the recognition accuracy rate and facility policy. The YouTube video clip below illustrates the use of speech recognition by a physician.

The quality of transcription is higher with speech recognition (if the software recognizes the words correctly). Once physicians are comfortable with the use of speech recognition software, it may be less time consuming than dictation. Also, long-term costs are lower, since in most instances the

Speech recognition technology
Software that recognizes the words being said by the person dictating and digitally converts the speech to text; as it is used it "learns" the dictator's voice, and therefore improves the accuracy of the transcription.

Voice recognition technology
Software that uses a person's voice to verify that they are who they say they are. A sample of a person's speech is recorded, and those speech patterns are tested against a database to verify that their voice matches their claimed identity.

for your information **fyi**

Nuance is a popular service provider of speech recognition technology. This YouTube video gives an example of dictation and transcription shared by the healthcare team: https://www.youtube.com/watch?v=d7vgd-INWBM.

transcription costs are lower (especially if a transcription service rather than transcriptionists employed by the office or hospital had been utilized in the past). The greatest advantage, though, is the speed of documentation. With traditional transcription, days could pass between the time a report was dictated and the time it was transcribed (known as turn-around time). With speech recognition, the documentation is instant—as the words are spoken, they are documented in the record. Of course, the record should be reviewed for quality and accuracy and then edited before the care provider authenticates (signs) the note, but the fact that there is a draft copy in the record so quickly is a strong benefit.

Many EMR/EHR software solutions have a speech recognition application.

5.7 Electronic Prescribing (ePrescribing)

ePrescribing Electronically transmitting prescriptions from care provider to pharmacy.

Point of care (POC) Documentation, dictation, and ordering of tests and procedures that occur at the same time the patient is being seen.

ePrescribing software is another component of the original Meaningful Use requirements of HITECH. With ePrescribing, the care provider sends prescriptions to the patient's pharmacy electronically, at the **point of care (POC)** (occurring at the time the patient is being seen). Electronically sending prescriptions speeds up the process for the patient, as opposed to the traditional method in which the care provider hands the patient a written prescription and the patient takes it to the pharmacy and waits for it to be filled (or returns at a later time). Even if the office calls in the prescription, the process takes longer than using ePrescribing.

Most important, quality of care is greatly improved with electronic prescribing; not only does the prescription itself go directly to the pharmacy, but also the patient demographics, insurance information, allergies, and medication history are sent as well. Care providers and pharmacists are alerted to possible food and drug interactions between medications that are currently prescribed or that the patient is already taking, and drug allergies and sensitivities are flagged. Also, medication dosing errors are avoided—for instance, if the care provider orders 250 mg of a particular drug for a 15-year-old patient, but the recommended dosage for that drug is 25 mg for a 15-year-old, an alert message automatically appears, so that the care provider can make the correction before the prescription is sent through to the pharmacy. Prescription renewal requests are handled more efficiently, too, since they are received electronically, with no need to manually update the patient's chart. And, of course, there are no more legibility issues—pharmacists do not have to make phone calls to the office to ask what the care provider had written, and the office staff does not have to take the time to track down the care provider or chart.

EXERCISE 5.4 **EHR**

Go to https://connect.mheducation.com to complete this exercise. To see instructional notes with the steps, visit the eBook in Connect or download them from www.mhhe.com/iehr4.

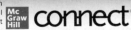

Using ePrescribe

Before we look at the steps involved in using ePrescribe, we will cover the parts of a prescription. They are

Drug name: The name of the drug in brand or generic form. For instance, HydroDIURIL is a brand name for hydrochlorothiazide (the generic name).

Dosage: The measurement of the amount of drug that is being administered. HydroDIURIL is prescribed in 25 or 50 mg doses to treat adult hypertension.

Sig: The "label," or instructions that the pharmacist needs to list on the prescription label. A common Sig for HydroDIURIL is "Take one tablet by mouth, once daily."

In our scenario for ePrescribe, Alfredo J. Garza called in for a refill of his prescription for Caduet (a medication for high blood pressure and angina) on May 9, 2022.

Since this information is found in the clinical part of the chart, Alfredo J. Garza's facesheet is first accessed, then the Medication List. The care provider typically carries out these steps unless he or she has given the healthcare professional a verbal order to do so.

Dr. Ingram has reviewed Mr. Garza's chart and authorizes you to submit a quantity of 30 tablets with two refills. He also asks you to add *Caduet (generic: amlodipine-atorvastatin) 10-10 mg, one tablet daily* to the drug database for future prescribing.

Follow these steps to complete the exercise on your own once you have watched the demonstration and tried the steps with helpful prompts. Use the information provided in the scenario to complete the information.

1. Click on 'Manage reports' button.
2. Click on 'Patient charts and graphs' button.
3. Click on 'Search by patient first name/last name/chart number/SSN' field and enter 'gar'.
4. Click on 'Alfredo Garza's' info.
5. Click on 'Add medication list' button.
6. Click on 'Status' button and select 'Active'.
7. Click on 'Drug type' button and select 'Rx'.
8. Click on 'Drug name' input field and enter 'Caduet'.
9. Click on 'Dosage' input field and enter '10-10 mg'.
10. Click on 'Quantity' input field and enter '30'.
11. Click on 'Drug form' drop-down and select 'Tablet'.
12. Click on 'Route' dropdown and select 'Oral'.
13. Click on 'Frequency' input field and enter 'Once daily'.
14. Click on 'Duration' input field and enter '30'.
15. Click on 'Last refill date' field and enter '05/09/2022'.
16. Click on 'Number of refills' input field and enter '2'.
17. Click on 'Diagnosis' input field and enter 'Angina'.
18. Click on 'Default provider' input field and enter 'Ingram'.
19. Click on 'Done' button.
20. Click on 'Chart and graphs' cancel button.
21. Click on 'Tools' module.
22. Click on 'Manage practice data' button.
23. Click on 'Drug database' button.
24. Click on 'Add new drug' button.
25. Click on 'Drug name (generic)' input field and enter 'amlodipine-atorvastatin'.
26. Click on 'Drug name (brand)' input field and enter 'Caduet'.
27. Click on 'Dosage 1' input field and enter '10-10 mg, one tablet daily'.
28. Click on 'Add drug' button.

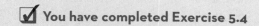 **You have completed Exercise 5.4**

5.8 Computerized Physician Order Entry (CPOE)

Computerized physician order entry (CPOE) Entering physician orders electronically rather than on paper. The order is transmitted directly to the appropriate department; for instance, an order for an x-ray goes directly to the radiology department, and an order for a CBC goes directly to the laboratory.

Interface The ability of one computer system or component to accept or send data to another system without loss of integrity or meaning.

No treatment, diagnostic test, or medication administration is performed on any patient without a care provider's order. Patients cannot be admitted or discharged without a care provider's order. Using paper records, orders were traditionally either written by the care provider or given verbally and written in the patient's record by a nurse. Orders may be in written form or electronically submitted via **computerized physician order entry (CPOE)**. Through this function, orders can be printed or electronically submitted to an outside laboratory, a medical equipment company, or a hospital with **interface** capabilities in EHRclinic. The interface capability means that one computer system (or component) can accept and receive data from another system. The systems may be at different locations or within the same facility. Your office may have EHRclinic software for PM and EHR, but your laboratory system may be designed and manufactured by a different vendor. If the computer programs for each are configured to exchange data without having to re-enter the data, orders can flow directly to the laboratory system and the results can flow directly back to the EHR in EHRclinic.

A major advantage of CPOE functionality is built-in clinical decision support. Alerts appear when orders are entered for medications or treatment that may cause an adverse reaction to a drug or drugs previously ordered for that patient. The same applies to dosing errors. If a care provider has ordered 250 mg of a drug for a 10-year-old patient, but the maximum dosage is 100 mg for that age group, then an alert appears, and a potentially serious situation is averted because the alert occurs before the drug is administered. Through the use of CPOE, as long as the facility's data dictionary includes a comprehensive listing of medications and abbreviations used, the probability of medication errors occurring is greatly reduced.

Regarding orders for diagnostic tests, once the order is carried out—for instance, a complete blood count (CBC)—the results are electronically sent to the care provider who ordered the lab test. Using CPOE is safer in this case as well, because there is no questionable handwriting or error in transcribing physicians' verbal orders, improving overall patient care.

5.9 Tracking Physicians' Orders

If a test is important enough to order, then learning the results of that test is equally important. Tests that are not carried out and reported in a timely manner can delay necessary care and cause inefficiency in the business processes of an office. Having the ability to track (determine which step of the process) the order status in an EHR system prevents communication breakdowns and unnecessary rework.

When an order has been completed and the results are ready for the care provider's review, he or she receives notification in the Tasks area. Depending on the EHR software vendor, providers will access labs/imaging by going into the Lab and Imaging reports in the facesheet, as shown in Figure 5.7. Others may have a Lab Flowsheet, and most include alerts to the care providers when actual lab values are critically outside the normal range.

Once the care provider clicks the Labs tab, all resulted orders will appear on the screen. In Figure 5.8, you can see that one order has been resulted, and it is for physical labs on Dr. Ingram's patient James Phillips.

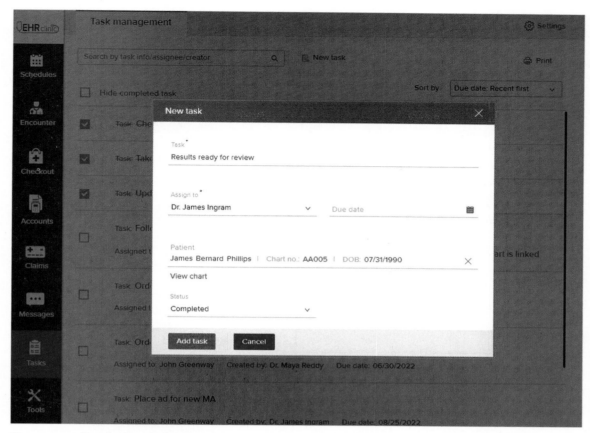

Figure 5.7   Results Ready for Review

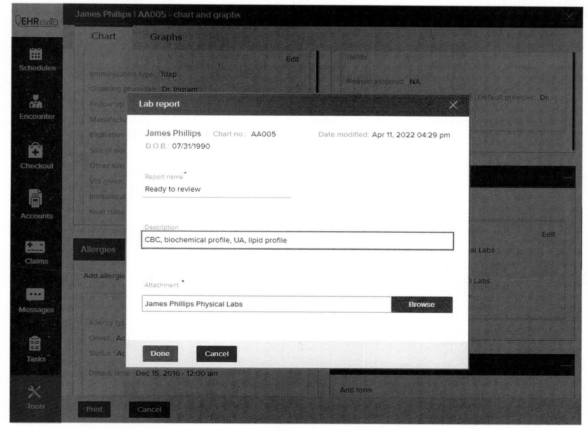

Figure 5.8   Resulted Order

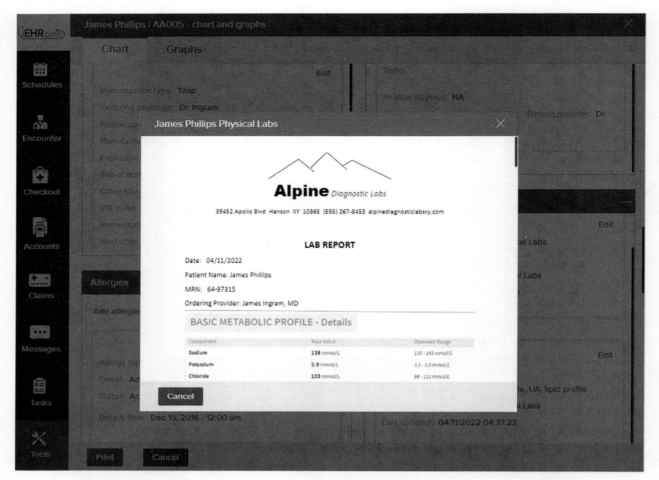

Figure 5.9   Order Details Screen

If, based on the results of the lab test, Dr. Ingram wants to order additional tests, prescribe a particular medication, or follow up with the patient soon, he will give additional orders to the healthcare professional to handle the situation accordingly.

Figure 5.9 represents the final screen the care provider sees. From it, he or she can note whether the results were normal or abnormal or were a specific assessment. The care provider can also send a follow-up task to one of the healthcare professionals in the office or to another care provider in the practice for review. These tasks can be done directly from the Lab screen without having to exit that function and find another.

EXERCISE   5.5   EHR

Go to https://connect.mheducation.com to complete this exercise. To see instructional notes with the steps, visit the eBook in Connect or download them from www.mhhe.com/iehr4.

Mc Graw Hill **connect**

Locate the Status of an Order

In this exercise, Dr. Ingram is asking you about the results of Alfredo Garza's lab and radiology work. You will again go to the facesheet of Alfredo J. Garza and review the Labs area, since your goal is to find out if Alfredo had the tests done and if the results are in his chart.

Upon reviewing the lab section of Mr. Garza's facesheet, you see that his lab and radiology tests are complete, but they have not yet been linked to the chart for review. You will add the physical lab and chest x-ray results to the chart and create a task alerting Dr. Ingram that they are ready for review.

Once you have accessed the facesheet, follow these steps to complete the exercise on your own once you have watched the demonstration and tried the steps with helpful prompts.

1. Click on 'Manage reports' button.
2. Click on 'Patient charts and graphs' button.
3. Click on 'Search by patient first name/last name/chart number/SSN' field and enter 'gar'.
4. Click on 'Alfredo Garza's' info.
5. Click on 'Add lab reports' button.
6. Click on 'Report name' input field and enter 'Chest x-ray'.
7. Click on Attachment 'Browse' button and select 'Alfredo Garza Chest X-Ray'.
8. Click on 'Choose' button.
9. Click on 'List of lab reports done' button.
10. Click on 'Add lab reports' button.
11. Click on 'Report name' input field and enter 'Physical labs'.
12. Click on Attachment 'Browse' button and select 'Alfredo Garza Physical Labs'.
13. Click on 'Choose' button.
14. Click on 'List of lab reports done' button.
15. Click on 'Chart and graphs' cancel button.
16. Click on 'Tasks' module.
17. Click on 'New task' button.
18. Click on 'Task' field and enter 'Review labs for Alfredo Garza'.
19. Click on 'Assign to drop down' button and select 'Dr. James Ingram'.
20. Click on datepicker icon in 'Due date' field and select 'April 13 2022' date.
21. Click on 'Search patient by first name/last name/chart no./DOB (mm/dd/yyyy)' field and enter 'gar'.
22. Click on 'Alfredo Garza' patient.
23. Click on 'Add task' button.

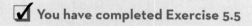 **You have completed Exercise 5.5**

5.10 The Problem List

Another requirement of Meaningful Use (now Promoting Interoperability) is an up-to-date **problem list** of current and active diagnoses. Providing quality care means following current diagnoses or conditions on an ongoing basis until the problems are resolved, or at least until they are stable. Of course, some medical conditions, such as asthma or coronary artery disease, may never resolve completely, but the care provider must ensure that the patient is stable and that his or her condition is not worsening. With the use of a problem list, as long as it is kept current, necessary testing or assessment of the condition does not "fall through the cracks." For instance, a patient may be seen today because of an upper respiratory infection but has also been treated

Problem list A listing kept in the patient's health record of all of his or her current (active) and resolved medical conditions.

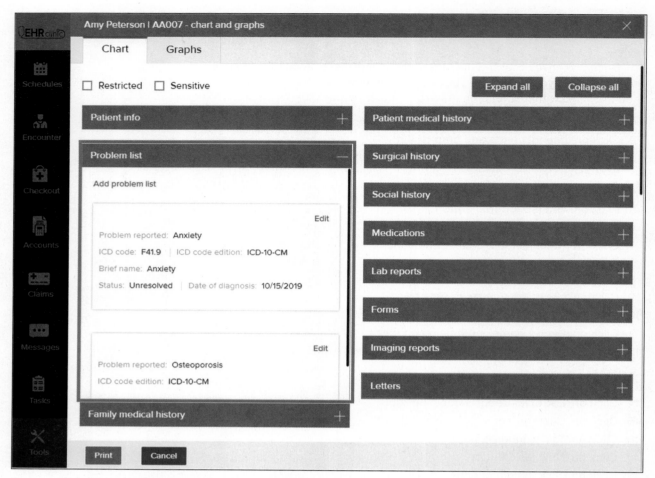

Amy Peterson | AA007 - chart and graphs

Chart   **Graphs**

☐ Restricted   ☐ Sensitive   [Expand all]   [Collapse all]

Patient info   +   **Patient medical history**   +

Problem list   —   **Surgical history**   +

Add problem list   **Social history**   +

                                    Edit   **Medications**   +

Problem reported: **Anxiety**
ICD code: **F41.9** | ICD code edition: **ICD-10-CM**   **Lab reports**   +
Brief name: **Anxiety**
Status: **Unresolved** | Date of diagnosis: **10/15/2019**   **Forms**   +

                                    Edit   **Imaging reports**   +

Problem reported: **Osteoporosis**
ICD code edition: **ICD-10-CM**   **Letters**   +

Family medical history   +

[Print]   [Cancel]

Figure 5.10 **Example of a Problem List**

by the care provider for hypertension, and on today's visit the care provider notes that the patient's blood pressure is elevated. By clicking on Hypertension in the problem list of diagnoses, the care provider is quickly able to see the patient's treatment history and prior blood pressure readings and then proceed accordingly. (See Figure 5.10 for an example of a problem list.)

Sometimes the information in a problem list is helpful to the patient as well as the care provider. The patient may have told the care provider something about his or her treatment or hospitalizations but later forgot the details. By having this complete history, the medical office has the information readily available when needed.

EXERCISE   5.6   EHR

Go to https://connect.mheducation.com to complete this exercise. To see instructional notes with the steps, visit the eBook in Connect or download them from www.mhhe.com/iehr4. Mc Graw Hill **connect**

Utilizing the Problem List

In the scenario we are about to view, Alfredo J. Garza has been treated for angina over the past few years. He was first diagnosed in 2012 and has been hospitalized at Memorial Hospital twice for it—once on June 15, 2014, and once on August 10, 2015. Mr. Garza has asked the office staff to complete a form he must give his employer, who needs to know if Mr. Garza has ever been hospitalized for angina and, if so, when. He does not recall the dates

112

but does remember giving that information to Dr. Ingram on his last visit, so he hopes the information can be found in his record.

Mr. Garza also states that he saw a rheumatologist on April 8, 2022, and was diagnosed with rheumatoid arthritis at that time.

From the facesheet of Alfredo J. Garza, the healthcare professional will locate angina from the Problem List area in order to get Mr. Garza the information he needs. The new diagnosis of rheumatoid arthritis will also be added to the Problem List, so that it will be in his chart at Summit Bay Health Center.

Once the facesheet of the patient's chart is accessed, follow these steps to complete the exercise on your own once you've watched the demonstration and tried the steps with helpful prompts.

1. Click on 'Patient charts and graphs' button.
2. Click on 'Search by patient first name/last name/chart number/SSN' field and enter 'gar'.
3. Click on 'Alfredo Garza's' info.
4. Click on 'Add problem list' button.
5. Click on 'Problem reported' input field and enter 'Rheumatoid arthritis'.
6. Click on 'ICD code edition' button and select 'ICD-10-CM'.
7. Click on 'Search by ICD code or generic diagnosis name' input field and enter 'rheu'.
8. Click on 'M06.9 Rheumatoid arthritis' procedure code.
9. Click on 'Diagnosis date' input field and enter '04/08/2022'.
10. Click on 'Status' button and select 'Unresolved'.
11. Click on 'Done' button.
12. Click on 'Chart and graphs' cancel button.

 You have completed Exercise 5.6

APPLYING YOUR SKILLS

In this chapter, we covered the usual contents of a SOAP note. Following are random sentences likely to be found in a provider's office note. After each sentence, note whether the sentence should be in the **S**ubjective, **O**bjective, **A**ssessment, or **P**lan portion of the office note. Again, these are random sentences and will not come together to form a note for one particular patient.

1. A chest x-ray performed in the office showed an infiltrate in the right lower lobe of the lung.
2. Grace has been complaining of a pain in her right side, which is stabbing in nature.
3. The patient was given an order for an ultrasound of the kidneys and bladder, which she should have done in the next week or so.
4. Nephrolithiasis
5. The patient's blood pressure is 145/95.
6. "I am here because I've had a headache for three days that just won't go away."
7. The patient should continue physical therapy for two more weeks.
8. Right lower lobe pneumonia
9. Both pupils are equal and reactive.
10. The patient states she has tried Aleve, but her right knee pain has not improved.

chapter 5 **summary**

LEARNING OUTCOME	CONCEPTS FOR REVIEW
5.1 Explain each element of a SOAP note.	– Subjective—the patient's description of the problem – Objective—the care provider's results of physical examination – Assessment—the diagnosis or diagnoses – Plan—the diagnostic tests or treatment plan for the patient
5.2 Identify elements of the history of present illness (HPI).	– Location of the condition (abdomen, arm, leg, head, etc.) – Quality of the symptoms – Severity of the symptoms – Duration/timing of the symptoms – Context under which symptoms occur – Modifying factors – Associated signs and symptoms
5.3 Identify elements of the review of systems (ROS).	– Body-system-by-body-system assessment of any signs or symptoms the patient is experiencing that may or may not be related to the reason for his or her visit – Not the same as the physical exam
5.4 Identify elements of the physical exam (PE).	– The extent of the exam is dependent on the patient's presenting symptoms (the chief complaint). – The physical exam relates to the findings of the care provider, not the patient, as in the ROS; for example, the patient complains of pain in the right lower abdomen, yet when the care provider presses on the right lower abdomen, the patient does not express feelings of pain – The advantages of using a scribe, particularly during the physical exam
5.5 Describe the process of traditional dictation and transcription.	– The physician dictates medical notes into a recording device – A transcriptionist types the words using word processing software – Often takes days for the transcribed report to be filed in the patient's record
5.6 Illustrate the advantages of speech recognition technology.	– The provider's documentation immediately appears in the patient's record, with no lag time between dictation and transcription – In the long term, it may be less expensive than traditional dictation and transcription – Quality is higher than with traditional transcription (in most cases)
5.7 Outline the benefits of ePrescribing.	– Less chance for medication errors – Potential food/drug interactions identified – Fewer man-hours to complete the process – More convenient and less wait time for patients – Overall, better-quality care

LEARNING OUTCOME	CONCEPTS FOR REVIEW
5.8 Evaluate the benefits of computerized physician order entry (CPOE).	- Fewer errors in carrying out orders because they are no longer handwritten - Orders sent directly from the office to the laboratory or hospital - Safer for the patient—the order is sent by the care provider rather than verbally given to another healthcare professional to send on to the laboratory or hospital - If an interface exists, the results automatically come back to the ordering physician
5.9 Support the necessity to track physicians' orders.	- Patient care—knowing the results of the test in a timely manner, proper treatment can be started quickly
5.10 Examine the benefits of a problem list.	- Timely follow-up of conditions - Serves as a reminder to the care provider to address problems on the patient's problem list - Information about each problem located in one place

chapter review

MATCHING QUESTIONS

Match the terms on the left with the definitions on the right.

_____ 1. **[LO 5.1]** SOAP note

_____ 2. **[LO 5.8]** interface

_____ 3. **[LO 5.4]** scribe

_____ 4. **[LO 5.6]** voice recognition technology

_____ 5. **[LO 5.8]** computerized physician order entry (CPOE)

_____ 6. **[LO 5.2]** history of present illness (HPI)

_____ 7. **[LO 5.7]** point of care (POC)

_____ 8. **[LO 5.10]** problem list

_____ 9. **[LO 5.7]** ePrescribing

_____ 10. **[LO 5.6]** speech recognition technology

a. patient's description of current symptoms

b. EMR feature that is part of HITECH's original Meaningful Use requirements

c. recognizes the words being dictated then digitally converts speech to text

d. immediate, real-time documentation of patient procedures

e. comprehensive record of a patient's complaints and conditions

f. documentation format that allows healthcare professionals to capture all aspects of a patient encounter

g. ability to access another provider's practice management software for patient care purposes

h. assistant who enters the dictation of a care provider into a patient record

i. uses a person's voice to verify their claimed identity

j. electronic entry of care provider orders for direct transmission to appropriate departments

MULTIPLE-CHOICE QUESTIONS

Select the letter that best completes the statement or answers the question:

1. **[LO 5.2]** Which of the following statements would NOT be included in the history of present illness?
   a. Blood pressure is 130/84, right arm, sitting.
   b. Pain radiates down the left leg.
   c. Patient c/o productive cough for one week.
   d. Symptoms improved after taking ibuprofen.

2. **[LO 5.3]** Which of the following would most likely require a complete review of systems?
   a. annual exam
   b. headache
   c. mole on back
   d. sore throat

3. **[LO 5.1]** Notes about a prescription ordered for a patient would appear in the _____ section of a SOAP note.
   a. subjective
   b. objective
   c. assessment
   d. plan

4. **[LO 5.3]** An ROS covers information likely documented in the
   a. history of present illness.
   b. medical history form.
   c. physical exam.
   d. SOAP note.

5. **[LO 5.9]** Dr. Henderson ordered liver function studies on Roberta Ware two weeks ago but has not yet seen the results. Curious as to why she does not have these results yet, Dr. Henderson accesses the electronic health record and sees that Mrs. Ware just had the test performed an hour ago. This is an example of
   a. computerized order entry.
   b. one of the most valuable uses of an electronic health record.
   c. a query.
   d. order tracking.

6. **[LO 5.6]** The biggest advantage of speech recognition software over manual transcription is
   a. clarity.
   b. cost.
   c. ease.
   d. speed of turn-around time.

7. **[LO 5.1]** Information gathered during a provider's physical exam would appear in the _____ section of a SOAP note.
   a. subjective
   b. objective
   c. assessment
   d. plan

8. **[LO 5.6]** The more speech recognition software is used, the
   a. faster it corrects mistakes.
   b. quicker it gets.
   c. more it learns the dictator's voice, and the more accurate it becomes.
   d. slower it gets.

9. **[LO 5.8]** There must be a _____ to perform any tests or treatments.
   a. diagnosis
   b. referral
   c. care provider order
   d. SOAP note

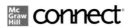

Enhance your learning by completing these exercises and more at **https://connect.mheducation.com**!

10. **[LO 5.5]** A person hired to manually record a physician's spoken words is known as a
    a. dictator.
    b. recorder.
    c. stenographer.
    d. transcriptionist.

11. **[LO 5.2]** Which of the following elements of an HPI are collected at a visit?
    a. all of them
    b. duration, quality, and severity
    c. location and severity
    d. only those that apply to the patient's chief complaint

12. **[LO 5.4]** The extent of a physical exam largely depends upon which of the following?
    a. age of the patient
    b. amount of time available
    c. patient's chief complaint
    d. patient's medical history

13. **[LO 5.10]** Promoting Interoperability (Meaningful Use) regulations require the keeping of an up-to-date
    a. exam registry.
    b. order queue.
    c. problem list.
    d. provider note.

14. **[LO 5.7]** The use of ePrescribing is part of the requirements for
    a. HIPAA.
    b. HITECH.
    c. HIM.
    d. HPI.

SHORT-ANSWER QUESTIONS

1. **[LO 5.2]** List the typical elements of a history of present illness.

2. **[LO 5.5]** List at least three drawbacks of handwritten patient charts.

3. **[LO 5.3]** In order for a practice to receive reimbursement for an ROS, what must happen?

4. **[LO 5.4]** Explain the factors that might influence the extent of a physical exam.

5. **[LO 5.1]** List the four sections of a SOAP note and give an example of each.

6. **[LOs 5.5, 5.6]** Why is there still a need for medical transcriptionists in an age of speech recognition software?

7. **[LO 5.3]** List the typical organs and body systems that would be covered in a complete review of systems.

8. **[LO 5.10]** List one reason a provider might use a patient's problem list.

9. **[LOs 5.3, 5.4]** Contrast an ROS with a PE.

10. **[LO 5.4]** List four types of medical providers who might perform a physical exam.

11. **[LO 5.8]** Explain what it means to have interface capabilities with EHRclinic. What benefits does interfacing have?

12. **[LO 5.9]** List three benefits of electronic health record order tracking capabilities.

13. **[LO 5.4]** Based on Alexis Shaw's physical exam as documented in the text, what is her chief complaint?

14. **[LO 5.6]** Contrast voice recognition with speech recognition.

APPLYING YOUR KNOWLEDGE

1. **[LOs 5.1, 5.2, 5.3, 5.4]** Patient James Frank presents for his appointment. He is complaining of fatigue and headaches. When Dr. Ingram examines him, he finds that James has an enlarged lymph node on the right side of his throat; his lungs are clear; his blood pressure is a little low at 100/68. Dr. Ingram suspects anemia or an underactive thyroid as the causes of James' fatigue, so he orders that a comprehensive blood panel be done. Create a SOAP note that properly documents each piece of James Frank's visit with Dr. Ingram.

2. **[LO 5.6]** Your office is preparing to implement new speech recognition technology, and you have been tasked with creating some talking points and benefits to share with your peers. How could you go about explaining the benefits of speech recognition software?

3. **[LOs 5.7, 5.10]** Why would ePrescribing and an up-to-date problem list be addressed under Promoting Interoperability (Meaningful Use) requirements?

4. **[LOs 5.7, 5.8, 5.9, 5.10]** Of the following electronic capabilities—ePrescribing, CPOE, order tracking, and the problem list—which do you think is the most beneficial? Explain your answer.

5. **[LO 5.7]** Create two flowcharts: one that shows the progression of a manually written prescription and one that shows the progression of a prescription entered using ePrescribing.

6. **[LO 5.4]** What are the benefits of using a scribe to document a patient's visit?

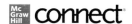 Enhance your learning by completing these exercises and more at **https://connect.mheducation.com!**

chapter references

American Health Information Management Association (AHIMA). (2012, November). Using Medical Scribes in a Physician Practice. *Journal of AHIMA, 83*(11): 64–69 [expanded online version].

Recording History: The History of Recording Technology. Retrieved from http://www.recording-history.org/HTML/dicta_tech5.php.

Recording History: The History of Recording Technology. The 1970s and the Decline of Dictation. Retrieved from http://www.recording-history.org/HTML/dicta_biz7.php.

Recording History: The History of Recording Technology. Retrieved from http://www.recording-history.org/HTML/dicta_tech2.php.

Shultz, C. G., and Holmstrom, H. L. (2015, May–June). The Use of Medical Scribes in Health Care Settings: A Systematic Review and Future Directions. *Journal of the American Board of Family Medicine, 28*: 371–381.

Wiedemann, Lou Ann. (2010, October). CPOE Lessons Learned. *Journal of AHIMA, 81*(10): 54–55.

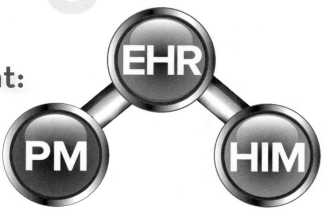

chapter six

Financial Management: Insurance and Billing Functions

Learning **Outcomes**

At the end of this chapter, the student should be able to

6.1 Illustrate the need for a claims management process.

6.2 List the information contained in an encounter form (Superbill).

6.3 Apply procedures to update a patient's account in EHRclinic.

6.4 Demonstrate coding using ICD-10-CM/ PCS and CPT® codes in EHRclinic.

6.5 Examine the correlation between documentation and code assignment.

6.6 Describe Accountable Care Organizations.

6.7 Describe the information contained in a remittance advice and an explanation of benefits.

6.8 Apply procedures to manage accounts receivable in EHRclinic.

6.9 Demonstrate the need for a compliance plan.

Key **Terms**

Abuse

Accounts payable

Accounts receivable

Adjudication

Affordable Care Act (ACA)

Chargemaster

Code linkage

Coinsurance

Compliance plan

Co-payment (co-pay)

Deductible

Encounter form (Superbill)

Evaluation and Management (E&M)

Explanation of Benefits (EOB)

Fee schedule

Fraud

Healthcare Common Procedure Coding System (HCPCS)

Insurance plan

Insurance verification

Managed care plan

Medical necessity

Principal diagnosis

Remittance advice (RA)

Subscriber

Transactions

What You Need to Know and Why You Need to Know It

Physicians, hospitals, and any other healthcare facilities are in business to take care of patients, first and foremost. However, they are also businesses. They have bills to pay, just like any other business—payroll, rent or mortgage, utilities, supplies, insurance, and, yes, the providers themselves need to be paid. The efficiency we have discussed in terms of providing patient care also applies to collecting monies owed to the office. The billing and collections process will be discussed in this chapter. Remember, though, that this is not a course on billing procedures. From this chapter, you will gain an awareness of how billing and EHR applications are intermeshed using EHRclinic. The specifics of *how* to complete and file insurance claims, manage accounts, collect unpaid bills, and handle financial management, in general, will be covered in another course. The coding of diagnoses and procedures will also be covered in other classes, but when you finish this chapter, you will understand how documentation, coding, and reimbursement are related.

6.1 Claims Management—Why and How

Every patient seen in a healthcare facility is charged for the care he or she receives. Yes, some accounts are "written off"; in other words, the patient does not pay, but there still needs to be an accounting of the visit and the charges that were incurred for the encounter (visit). If this is not done, the business profile of the office or facility will show an inaccurate picture of the number of patients seen, the procedures carried out, the charges incurred, and the amount of money collected. In other words, the statistics collected for that healthcare facility will not be valid, because not all of the patients are included in the database.

The financial well-being of a medical practice or any other healthcare facility is of great importance if the facility is to stay in business. Therefore, a process—or, to be specific, a written claims management process—is necessary. Each step of the process must be carried out efficiently and effectively. This process includes written policies—how much is charged per service, known as the **fee schedule**, the timing of filing claims, follow-up on unpaid claims, and collections procedures when claims are not paid must all be in writing. The importance of written policies will be addressed in the compliance section of this chapter.

In a physician's practice, which is what we will concentrate on in this worktext, the use of practice management (PM) software greatly improves the efficiency of a claims process, because it allows for more accurate capturing of charges, submits automatic reminders, offers a variety of reporting options, and provides automatic follow-up of each account. There is far less chance of missed charges, missed payments, and payments posted to the wrong account with a computerized system than with a manual one. Just the ability to run reports on daily charges, daily payments, and accounts in collections increases the efficiency of the business processes. In other settings—hospitals, long-term care facilities, and so on—similar software is in use because the end result is the same: getting paid!

Remember that each patient is entered only once in the practice's database of patients, but each patient may have more than one encounter (visit) attached to that master entry (Figure 6.1). Each encounter has an account

Fee schedule The amount charged for services rendered in a physician's office by Current Procedural Terminology (CPT®) code.

ICD-10-PCS is the coding system used to code procedures for inpatients in the hospital setting. The table below shows examples of ICD-10-PCS codes.

Splenectomy (removal of spleen)	07TP4ZZ
Salpingectomy (removal of fallopian tubes), bilateral	0UT74ZZ
Cholecystectomy (removal of gallbladder)	0FT40ZZ

HCPCS Level 2 codes are used to show tangible items provided to the patient, such as suture kits, ambulance services, and orthotic devices (cane, splint, etc.). Level 2 codes are used in any healthcare setting and are part of the chargemaster.

The following table shows examples of HCPCS Level 2 codes.

Code	Description
A0998	Ambulance response and treatment without transport
E0105	Cane, triple or quad
A6453	Self-adherent elastic bandage, 3" width

6.5 The Relationship between Documentation and Coding

Services rendered to a patient—whether they involve the face-to-face time with the physician, treatment, or diagnostic tests and procedures—cannot be billed to insurance unless they are medically necessary. That is to say, there must be sufficient signs, symptoms, or history to warrant the services given. Again, this is the purpose of code linkage in the billing process. In addition to demonstrating the relationship between diagnosis and procedure codes, the documentation in the record must support the need for any and all services and procedures. The EHR has been instrumental in making it possible for care providers to spend beneficial face-to-face time with their patients rather than spend time completing their records. Of course, documenting the patient's record while the patient is in the room also takes some finesse. The provider does not want to appear to be paying more attention to the computer screen than to the patient, but the more the provider uses the computer to document, the more easily he or she will be able to document, listen attentively, and converse with her patients at the same time. As mentioned in the previous chapter, care providers often use scribes, so that their attention is on the patient and the scribe's attention is on entering health data into the health record.

Performing services that are not necessary and coding services that were not actually performed constitute insurance (including Medicare and Medicaid) **fraud**. Fraud is intentional deception, which in healthcare takes advantage of a patient, an insurance company, Medicare, or Medicaid.

Whether you are studying to become a health information professional, a medical assistant, or a medical coder and biller, you will take courses that are specific to coding, and you will spend a significant amount of time discussing accurate, appropriate coding, as well as the guidelines that apply to the coding and billing functions—in particular, guidelines stating that only documented diagnoses and procedures/services should be coded!

Fraud Intentional deception, which in healthcare takes advantage of a patient, an insurance company, Medicare, or Medicaid.

Go to https://connect.mheducation.com to complete this exercise. To see instructional notes with the steps, visit the eBook in Connect or download them from www.mhhe.com/iehr4.

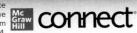

Maintain the ICD-10-CM and CPT® Databases

Typically, electronic health record software has databases for ICD-10-CM and CPT® codes. These databases allow users to easily select diagnostic and procedure codes without having to look them up with each patient encounter. Once the codes have been selected, the practice management software uses the codes for claim generation and submission.

As previously mentioned, the ICD-10-CM and CPT® codes are updated annually. Most diagnostic and procedure codes remain the same; however, there are some that may change and new ones that are added. To ensure that the practice is using the most up-to-date codes, it is necessary to maintain the databases by revising existing codes and manually adding new ones.

Dr. Ingram has decided that he will be performing abdominal ultrasound imaging procedures in the clinic. Since this is a new procedure for the office, the CPT® code 76700 for US Abdomen, Complete ($230) will need to be added as a procedure to the database. Additionally, Dr. Ingram has identified that the ICD-10-CM code for acute appendicitis is not in the database. This code, K35.80 Unspecified acute appendicitis, will need to be added to the database as well.

Follow these steps to complete the exercise on your own once you have watched the demonstration and tried the steps with helpful prompts in practice mode. Use the information provided in the scenario to complete the information.

1. Click on 'Manage practice data' button.
2. Click on 'CPT® codes' button.
3. Click on 'Search by code/description' field and enter 'abd'.
4. Click on 'Add new CPT® code' button.
5. Click on 'Edition' drop-down and select '2018'.
6. Click on 'Code' input field and enter '76700'.
7. Click on 'Type description' drop-down and select 'Imaging'.
8. Click on 'Description' input field and enter 'US Abdomen, Complete'.
9. Click on 'Amount - Need fee schedule' input field and enter '230'.
10. Click on 'Add CPT® code' button.
11. Click on 'Information management' button.
12. Click on 'ICD codes' button.
13. Click on 'Search by code/description' field and enter 'app'.
14. Click on 'Add new ICD code' button.
15. Click on 'Edition' drop-down and select 'ICD-10-CM'.
16. Click on 'Code' field and enter 'K35.80'.
17. Click on 'Description' field and enter 'Unspecified acute appendicitis'.
18. Click on 'Add ICD code' button.
19. Click on 'Information management' button.

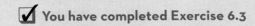

✓ **You have completed Exercise 6.3**

In the next exercise, you will see how ICD-10 and CPT® codes are assigned using the EHRclinic software.

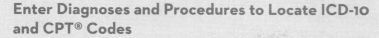

Enter Diagnoses and Procedures to Locate ICD-10 and CPT® Codes

Once a patient has been seen and examined by the care provider, a diagnosis is made. The written diagnosis is then transformed into a numeric code. In our example, it is done using a function of EHRclinic, but it can also be done manually, using code books. As mentioned earlier, the diagnosis coding is done using ICD-10-CM, and the procedures or services are coded using CPT® and/or HCPCS Level 2.

In the example that follows, Dr. Ingram has just seen a patient, Mark Robinski on April 4, 2022. Remember, only the care provider can make a diagnosis. So from the Patient Encounter screen, Dr. Ingram will be using the Assessment field (found within the encounter) to add a diagnosis for Mark Robinski.

Mark Robinski's diagnosis is diabetes mellitus, type 2, and Dr. Ingram orders a fasting blood sugar and urinalysis. A diagnosis code (ICD-10-CM) and a procedure code (CPT®) will be assigned in the following exercise. The software will automatically assign the codes, but it is important to read the description of the codes and compare it to the narrative diagnosis the care provider has made. One should never code more than what the care provider has documented, and if information is missing in the documentation, it is important to query the provider to determine if the documentation is accurate or if a procedure should not be billed for.

While the healthcare professional is completing the details for Mr. Robinski's encounter, Dr. Ingram decides to provide some diabetic education and states that Mr. Robinski should follow up in one month. The tests must be ordered, along with a venipuncture procedure, and the tasks must be documented within the patient's encounter.

Follow these steps to complete the exercise on your own once you have watched the demonstration and tried the steps with helpful prompts in practice mode. Use the information provided in the scenario to complete the information.

1. Click on 'Provider encounter' section.
2. Click on 'Mark Robinski's' appointment.
3. Click on 'Chief complaint' field.
4. Click on 'Follow-up Visit'.
5. Click on 'Present illness' field and enter 'Patient reports elevated blood sugar levels, thirst/dry mouth, increased urination, and fatigue'.
6. Click on 'Review of systems' field.
7. Click on 'ROS-Normal: remainder of ROS reviewed, and generally unremarkable except as noted in HPI'.
8. Click on 'GENERAL: No weight change, fever, chills, night sweats, generalized weakness'.
9. Click on 'EYES: No diplopia, tearing, eye pain, blind spots, light sensitivity, excessive blinking'.
10. Click on 'HEENT: No headache, dizziness, lightheadedness, diplopia, tearing, eye pain, blind spots, excessive blinking, tinnitus, ear pain or discharge, nose bleeding, nasal obstruction, nasal discharge, gingival bleeding, dental problems, sore throat, hoarseness, difficulty swallowing, neck stiffness, neck pain'.
11. Click on 'Examination' field.

(continued)

12. Click on 'GENERAL: Well developed. Well nourished. Alert. Oriented to person, place, and time. In no apparent distress'.
13. Click on 'HEENT: PERRLA. TM Right Clear. TM Left clear'.
14. Click on 'NOSE: Clear. Nasal mucosa is moist and normal in appearance, slight deviation of septum noted, turbinates normal'.
15. Click on 'MOUTH/THROAT: Clear. Dentition good. Normal mucosa, tongue, gingiva, and oropharynx. Palate elevates in midline. No thrush, erythema, or exudate'.
16. Click on 'Add diagnosis' button.
17. Enter 'dia' in 'Search' field and select 'Diabetes (Type 2, controlled)'.
18. Click on 'Add lab' button and select 'Venipuncture (blood draw)', 'Fasting blood glucose', and 'Urinalysis'.
19. Click on 'Follow up required' drop-down and select 'Yes'.
20. Click on 'Follow-up timeline' field and enter '1'.
21. Click on 'Add attachments' button and select 'Diabetes and You'.
22. Click on 'Ready for treatment' button and click on 'Proceed'.
23. Click on 'Password' field and enter '123456'.
24. Click on 'Done' button.
25. Click on 'Okay' button.

✓ **You have completed Exercise 6.4**

6.6 Accountable Care Organizations

The model of healthcare reimbursement for patients enrolled in the original Medicare program was fee-for-service for years, although Medicare introduced managed care models over the past several years. In a fee-for-service model, services are rendered and hospitals and physicians are paid as long as the services are considered medically necessary. In healthcare reform legislation, through a portion of the **Affordable Care Act (ACA)**, providers and hospitals are required to show that they are providing high-quality, coordinated care and are seeking patient input regarding their experience. In addition, positive patient outcomes and less redundancy of services are expected. In other words, reimbursement is tied to quality and the efficient use of healthcare services, as well as overall patient satisfaction.

When hospitals, doctors, and other healthcare providers formally work together to provide high-quality care, the result is an Accountable Care Organization (ACO). Accountable Care Organizations are groups of doctors, hospitals, and other healthcare providers (home health agencies or durable medical equipment companies, for example) who form a voluntary partnership that results in coordinated, high-quality care to their Medicare patients.

There are several types of Accountable Care Organizations, the first of which is the Shared Savings type, in which providers share in any financial savings, along with Medicare beneficiaries, if they meet quality and cost benchmarks, and it is a fee-for-service model. The Medicare Shared Savings ACO is known as the Medicare Shared Savings Program. The second type is an Investment Model ACO, for organizations that are interested in a prepaid shared savings program; this type of ACO targets healthcare organizations in rural and under-served areas. The third type of ACO is for Medicare beneficiaries on dialysis, and it is known as the Comprehensive ESRD Care Initiative.

The fourth type of ACO is the Next Generation ACO Model, which is managing specific populations of Medicare patients throughout the country where providers already have significant experience working with an ACO model. In the Next Generation ACO, predictable financial targets are set; providers and beneficiaries are given greater opportunities to coordinate care and are given the opportunity to attain the highest quality standards of care. The fifth ACO type, the Pioneer ACO, is available to providers and healthcare organizations that have experience working within an ACO model, meaning that they are used to coordinating care across different care settings. They are poised to move from a shared savings payment model to a population-based payment model, which is similar to the Medicare Shared Savings Program (Accountable Care Organizations: General Information. cms.gov).

Participation in an ACO is voluntary, and Medicare patients will not see any changes to their coverage because of a physician's or hospital's choice to become part of an ACO.

For the quality and efficiency of the delivery of healthcare to be measurable, access to structured data (through ICD-10, CPT®, and HCPCS codes) is necessary. The delivery of care must be "coordinated," thus, hospital(s), provider(s), and ancillary service providers within an ACO must be able to share patient information. The EHR and interoperable systems make the sharing of data possible. Quality measures are monitored and are related to the patient's experience, care coordination, and patient safety. The higher the quality of care delivered, the higher the shared savings earned by the ACO.

6.7 Accounts Receivable—Getting Paid

You may have heard the terms **accounts payable** and **accounts receivable** at some point in time. Accounts payable is money going out—paying the bills. Accounts receivable, on the other hand, is money coming in—in this context, the insurance companies' payment of claims that have been filed by Summit Bay Health Center and any monies owed by patients. Of course, it is imperative that what is billed is paid and that there is an accurate accounting of all **transactions**. Transactions are the posting of charges and the payment of claims.

Before insurance companies will pay for procedure charges, the healthcare practice must generate and submit a claim for each encounter to bill the insurance company.

Accounts payable Monies being paid from the medical practice—for instance, to pay for supplies, rent, utilities, payroll, etc.

Accounts receivable Monies coming into a medical practice—for instance, insurance payments or payments made by patients.

Transactions Posting of charges and the payment of claims in the practice management system to update patients' accounts.

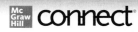 Go to https://connect.mheducation.com to complete this exercise. To see instructional notes with the steps, visit the eBook in Connect or download them from www.mhhe.com/iehr4.

 EXERCISE 6.5

Generate a Claim and Submit It to the Insurance Company

Recall that Dr. Ingram saw Mark Robinski (chart number AA009) on April 4, 2022, for a diabetes follow-up. During the visit, Dr. Ingram also ordered a fasting blood sugar and urinalysis. The diagnosis and procedure codes were entered as part of Mr. Robinski's encounter. A claim must be generated for the visit, and these services must now be billed to the insurance company.

Mr. Robinski paid his co-payment for this visit on his way out, with his VISA credit card for $25.00.

(continued)

Follow these steps to complete the exercise on your own once you have watched the demonstration and tried the steps with helpful prompts in practice mode. Use the information provided in the scenario to complete the information.

1. Click on 'Checkout' module.
2. Click on 'Search by patient first name/last name/chart number' field and enter 'rob'.
3. Click on 'Mark Robinski's 04/04/2022' charge capture.
4. Click on 'Add diagnostic codes (ICD Codes) option for procedure' 80048 and select 'E11.9 Diabetes (Type 2, controlled)'. Click 'Close'.
5. Click on 'Add diagnostic codes (ICD Codes) option for procedure' 82947 and select 'E11.9 Diabetes (Type 2, controlled)'. Click 'Close'.
6. Click on 'Add diagnostic codes (ICD Codes) option for procedure' 36415 and select 'E11.9 Diabetes (Type 2, controlled)'. Click 'Close'.
7. Click on 'Add diagnostic codes (ICD Codes) option for procedure' 99203 and select 'E11.9 Diabetes (Type 2, controlled)'. Click 'Close'.
8. Click on 'Ready for payment' button and click 'Proceed'.
9. Click on 'Add payment' button.
10. Click on 'Payment information' field.
11. Enter 'cop' in 'Payment information' field and select 'COPAY'.
12. Click on 'Amount' field and enter '25'.
13. Click on 'Payment method' button and select 'credit card'.
14. Click on 'Check no' field and enter '1439'.
15. Click on 'Apply payment' button.
16. Click on 'procedure code 99203 payment' and enter '25'.
17. Click on 'Save payments' button.
18. Click on 'Cancel' button.
19. Click on 'Claims' module.
20. Click on 'Generate claim' button.
21. Click on 'Chart number range from' field and enter 'AA009'.
22. Click on 'AA009'.
23. Click on 'Generate claim' button.
24. Click on 'Okay' button.
25. Click on 'Mark Robinski's CLA00001' Submit claim button.
26. Click on 'Okay' button.

✓ **You have completed Exercise 6.5**

Remittance advice (RA) A detailed accounting of the claims for which payment is being made by an insurance company. The remittance advice accompanies the payment from the insurance company.

Explanation of benefits (EOB) An explanation of the charges for services, the amount paid by the insurance company, and the amount due by the subscriber, which is sent to the subscriber (and to the provider, in some instances).

Subscriber The primary person covered by an insurance plan.

Insurance companies submit payments to care providers and hospitals electronically (electronic claims transactions or submissions), by check, or by automatic deposit into the bank account of the office/hospital. But the amount of the payment may be for more than one patient's care. The insurance company submits the payment with a detailed accounting of the claims for which payment is being made. The document that accompanies the payment to the provider is called a **remittance advice (RA)** (Figure 6.7). A similar document is called an **explanation of benefits (EOB)** and is sent to the **subscriber**, who is often the patient (unless the patient is a

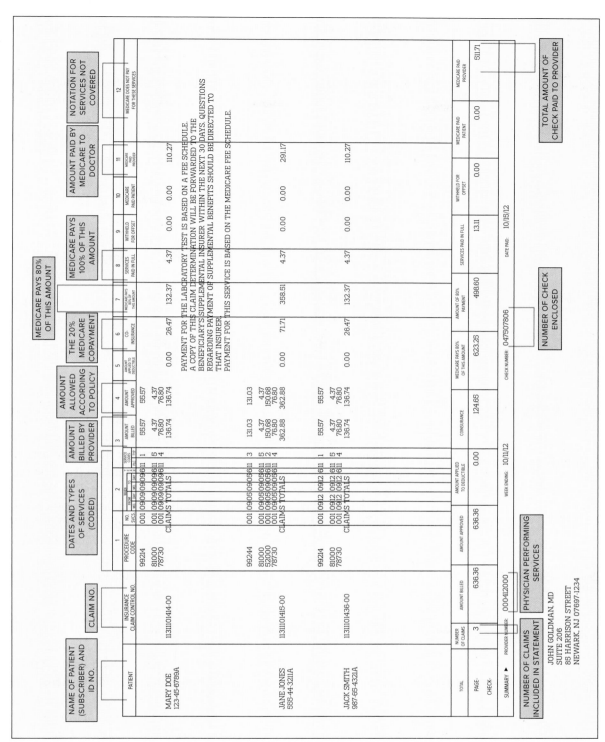

Figure 6.7 Remittance Advice

Source: Booth, K.A., Whicker, L.G., Wyman, Terri D., and Moany Wright, Sandra. (2011). *Medical Assisting* (4th ed.). New York: McGraw-Hill Companies. Reprinted by permission.

spouse or a child of the patient) notifying him or her of what was billed, what was paid, and what the subscriber owes.

The following information is typically included on an RA or EOB. Again, this is not a billing class; there will be more than one patient included, typically, and many insurance companies include more information than is listed here.

- Provider's name and National Provider Identification (NPI) number
- Patient's name

- Claim number
- Medical record number
- Date(s) of service
- Claim status (open, denied, more information needed, paid, etc.)
- Electronic Transaction Number (if RA and payment have been sent via electronic means)
- Service detail
    - Each CPT® code billed (as submitted on the claim form)
    - Amount charged for each code
    - Allowed amount (amount the insurance carrier has agreed to pay) for each code
    - Co-pay paid by the patient
    - Adjusted amount (difference between what was charged and the allowed amount)
- Recap of charges and payments
    - Total reported charges amount
    - Charges not covered amount
    - Charges denied amount
    - Covered charge amount
    - Glossary of explanation codes

It is important to have a good understanding of the entire process involved in submitting an insurance claim and receiving payments. The process begins after the patient has completed services or procedures. A healthcare professional completes the insurance claim, based on the information listed on the Superbill (also known as a routing slip or encounter form), as well as the provider's documentation, paying special attention to ensuring that the procedure codes are appropriately linked to the diagnostic codes (code linkage) to demonstrate medical necessity. Once the claim is completed and double-checked for accuracy, it is submitted to the insurance carrier.

Adjudication The process of reviewing claims by the insurance carrier to determine payment.

After the insurance carrier receives the claim, it undergoes **adjudication**. Adjudication is the process in which claims are reviewed to determine if the services are covered under the patient's plan and therefore should be paid, denied, or partially paid based on the completeness, accuracy, and code linkage of the claim. Once a determination of payment has been made, the insurance carrier will send a payment to the provider, along with a remittance advice (RA) that identifies the payment decisions and any items that may need to be resubmitted or corrected. When the practice has received the RA with the payment, the practice must post the payments to specific charges (CPT® codes) in the patient's account. Any unpaid charges or remaining balances, such as coinsurance charges, will then be sent to the patient in a statement. In some cases, the patient may have a secondary insurance that will be billed for excess charges before the patient statement is generated.

Ensuring that claims are correct before sending them to insurance carriers provides the best payment results and saves the practice the time and expense required to correct and resubmit them. Understanding the claims process is essential to maintaining a healthy revenue and positive cash flow for the practice.

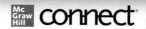
Investigate an Unpaid Insurance Claim

On May 18, 2022, Mark Robinski calls the billing office because he has received an EOB from his insurance company that his office visit of April 4, 2022, was not covered and therefore the charges are his responsibility to pay. He contacted his insurance company and was told that the diagnosis submitted was for history of fatigue (R53.83) and is not covered. He recalls that his office visit on April 4 was for a follow-up of his diabetes mellitus. He asks the biller to check the account. The biller finds that, indeed, the documentation on his record shows that his chief complaint was for follow-up of diabetes, which should be a first-listed diagnosis on the claim for April 4. This exercise will take you through looking up the diagnosis codes that were filed on the insurance claim for the April 4 visit and correcting the first-listed diagnosis to read E11.9, diabetes mellitus, type 2.

Follow these steps to complete the exercise on your own once you have watched the demonstration and tried the steps with helpful prompts in practice mode. Use the information provided in the scenario to complete the information.

1. Click on 'Checkout' module.
2. Click on 'Search by patient first name/last name/chart number' field and enter 'rob'.
3. Click on 'Mark Robinski's 04/04/2022' charge capture.
4. Click on 'R53.83's delete icon' for procedure '99203'.
5. Click on 'Add diagnostic codes (ICD Codes) option for procedure' 99203 and select 'E11.9 Diabetes (Type 2, controlled)'.
6. Click on 'Close' button.
7. Click on 'Save changes' button.

A corrected claim may now be sent to the insurance company.

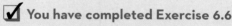 **You have completed Exercise 6.6**

6.8 Managing Accounts Receivable in EHRclinic

The management of patient accounts, from charging patients for services to tracking accounts receivable and collections, begins by setting up the parameters of each insurance carrier and each plan within the insurance. The plan is the extent of coverage offered. For instance, 400 patients in your office have Blue Cross/Blue Shield insurance, but for those 400 patients, there are more than 20 plans. Plans differ regarding

- Co-pay and coinsurance requirements. Some plans require a co-pay or coinsurance, others do not, and the dollar amounts vary by plan. Let's look at an example. Neil Holt is an engineer for Johnsontown Analytics, and his insurance is McGraw-Hill Prime. He is responsible for a $20 co-pay, and he is responsible for 20% of all outpatient service charges. Lisa Haver also works for Johnsontown Analytics; she, too, has McGraw-Hill insurance, but she works at a different location in a different state, and her plan requires a $25 co-pay, plus 20% of all outpatient services.

- Extent of coverage and whether or not services are covered at all. For example, Neil Holt's plan covers outpatient mental health services, whereas Lisa Haver's does not.
- Rules regarding filing of claims. These rules may differ from plan to plan, and they certainly differ from insurance company to insurance company.

Because of these differences, it is imperative that a medical office or hospital use a system that efficiently applies the various policies to the correct patients.

When a medical office purchases any type of software, such as PM software, an administrative staff member (often the office manager, office administrator, or business manager) works with an installation specialist from the software company to build libraries and databases that are used to perform functions within the various applications (accounts receivable, patient chart, etc.). Common libraries include

- Insurance company library—includes all the insurance companies and the individual plans that are represented by the patients in the practice. These can be created, edited, or deleted within EHRclinic.
- ICD-10-CM, CPT®, and HCPCS Level 2 code tables—must be maintained every year to account for additions, deletions, and amendments to codes. In order to get paid in a timely manner, a practice must submit only active, valid codes; otherwise, the claim will be rejected.
- Fee schedule—listed by CPT® code and done for Medicare, for group insurance, and by individual contracts for managed care plans. The charge for each service is documented in a fee schedule.
- Reports—in particular, aging reports (length of time a claim has remained unpaid) are set up to allow for timely tracking and follow-up of claims.
- Alerts—reminders to the office staff related to the billing functions. Some examples are co-pay alerts, write-offs, and overdue balances. Alerts assist the staff in collections processes in particular.

Using PM software to accomplish the filing, follow-up, and collection of claims also allows for the electronic remittance of claims, as well as electronic receipt of payment from insurance carriers. The healthcare professional can see at a glance exactly what is happening with a claim or claims at any time in the process. Collections procedures are also streamlined using PM software. Many offices use an outside collections agency to collect overdue balances. With the use of PM software, a report of accounts ready for collections is sent electronically, the office is able to see the status of the account, and paid claims are sent to the office, often electronically. The longer an account "ages," the longer it takes for a practice or any other healthcare facility to be paid, whether the payment is coming from a patient or an insurance carrier.

Greater billing accuracy is an advantage of using PM software, and there is less chance of lost charges and therefore lost revenue. Each time a patient is seen, and the care provider documents the progress note in EHRclinic and orders tests that are done on-site, he or she is prompted to select the ICD-10 code and the CPT® codes that correspond to the diagnosis and procedures (code linkage).

The face-to-face time between a patient and the care provider is charged with a CPT® code known as an **Evaluation and Management (E&M)** code. E&M codes are only used in the physician practice setting. It is generated based on documentation made by the care provider. The E&M code is dependent on whether the patient is new to the practice (not seen by any provider in the practice within the past three years) or an established patient (seen by any provider in the practice within the last three years); the level of history (including chief complaint and review of systems); the level of physical exam performed; the depth of medical decision making necessary; and other contributory factors.

Two examples of E&M codes are

99213 An office visit for an established patient, 20 years old, who was seen for exercise-induced asthma

99203 Initial office visit for a 30-year-old patient who has recently been complaining of rectal bleeding

In your CPT® coding class, you will learn the intricacies of assigning E&M codes, but at this point it is important to know that E&M codes are CPT® codes that reflect the professional services rendered to a patient.

Evaluation and Management (E&M)
The CPT® codes used to capture the face-to-face time between a patient and the care provider; takes into consideration the extent of the history, the extent of the physical exam, and the level of medical decision making required.

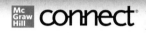

Go to https://connect.mheducation.com to complete this exercise. To see instructional notes with the steps, visit the eBook in Connect or download them from www.mhhe.com/iehr4.

PM **EXERCISE 6.7**

Use Documentation to Alter E&M Coding Level

The level of E&M code, and therefore the amount charged for the face-to-face time of a visit, is tied to the extent of history, review of systems, and physical exam documented as structured data in EHRclinic. Mark Robinski's current E&M code is 99203, which indicates that he is being charged as a new patient with a 30-minute visit. The documentation in his encounter, however, indicates that he is an established patient being seen for a follow-up visit of approximately 25 minutes. In this exercise, the level of E&M code will need to be updated to 99214 based on the documentation in Mark Robinski's medical record.

Follow these steps to complete the exercise on your own once you have watched the demonstration and tried the steps with helpful prompts in practice mode. Use the information provided in the scenario to complete the information.

1. Click on 'Checkout' module.
2. Click on 'Search by patient first name/last name/chart number' field and enter 'rob'.
3. Click on 'Mark Robinski's 04/04/2022' charge capture.
4. Click on 'Close' icon (X) for procedure 99203.
5. Click on 'Search procedure code' input field and enter '99214'.
6. Click on '99214 EP Intermed L4 Detailed' procedure code.
7. Click on 'Add diagnostic codes (ICD Codes)' option for procedure 99214 and select E11.9 Diabetes (Type 2, controlled).
8. Click on 'Close' button.
9. Click on 'Save changes' button.

☑ **You have completed Exercise 6.7**

Once the claim has been filed and payment has been sent to the office (either by mail, by direct deposit into the practice's account, or electronically), the payment for each procedure is posted to the patient's record for that date of service.

We will now follow the steps to post a payment using EHRclinic.

Go to https://connect.mheducation.com to complete this exercise. To see instructional notes with the steps, visit the eBook in Connect or download them from www.mhhe.com/iehr4.

 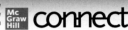

EXERCISE 6.8 PM

Post an Insurance Payment to an Account

In our scenario, Dr. Ingram's office has received an RA, which includes payment to cover the claim for Mark Robinski for date of service April 4, 2022. There are four charges for this account. They are CPT® code 99214, which is an Evaluation and Management code for the face-to-face time he spent with the doctor; code 36415 for a venipuncture (blood draw) procedure; code 82947 for a fasting blood sugar test; and code 81000 for urinalysis testing.

The total amount of the remittance for Mark Robinski is $189, with the following amounts allocated to each procedure:

- $91.00 was paid for E&M procedure 99214 (EP Intermed L4 Detailed).
- $15.00 was paid for lab procedure 36415 (venipuncture).
- $15.00 was paid for lab procedure 81000 (urinalysis).
- $68.00 was paid for lab procedure 82947 (fasting blood glucose).

We will be working in the Accounts module under the insurance transactions function. The objective is to mark each service as paid, based on the amount of money received.

Follow these steps to complete the exercise on your own once you have watched the demonstration and tried the steps with helpful prompts in practice mode. Use the information provided in the scenario to complete the information.

1. Click on 'Search by patient first name/last name/chart number' field and enter 'rob'.
2. Click on 'Mark Robinski's 04/04/2022' charge capture.
3. Click on 'Ready for payment' button.
4. Click on 'Proceed' button.
5. Click on 'Add adjustment' button.
6. Click on 'Reason code' field.
7. Enter 'adj' in 'Reason code' field and select 'ADJCHK'.
8. Click on 'Amount' field and enter '189'.
9. Click on 'Apply adjustment' button.
10. Click on 'Procedure code 36415 adjustment' and enter '15'.
11. Click on 'Procedure code 82947 adjustment' and enter '68'.
12. Click on 'Procedure code 81000 adjustment' and enter '15'.
13. Click on 'Procedure code 99214 adjustment' and enter '91'.
14. Click on 'Save adjustment' button.
15. Click on 'Checkout' button.
16. Click on 'Proceed' button.
17. Click on 'Okay' button.

✓ **You have completed Exercise 6.8**

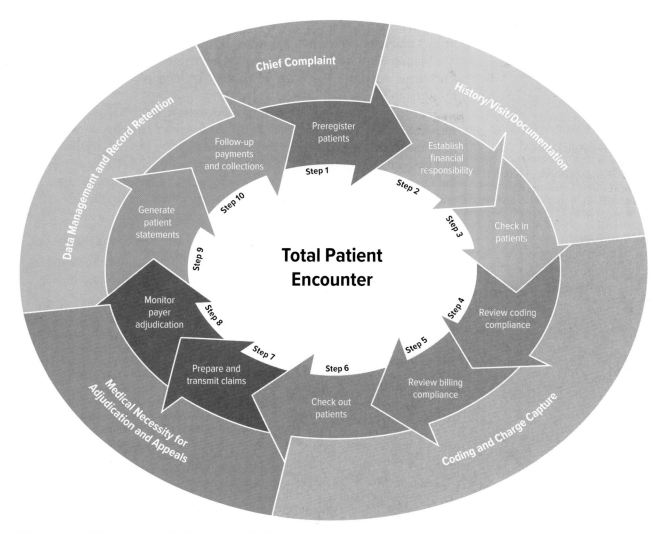

Figure 6.8   The Revenue Cycle with Medical Documentation

Source: McGraw Hill Education

The typical revenue cycle within an ambulatory healthcare setting is shown in Figure 6.8. Some steps may be repeated two or three times, but the goal is payment of the claim.

6.9 | Compliance

Medicare, Medicaid, TRICARE, Workers' Compensation, group health insurance, and managed care plans are all examples of types of insurance coverage. Each has rules and regulations related to the coding, billing, and collection of healthcare claims. Intentionally not following those rules and regulations can result in allegations of fraud or, at the very least, **abuse**. Abusive coding and billing practices are inconsistent with typical coding and billing practice. Being found guilty of either can result in monetary fines or, in the worst-case scenario, a sanction from any one or more insurance plans. If a care provider is sanctioned by Medicare, the provider is forbidden to accept Medicare patients into his or her practice. In an internal medicine practice, Medicare enrollees most likely make up a good percentage of

Abuse Coding and billing that is inconsistent with typical coding and billing practices.

the patient population. Needless to say, being sanctioned by Medicare will impact a practice to the point that it may put the provider out of business.

Managed care plans that find a care provider or practice engaging in fraudulent activity may drop that office from their preferred provider list, resulting in a negative impact on the practice's income.

For federal programs, the Office of Inspector General (OIG) investigates suspected cases of fraud. In order to defend the practice in the event of a visit from the OIG, a **compliance plan** should be in place in every medical office and hospital. Not only should it be in place, but it should also be followed. If the OIG does audit your practice, showing that you have a compliance plan and demonstrating that it is followed will be an advantage; having one and *not* following it may not be. The requirements of a compliance plan are

- Conducting audits and monitoring work performed by the office staff
- Developing and implementing standards of practice to be followed by office staff (including care providers) that are uniformly and consistently applied
- Appointing a compliance officer
- Training new staff immediately after hire on office policies and procedures and offering periodic in-services to all staff (including care providers)
- Fixing any problems that are found, investigating the reason for problems, and retraining staff as necessary
- Encouraging staff to bring any compliance issues to the office administration
- Enforcing the office's policies and procedures and not making exceptions

Having, following, and referencing a practice's written policies, procedures, and compliance plan will assure sound fiscal practices within a practice or facility and may be a sound defense, should the practice ever be involved in fraud or abuse allegations.

Compliance plan A formal, written document that describes how the hospital or physician's practice ensures rules, regulations, and standards are being adhered to.

APPLYING YOUR SKILLS

Accountable Care Organizations are part of the largest healthcare reimbursement reform in years. You have been given basic information about ACOs. Now, research on your own to find the following answers.
1. The Centers for Medicare & Medicaid Services (CMS) is responsible for ACOs. Describe one of the types of ACOs available to providers.
2. Why is it so important to accurately code diagnoses and procedures as this relates to ACOs?
3. Do an Internet search of Accountable Care Organizations and describe an ACO that you find.

chapter 6 summary

LEARNING OUTCOME	CONCEPTS FOR REVIEW
6.1 Illustrate the need for a claims management process.	- Though the primary purpose of a medical office is to provide patient care, it is still considered a business - Written policies are necessary to run the office effectively and efficiently - Use of **PM** software improves efficiency - A patient account for an encounter begins when the appointment is made - Insurance verification should be completed—either before the day of the visit or when the patient arrives (beforehand is preferred) - Patient check-out occurs once the visit is complete

6.2 List the information contained in an encounter form (Superbill).	- A Superbill is otherwise known as an encounter form or a routing slip and includes at least
	  • Name and address of medical practice
	  • NPI number
	  • Patient's name
	  • Patient's chart number
	  • Date and time of visit
	  • CPT® codes
	  • Diagnosis narrative by care provider
	  • ICD-10-CM diagnosis codes
	- It can be hard copy or electronic
	- The information on the Superbill transfers to the CMS-1500 claim form
	- It includes some identifying information about the encounter as well as the diagnosis and procedure codes using ICD-10 and CPT® code sets
	- Code linkage is the relationship between the diagnosis and procedure codes to demonstrate medical necessity

6.3 Apply procedures to update a patient's account in EHRclinic.	- Patients share costs with insurance carriers by paying co-payments and coinsurance - Co-payments are fixed amounts that are paid for at each encounter - Coinsurance payments are based on a percentage of the patient's healthcare costs - Co-payment may be collected at the time of check-in or check-out, depending on office policy - Financial alerts appear when the patient is checked into EHRclinic at the time of arrival; the insurance plan entered in the system determines which, if any, alerts appear - Once paid, the co-pay is immediately posted in EHRclinic - Charges start to accrue once the patient is taken to the examining room and is seen by a healthcare professional - Insurance status may be looked up at any time

(continued)

LEARNING OUTCOME	CONCEPTS FOR REVIEW
6.4 Demonstrate coding using ICD-10-CM/PCS and CPT® codes in EHRclinic.	– The provider's assessment is otherwise known as the diagnosis (or diagnoses, plural) – Services rendered may be diagnostic (x-rays, lab tests) or therapeutic (sutures, cleansing of a wound, injections) – Diagnoses are coded using the ICD-10-CM code set; a diagnosis or diagnoses must be recorded at the end of every visit and coded using ICD-10-CM in both hospital and outpatient (physicians' offices) settings – The first-listed diagnosis is the one most closely related to the reason the patient was seen – Any conditions that were diagnosed, were treated, or required more nursing or provider attention should be documented – Procedures are coded using CPT® in the physician's office – Procedures are coded using ICD-10-PCS in the hospital setting – Code linkage shows the relationship between the procedure code and the diagnostic code to demonstrate medical necessity – HCPCS Level 2 codes are used to code equipment and supplies – Coding is done for statistical and reimbursement purposes
6.5 Examine the correlation between documentation and code assignment.	– All services and procedures performed must be medically necessary – The diagnoses support the medical necessity for the procedure(s) and service(s) through code linkage – Performing services that aren't medically necessary and billing for them are considered fraud
6.6 Describe Accountable Care Organizations.	– New reimbursement model for Medicare patients – Came about through the Affordable Care Act (ACA) – Goals are high-quality care, patient satisfaction, decreased redundancy of services, and coordination of care – Voluntary partnership among physicians, hospitals, and other healthcare providers – Models: Medicare Shared Savings Program; ACO Investment Model; Advance Payment ACO Model; Comprehensive ESRD Care Initiative; Next Generation ACO Model; Pioneer ACO Model – Dependent on measurable outcomes through reporting based on ICD-10, CPT®, and HCPCS codes as well as the ability to share patient information between and among members of the ACO

LEARNING OUTCOME	CONCEPTS FOR REVIEW
6.7 Describe the information contained in a remittance advice and an explanation of benefits.	– Accounts receivable—money paid to the office by insurance carriers – Transactions—documentation of all money paid and applying it to the correct patient's balances – Remittance Advice (RA), also referred to as an explanation of benefits (EOB) when this document is sent to patients, accompanies the payment and explains the claims to which the payments apply – The subscriber is the person who is covered under the group insurance plan
6.8 Apply procedures to manage accounts receivable in EHRclinic.	– Efficiency and effectiveness of managing the financial aspects start with accurately setting up the parameters of each insurance carrier and the plans within each in the PM software – The type of plan a patient has determines the extent of coverage and the co-pay requirements – Each insurance carrier (and the plans within) has rules and regulations regarding filing of claims – Libraries are built within the PM software for each insurance carrier – The Revenue Cycle with Medical Documentation demonstrates the process for sending claims and receiving payments

6.9 Demonstrate the need for a compliance plan.	– All offices should have written policies and procedures for all processes in the office but, in particular, for the financial aspects
	
	– All policies should be complied with uniformly and consistently
	
	– Each insurance carrier has rules and regulations that must be followed
	
	– Not following the rules and regulations may constitute fraud or abuse
	
	– The Office of Inspector General enforces the rules and regulations set forth by any federal insurance plans
	
	– The office should have a compliance plan to ensure that all rules and regulations are being followed; the plan should include
	
	  • Conducting internal audits of work performed
	
	  • Developing standards of practice
	
	  • Appointing a compliance officer
	
	  • Training new personnel, updates for experienced personnel
	
	  • Correcting any known problems, retraining staff as necessary
	
	  • Encouraging open communication from staff regarding compliance issues
	
	  • Enforcing all policies and procedures

chapter review

MATCHING QUESTIONS

Match the terms on the left with the definitions on the right.

_____ 1. **[LO 6.5]** fraud

_____ 2. **[LO 6.7]** transaction

_____ 3. **[LO 6.1]** managed care plan

_____ 4. **[LO 6.7]** accounts receivable

_____ 5. **[LO 6.8]** Evaluation and Management

_____ 6. **[LO 6.1]** fee schedule

_____ 7. **[LO 6.7]** subscriber

_____ 8. **[LO 6.9]** compliance plan

_____ 9. **[LO 6.3]** co-payment

_____ 10. **[LO 6.7]** explanation of benefits (EOB)

_____ 11. **[LO 6.3]** coinsurance

_____ 12. **[LO 6.2]** code linkage

a. list of how much is charged per service by CPT® code

b. document sent from an insurance company to a subscriber outlining payment decisions

c. portion of a bill that is usually the responsibility of the patient, typically collected upon check-in

d. primary individual covered under an insurance plan

e. formal, written guidelines that describe how a healthcare office intends to follow established rules and regulations

f. actions, such as posting payments or processing claims, done in a practice management system to update patient accounts

g. codes representing the face-to-face time spent with a provider

h. monies coming into a medical practice

i. act of deception that takes advantage of another person or entity

j. form of insurance that monitors patients, care, and performance to ensure quality

k. using the diagnostic and procedure codes together to show medical necessity

l. form of cost-sharing with an insurance carrier in which the patient pays a percentage of medical expenses

MULTIPLE-CHOICE QUESTIONS

Select the letter that best completes the statement or answers the question:

1. **[LO 6.2]** The information contained in an encounter form is eventually transferred to the _____ for submission.
   a. claim form
   b. encounter form (Superbill)
   c. insurance form
   d. registration form

2. **[LO 6.5]** Only services deemed medically _____ can be billed to insurance.
   a. necessary
   b. progressive
   c. restorative
   d. useful

3. **[LO 6.4]** What does the "CM" stand for in ICD coding?
   a. care management
   b. clinical modification
   c. code management
   d. coding methodology

4. **[LO 6.8]** The amount of a patient's co-pay may vary by
   a. care provider.
   b. insurance plan.
   c. office location.
   d. visit type.

5. **[LO 6.3]** Charges begin to accrue once the
   a. appointment is made.
   b. patient checks in at the reception area.
   c. medical assistant or care provider interacts with the patient.
   d. claim has been filed.

6. **[LO 6.7]** A remittance advice is typically given to a/an _____, whereas an explanation of benefits is typically given to a/an _____.
   a. patient; provider
   b. provider; patient
   c. insurance company; patient
   d. provider; insurance company

7. **[LO 6.2]** When submitting claims to insurance carriers, providers show medical necessity by
   a. including a glossary of terms in the claim.
   b. using code linkage.
   c. writing a claim summary.
   d. sending copies of patient charts with the claim.

8. **[LO 6.9]** To avoid negative consequences, a compliance plan should be _____ in every hospital and medical office.
   a. ignored
   b. followed
   c. used as a suggestion
   d. discarded

9. **[LO 6.8]** The _____ is usually the person to set up information libraries within practice management software programs.
   a. care provider
   b. healthcare professional
   c. medical assistant
   d. office manager

Enhance your learning by completing these exercises and more at https://connect.mheducation.com!

10. **[LO 6.5]** Who is the only person authorized to make a diagnosis?
    a. care provider
    b. healthcare professional
    c. medical assistant
    d. office manager

11. **[LO 6.3]** To check if a claim has been paid, which menu will the healthcare professional look at?
    a. Accounts Payable
    b. Accounts Receivable
    c. Claims Module
    d. Claim Updates

12. **[LO 6.6]** Which of the following is true of the Pioneer ACO model?
    a. It is based on fee for service.
    b. It applies to Medicaid only.
    c. Providers share in a greater percentage of savings, but they also share in a greater percentage of financial losses.
    d. It requires participation by hospitals and medical vendors.

13. **[LO 6.1]** Depending on the terms of a patient's insurance coverage, the balance remaining after insurance has paid may be
    a. written off as paid in full.
    b. removed from the Master Patient Index.
    c. sent to collections.
    d. written off as paid in full or sent to collections.

14. **[LO 6.1]** Expected methods of payment are discussed when a patient
    a. checks in.
    b. is seen by the provider.
    c. is discharged.
    d. makes an appointment.

SHORT-ANSWER QUESTIONS

1. **[LO 6.1]** List four ways practice management software improves claim management.
2. **[LO 6.7]** Contrast accounts receivable with accounts payable.
3. **[LO 6.8]** What is the difference between an insurance provider (carrier) and an insurance plan?
4. **[LO 6.2]** List at least five items that are typically included on a hard-copy Superbill.
5. **[LO 6.3]** What is an alert?
6. **[LO 6.5]** How have EHRs improved the face-to-face time between patients and care providers?
7. **[LO 6.2]** Explain how the symbols available in practice management software make claim management easier and more accurate.

8. **[LO 6.6]** Summarize the goal of Accountable Care Organizations in three or four sentences.

9. **[LO 6.5]** Explain fraud in terms of the healthcare profession.

10. **[LO 6.3]** List three reasons that you might need to check the status of an insurance claim.

11. **[LO 6.8]** What is an aging report?

12. **[LO 6.7]** What four items are included in the recap of charges and payments found on an EOB?

13. **[LO 6.4]** List the three types of codes used in a clinical setting and give an example of how each is used.

14. **[LO 6.4]** Discuss at least three benefits of moving to ICD-10.

15. **[LO 6.9]** What is the difference between fraud and abuse?

APPLYING YOUR KNOWLEDGE

1. **[LO 6.3]** Discuss why many healthcare practices refuse to see patients who do not pay their co-pays at the time of their visit.

2. **[LOs 6.5, 6.9]** Research two recent cases of medical/insurance fraud (an Internet search of medical insurance fraud will take you in the right direction) and discuss the outcome of each case. Provide specifics about your sources (Internet, medical journals, textbooks, etc.).

3. **[LOs 6.1, 6.8]** Why might an office need to use a collections agency to pursue overdue accounts?

4. **[LO 6.7]** Why is there so much information contained on an RA or EOB form?

5. **[LOs 6.4, 6.5, 6.9]** Anna Devlan is a healthcare professional who is responsible for claim completion and submission at Summit Bay Health Center. Recently, she was coding a patient's chart for a recent encounter and could not find a code that exactly matched the diagnosis made by the care provider, so she found the closest match and coded that. Did Anna commit fraud and/or abuse? Explain your answer.

6. **[LO 6.6]** Paul Donovan, a Medicare patient, suffers from Crohn's disease and rheumatoid arthritis. Recently, he presented to County Hospital complaining of hip pain. How will the interoperability offered under Accountable Care Organization models impact Mr. Donovan's care?

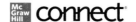

Enhance your learning by completing these exercises and more at **https://connect.mheducation.com!**

chapter references

Booth, K.A., Whicker, L.G., Wyman, Terri D., and Moany Wright, Sandra. (2011). *Administrative Procedures for Medical Assisting* (4th ed.). New York: McGraw-Hill Companies.

Centers for Medicare & Medicaid Services (CMS). *Accountable Care Organizations.* Retrieved from http://www.cms.gov/Medicare/Medicare-Fee-for-Service-Payment/ACO/index.html?redirect=/aco/.

Centers for Medicare & Medicaid Services (CMS). *Accountable Care Organizations (ACOs): General Information.* Retrieved from http://innovation.cms.gov/initiatives/aco/.

Centers for Medicare & Medicaid Services (CMS). *Medicare Shared Savings Program.* Retrieved from https://www.cms.gov/Medicare/Medicare-Fee-for-Service-Payment/sharedsavingsprogram/about.html.

Current Procedural Terminology. (2019). Chicago: American Medical Association.

Examples of CPT® codes based on CPT® 2019.

Examples of HCPCS codes based on HCPCS 2019.

Examples of ICD-9-CM codes based on ICD-9-CM 2013.

ICD-10-CM/PCS codes based on ICD-10: Version 2016.

ICD-10-CM Codebook. (2019). Salt Lake City, UT: Contexo Media.

ICD-9-CM, Volumes I, II, & III. (2013). Ingenix. Salt Lake City, UT.

Newby, C. (2010). *From Patient to Payment: Insurance Procedures for the Medical Office* (6th ed.). New York: McGraw-Hill Companies.

White, S., et al. (2011, June). An ACO Primer. *Journal of AHIMA*, *82*(6): 48–50.

World Health Organization. (2013). *International Classification of Diseases.* Retrieved from http://www.who.int/classifications/icd/en/.

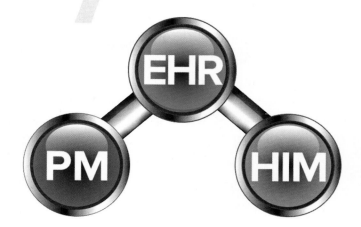

chapter **seven**

Privacy, Security, Confidentiality, and Legal Issues

Learning Outcomes

At the end of this chapter, the student should be able to

7.1 Identify HIPAA privacy and security standards.

7.2 Evaluate an EHR system for HIPAA compliance.

7.3 Describe the role of certification in EHR implementation.

7.4 Apply procedures to set up security measures in EHRclinic.

7.5 Follow proper procedures to access sensitive or restricted-access records.

7.6 Apply procedures to ensure data integrity.

7.7 Apply procedures to release health information using EHRclinic.

7.8 Account for data disclosures using EHRclinic.

7.9 Exchange information with outside healthcare providers for continuity of care using EHRclinic.

7.10 Outline the content of compliance plans.

7.11 Appraise the importance of disaster recovery planning.

Key Terms

Access report
Accounting of disclosures
American Health Information Management Association (AHIMA)
Audit trail
Blog
Breach of confidentiality
Computer virus
Confidentiality
Covered entity
Data integrity
Directory information

Disaster recovery plan
Firewall
Hardware
Healthcare Information and Management Systems Society (HIMSS)
Malware
Minimum necessary information
Notice of Privacy Practices
Password
Privacy
Social media
User rights

What You Need to Know and Why You Need to Know It

No matter what type of healthcare professional you become—a nurse, medical assistant (clinical or administrative), health information technician or manager, coder, biller, registration clerk, receptionist, or care provider—you will come in contact with patients' health information. In healthcare, and particularly with electronic healthcare, privacy and security are on everyone's mind—the patients', the providers', the media's, and the government's. There is concern that computer hackers and personnel who work in healthcare facilities will gain access to records that they have no legitimate need to access. The concern is justified, but even in a paper system, frequent privacy breaches have occurred. It is just as easy for a healthcare professional to look in a patient's chart at the nurses' station as it is to sit down at a computer that is left open to a patient's record and read it. The difference is that it is far easier to change information within the record or records without the change(s) being detected until it may be too late, and it is far easier to share that patient's or thousands of patients' health information without authorization and for unethical and unlawful reasons when an electronic health record system is hacked. In this chapter, we will discuss laws that protect privacy and security as well as methods to lessen the chances of privacy breaches occurring. It is the responsibility of all healthcare professionals and care providers to maintain patient privacy and confidentiality and to access health information only on a need-to-know basis.

7.1 The HIPAA Privacy and Security Standards

HIPAA was passed in 1996 and contains several rules, though, for our purposes in this chapter, we will be concentrating on the Privacy and Security Rules. In addition, in 2009, the Health Information Technology for Economic and Clinical Health Act (HITECH) went a step further, making the original Privacy and Security Rules under HIPAA more stringent. HITECH also gives more power to federal and state government authorities to enforce the Privacy and Security Rules.

On March 26, 2013, the Omnibus Final Rule to the HITECH Act went into effect, with compliance required in September 2013. Changes included more enhancements to protect patient privacy, additions to individual patient rights, and strengthening of the government's ability to enforce the law. HIPAA was expanded to give more control over any covered entity's business associates—for example, external coding consultants and software service providers. The Notice of Privacy Practices has been expanded, and the maximum civil penalty for knowingly violating HIPAA is $50,000 per violation up to a maximum of $1.5 million per violation category per year (HIPAA Journal). Related to HITECH, the breach notification standards have been enhanced. Examples of the enhancement in patient rights include the requirement that providers who utilize electronic health records must provide patients with their records in electronic form when requested. In addition, patients who are paying for their services in cash may instruct the provider not to bill their insurance and not to divulge any information about the services to the patient's health insurance carrier.

The intent of both is to ensure that protected health information (PHI) is kept private and secure. They give patients the right to determine who sees their health information but still give **covered entities** (healthcare providers,

for your information fyi

More information about HIPAA can be found at http://www.hhs.gov/ and then searching for "HIPAA for Professionals," and HITECH information can be found at https://www.healthit.gov/ and searching for "HITECH."

Covered entity Any healthcare entity that captures or utilizes health information. These include healthcare plans (insurance companies), clearinghouses that process healthcare claims, individual physicians and physician practices, any type of therapist (mental health, physical, speech, occupational), dentists, hospital staffs, ambulatory facilities, nursing homes, home health agencies, pharmacies, and employers.

clearinghouses, or health insurance plans) the leeway to access the PHI needed to care for patients, collect payment for services rendered, and operate a business. Protected health information is any piece of information that identifies a patient—it includes a patient's name, date of birth (DOB), address, email address, and telephone number; the patient's employer; any relatives' names; the patient's Social Security number and medical record number; account numbers tied to the patient's account; the patient's fingerprints; any photographs of the patient; and any characteristics about the patient that would automatically disclose his or her identity (for instance, "the governor of the largest state in the United States").

In addition, PHI includes the medical information that is tied to the person, including diagnoses, test results, treatments, and prognosis; documentation by the care provider and other healthcare professionals; and billing information.

HIPAA states (and HITECH enhances) that only persons who have a need to know may have access to a patient's PHI. And to take it a step further, they are entitled only access to the **minimum necessary information** required to do their jobs. An example is a covered entity, such as a health insurance company that is working on a claim for a patient who underwent coronary artery bypass three months ago. Unless the insurance company can prove otherwise, the minimum necessary information it needs is the supporting documentation related to the bypass surgery. The fact that the patient delivered a child in 1980 has nothing to do with the bypass surgery, and therefore the company does not need access to those records.

There are many ways that facilities protect the **privacy** and **confidentiality** of their patients. Privacy is the right to be left alone. In other words, no one should infringe upon a patient's time or personal space while the patient is being treated; that is why admissions departments and registration areas have partitions or cubicles so that the patient has some privacy. Confidentiality is keeping a secret; in healthcare, it means keeping information about a patient to oneself. Patients have the right to expect that their medical information is going to be kept confidential. Written policies and ongoing education of staff are two very important aspects of complying with the HIPAA and HITECH rules.

Every healthcare facility and office must have written privacy and confidentiality policies that address, at a minimum,

- Release (disclosure) of information to outside sources. PHI is released to outside entities only upon written authorization of the patient/legal representative (or as required by law), and release to inside sources (access) is only on a need-to-know basis. The policy should also address exceptions. Let's first look at internal access as an example. Cathy Hess was a patient on unit 3E of Memorial Hospital from May 3 to May 5. Suzanne Hess is a nurse who works at Memorial Hospital and is Cathy Hess' sister-in-law. She does not work on 3E and did not take care of Suzanne. She did not have, does not have, and will not have a need to access Cathy's health record. But let's say two months after Suzanne's hospitalization, Cathy is on a committee that is auditing records for a study and Suzanne's record happens to be one of the records in the sample. Cathy could ask one of the other reviewers to audit that particular record, but if Cathy does review Suzanne's record, she is accessing the record within the scope of her job, and she does

Minimum necessary information As required by the Health Insurance Portability and Accountability Act (HIPAA), releasing the minimum information to satisfy the reason the information is needed or the minimum necessary to perform a job function.

Privacy The right to be left alone; the right to expect that one's personal space is respected while undergoing healthcare.

Confidentiality The patient's right to expect that his or her health information will not be released to any person or entity without the patient/guardian's written authorization or as required by law or regulation.

have a need to know in that case. Internal access does not require authorization from the patient if there is a need to know.

- Outside access without the need for authorization of the patient/personal representative. This includes access by an insurance company (for payment of the bill), by public health officials in cases of mandatory reporting (infectious diseases, for example), and by licensing and accrediting agencies.

- Release of **directory information**. Directory information includes the fact that the patient is in the hospital (or is being treated at an ambulatory facility) and his or her room number. However, if a patient does not want certain individuals (or anyone) to know that he or she is in the hospital or the location within the hospital, then the patient/legal representative would sign a document stipulating who can and cannot have access to that information.

- Written guidelines and examples of what is considered minimum necessary information by reason for the request

- Faxing of documentation—information that can and cannot be faxed and the protocol to be followed, should information be faxed to the wrong location

- Computer access and lockdown. Policy requires staff to lock their computers down (sign out) if they are going to be away from their desks for any length of time.

- Password sharing—makes it a disciplinary offense to share one's password with another

- Computer screens—should be kept out of view of the public or anyone else who might have access to areas with computers

- Shredding any hard-copy documents (where applicable) rather than just discarding them in a wastepaper basket

- Signing by patients of a **Notice of Privacy Practices,** so that patients are aware of how their personal health information will be used. The Notice of Privacy Practices must be in writing and be signed by the patient/legal representative. It informs the patient how his or her health information will be used and the reasons it may be released, notifies the patient that he or she may view or have copies of the health record and may request amendments to it, and states the procedure for filing a complaint with the Department of Health and Human Services.

- Requirement that all staff (including care providers) sign a document committing themselves to keep private and confidential the information that is written, spoken, or overheard about any and all patients

Once a paper record is converted to an electronic one, the paper copy is no longer needed. It is best practice to destroy the paper copy if the electronic version is considered the legal document and the one upon which healthcare decisions are made. The paper record should be destroyed either by incineration or by shredding. An example of a shredding policy statement in an office that no longer keeps hard-copy records (a "paperless environment") is

The electronic health record is the legal health record at Summit Bay Health Center. Printed copies should only be made when there is a need to refer to the printed document rather than the computerized image.

Directory information The fact that a patient is an inpatient (or being treated as an outpatient) as well as his or her location within the facility.

Notice of Privacy Practices A requirement of the Health Insurance Portability and Accountability Act (HIPAA) that patients are made aware (in writing) of their rights under HIPAA, including the fact that the patient has the right to view/receive a copy of his or her own record, the fact that amendments to the documentation may be requested, the ways in which their health information will be used and released to outside entities, and the procedure to file a complaint with the Department of Health and Human Services.

Once the printed document is no longer needed, it is to be placed in one of the marked shred bins immediately. Shred bins are located in the business office and in the secure area of the front office. The only exception to this policy is the printed copies made for patients' requests, or that are to be mailed by the Release of Information Specialist.

In addition to the policies noted previously, security-specific policies should address

- Password protection. Every computer user must have a unique code or **password**, that is known (and used) only by the user. Passwords should not be easily discerned; for instance, the user's birthdate, spouse's name, child's name, phone number, and the like would not be secure passwords. Instead, the password should be a combination of numbers, letters, and special characters (symbols), no less than six and no longer than eight characters in length, and the system should be set up to prompt users to change their password at least every 90 days. Individual offices and facilities will set policies regarding their password configuration requirements. The software system in use will dictate some of the password constraints as well.

    Password A unique code, known only to the user, that is used to gain access to computer applications.

- Appointment of a security and/or privacy officer. Someone in the facility must be named as privacy and security officer, though these may be two individuals. The privacy/security officer is ultimately responsible for setting, monitoring, updating, investigating, and enforcing all privacy and security policies.

- Log-in attempts. The system setup should include automatic lock-out when a user attempts to log in a certain number of times (usually three) with the wrong password. The policy and procedure should also address how to regain access. No doubt you have already experienced this with online banking, a credit card company, or the learning management system at your college.

- Protection from **computer viruses** and **malware**. This should include the facility's policy on downloading music or other attachments that may carry viruses and malware. A virus is a "deviant program, stored on a computer floppy disk, hard drive, or CD, that can cause unexpected and often undesirable effects, such as destroying or corrupting data. Malware comes in the form of worms, viruses, and Trojan horses, all of which attack computer programs" (Williams and Sawyer). In early 2016, several hospitals were plagued by computer malware. Though patient records were not accessed, MedStar Health near Washington, DC, was affected and the system's users were not able to log in. This attack affected 250 outpatient locations and 10 hospitals. As a precaution, the health system sent patients to other facilities until the problem was resolved and the FBI was involved in the investigation (Cox, Turner, and Zapotsky).

    Computer virus A deviant program, stored on a flash drive, hard drive, or CD, that can cause unexpected and often undesirable effects, such as destroying or corrupting data.

    Malware Malware is short for malicious software and includes deviant software such as worms, viruses, and Trojan horses, all of which attack computer programs.

- Security audits. A policy should be in place and carried out that requires random security audits to monitor access to patients' records. This may be done on a rotating basis, so that all staff members (including providers) are audited periodically, or it may be done based on a random selection of patients in the database. Of course, the investigation of any rumored or known breaches should include a security audit. It is important that internal security audits be carried out since the

Officer of Inspector General (OIG) also carries out random audits of EHR system security vulnerabilities.

- Off-site access. With the use of current technology, many PMs and EHRs can be accessed via the Internet. Policies must dictate who can access remotely as well as what information can be viewed and/or edited remotely.

- Printing policies. The more information that is printed from the EHR or PM software, the greater the chance there is of unauthorized disclosure.

- Destruction policies. If paper copies of the electronic record are going to be made, then the destruction of those copies also needs to be addressed. The usual method of destruction is shredding, either externally by a destruction company or internally through the use of portable shredders. Regardless of which is used, a policy must be in place that states when paper copies are destroyed, how, by whom, and when.

- Detailed policies and procedures that address privacy or security incidents. Disciplinary action should be addressed in this policy as well.

- Staff education—the requirement that all staff (including care providers) participate in continuing education opportunities to reinforce the laws governing privacy and security.

- Email. It is a part of everyday life, not just in our personal lives but in our work lives as well. Anything written in an email is protected information. However, it is not a secure means of communication, and the facility should adopt policies related to the sending and receiving of email messages, including what, if any, patient-related information can be sent via email. Like faxes, emails can go to the wrong individual, constituting a privacy breach. There must be a policy regarding patient-related emails or emails to or from patients—are they a part of the patient's health record, and if so, how will the email become part of the record? Emails should be encrypted, which means the words are scrambled and can be read only if the receiver has a special code to decipher it, but encrypting still does not ensure total security. Encryption applies to any information that is electronically transmitted.

Firewall A system of hardware and/or software that protects a computer or a network from intruders by filtering activity over the network.

Hardware The tangible items that are used in automation (e.g., the processing unit, screen, keyboard, mouse, laptops, handheld devices).

Firewalls should also be used to deter access to the system by unauthorized individuals. Williams and Sawyer define a firewall as "a system of hardware and/or software that protects a computer or a network from intruders."

Hardware also has to be protected, and policies must be written to govern the security of hardware devices. Hardware includes desktop computers, laptop computers, handheld devices, and the like. These devices are always at risk for loss or theft. To protect the information on a device, follow these simple rules:

- Always lock down (sign out of) the device when it is unattended, and require a password to log on.

- Never store the passwords to any of your hardware devices or sites on the computer.

- Back up files onto a CD, an external hard drive, or a flash drive.

- Encrypt PHI if policy allows health records to be stored on the device.

- Use the portable devices in a secure area—using one in the cafeteria and walking away to freshen your coffee is not secure.

- Wipe the hard drives of any computers that are taken out of use before recycling them or placing them in the trash. This is typically the responsibility of the IT department.

Privacy and security need to be kept in mind at all times in any healthcare facility or practice. Not doing so, even unintentionally, may result in hefty fines. The new fines, as a result of the Omnibus Final Rule, are as follows:

Category of Violation	Fine per Violation	Total Violation When Breach Involved the Same Provision within the Same Calendar Year
Unknowing (unintentional)	$100–$50,000	$1,500,000
Reasonable cause	$1,000–$50,000	$1,500,000
Willful neglect (corrected)	$10,000–$50,000	$1,500,000
Willful neglect (not corrected)	Minimum of $50,000	$1,500,000

Healthcare organizations using an EHR must meet the HIPAA standards of privacy and confidentiality. In addition, states may have even more stringent rules. The American Recovery and Reinvestment Act of 2009 (ARRA), through HITECH, made the rules regarding privacy and security of electronic systems more stringent yet. **Accounting of disclosures** is a responsibility of healthcare facilities as a result of HITECH. Facilities must be able to provide a patient with a listing of disclosures, if requested. Also, facilities with an EHR must be able to provide a patient with a listing of people who had access to his or her protected health information internally. This is known as an **access report**. The access report must contain the names of the individuals who accessed that person's record as well as the names of persons who do not work at the facility who had access to the record. For instance, a hospital may grant a local nursing home admissions department the right to view the health record of a patient who is being considered for nursing home placement. This is required to assess whether or not the nursing home has the facilities needed to care for that patient, and it is part of the continuum of care; thus, it is a necessary release. The hospital would note, in the access report, that the patient's PHI was released to a certain nursing home but would not be able to supply the names of the individual(s) who accessed it at the nursing home.

Accounting of disclosures Providing the patient, upon request, with a listing of all disclosures of his or her health information, both internally and externally.

Access report A report of all persons (within the facility) who have had access to a patient's protected health information.

7.2 Evaluating an EHR System for HIPAA Compliance

According to the Office of the National Coordinator for Health Information Technology (ONC) website, "Health information technology (health IT) makes it possible for health care providers to better manage patient care through secure use and sharing of health information." Health IT includes the use of electronic health records (EHRs) instead of paper medical records to maintain people's health information.

To better manage patient care using electronic means, however, it is necessary to comply with certain regulations. The HIPAA rules that address electronic health information are listed in Table 7.1.

TABLE 7.1 Functionality of an EHR as Required by HIPAA Regulations

Functionality	Meaning
Password protection	Passwords must be assigned to all users of an electronic health record system and the passwords must meet certain criteria: length, properties, expiration intervals, and a number of log-in attempts before lock-out.
User identification	Each user must have a unique identifier to log in, often consisting of the person's first initial and last name. This allows for tracking and reporting of activity within the system by the user.
Access rights	Policies are written and adhered to regarding access to functionality within the EHR that is dependent on the person's (or position's) need to know.
Accounting of disclosures	Upon authorized request, an accounting of all disclosures from a patient's health record, going back a minimum of six years from the date of request, must be provided. The patient's health record must also be made available to the patient, or to an outside entity at the patient's request.
Security/ backup/ storage	A backup of the EHR database must be kept in a secure location, and restoration of the backup database must be possible at any given time. Other security requirements include controlled access to the database, use of passwords to access the database, use of firewalls, and antivirus programs.
Auditing	This task provides the ability to run reports by users or by patients that specify the menu, module, or function accessed; the date and time of the access; whether the information was viewed, edited, or deleted; and the user ID of the individual staff member.
Code sets	The EHR must use ICD-10 codes, CPT® codes, and HCPCS codes to store and transmit information.

Source: https://www.hhs.gov/hipaa/for-professionals/security/laws-regulations/index.html.

Regarding passwords, though longer passwords are more secure than shorter ones, the most secure passwords include a combination of letters (upper- and lowercase), symbols, and numbers. The password "summerday" is more secure than "summer," for example, yet "summer18$#" is even more secure. Healthcare organizations set their own policies regarding the length and configuration of passwords.

In a medical practice, it may be the office administrator who starts the search for EHR software and keeps in mind the requirements of a compliant system. Other individuals who should also be involved in researching, selecting, and implementing the EHR include a representative of care providers, a member of the front office (reception) staff, a clinical staff representative, health information staff, coding/billing staff, and an information technology (IT) professional who is an expert in the technological aspects of the software and hardware, networking, and interoperability of systems. This group should always keep in mind

- The required components of a compliant EHR
- The needs of the office or facility
- The intended budget for acquiring a system as well as yearly budget requirements
- Staff and training needs
- The intent of the EHR—is it to interface with the existing PM system, or will an entirely new system that accomplishes both be purchased?
- The timeline—what is the target date for implementation?

7.3 The Role of Certification in EHR Implementation

There are many agencies that certify EHR software. Both the information technology (IT) and the health information technology (HIT) aspects of an EHR system must be taken into consideration, and during the process of assessing various systems and vendors, looking at certified EHR systems is a good place to start.

CMS and the Office of the National Coordinator for Health Information Technology (ONC) have established standards and other criteria for structured data that EHRs must use in order to qualify for an incentive program to upgrade an existing EHR or purchase a new one. The ONC, through consultation with the Director of the National Institute of Standards and Technology, recognizes programs for this voluntary certification if they are in compliance with certification criteria (HHS: Proposed Establishment).

The **Healthcare Information and Management Systems Society (HIMSS)** is an independent, nonprofit organization with the mission "to lead healthcare transformation through the effective use of health information technology" (HIMSS: About HIMSS). HIMSS and the **American Health Information Management Association (AHIMA)** are professional associations that are highly respected in the fields of information technology (IT) and health information management (HIM). Each has myriad sources, references, guides, best practices, and practice briefs for use in the selection and implementation of an EHR, and both organizations highly value certification.

Healthcare Information and Management Systems Society (HIMSS) An association of health informatics and information professionals formed to promote a better understanding of healthcare informatics and management systems.

American Health Information Management Association (AHIMA) A professional association for the field of health information management.

Selecting a product that is certified is good business practice and will save the office administration much of the legwork necessary to ensure the selection of a product that not only meets the needs of the organization but has already been tested and proven to meet regulatory requirements.

7.4 Applying Security Measures

Assigning passwords, allowing access to only the functions that are necessary to perform a job, and following the other policies outlined in Section 7.1 all play a role in assuring the privacy, confidentiality, and security of the health information stored in your facility's PM and EHR systems.

The next two exercises apply basic security measures in EHRclinic. These functions will usually be set up by the office administrator or manager.

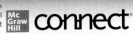
Add a New Clinical User

In this scenario, the office manager has just hired a new medical assistant
(MA), Patric Wilson, and she is going to set Patric up as a user in EHRclinic.
Certain information is needed from Patric before the office manager begins
the setup process.

Field	Value
Full name	Wilson, Patric
Username	pwilson
Email	pwilson@sbhc.com
Sex	Male
DOB	07/08/1980
Telephone number	419-555-2973 (cell)
Address	47132 Brookline Drive Carey, OH 43316
Soc. Security no.	363-92-4410
Hire date	03/22/2022
Position	Medical assistant
Credentials	CMA(AAMA)

Follow these steps to complete the exercise on your own once you
have watched the demonstration and tried the steps with helpful prompts in
practice mode. Use the information provided in the scenario to complete the
information.

1. Click on 'Manage practice data' button.
2. Click on 'Staff information' button.
3. Click on 'Add new staff' button.
4. Click on 'First name' input field and enter 'Patric'.
5. Click on 'Last name' input field and enter 'Wilson'.
6. Click on datepicker (calendar) icon in 'Date of birth' field.
7. Click on 'Select month' and select 'July'.
8. Click on 'Select year' and select '1980'.
9. Select 'July 08 1980' date.
10. Click on 'Gender' drop-down and select 'Male'.
11. Click on 'Street' input field and enter '47132 Brookline Drive'.
12. Click on 'City' input field and enter 'Carey'.
13. Click on 'State' drop-down and select 'Ohio'.
14. Click on 'Zip' input field and enter '43316'.
15. Click on 'Primary phone' input field and enter '419-555-2973'.
16. Click on 'Primary phone type' drop-down and select 'Cell'.
17. Click on 'Email' input field and enter 'pwilson@sbhc.com'.
18. Click on 'SSN' input field and enter '363-92-4410'.
19. Click on 'Employment start date' input field and enter '03/22/2022'.
20. Click on 'Position/Job title' drop-down and select 'Medical assistant'.

21. Click on 'Credentials' input field and enter 'CMA(AAMA)'.
22. Click on 'Add new staff' button.

Once Patric has been added to the staff database, a username, such as pwilson01, will be assigned to him. His default password will be "Clinic321," which is used in the initial setup of all new staff members. In the examples used throughout the worktext, the default password is "Clinic321." In an actual work setting, this default password would be changed to a password of the user's choice that met the practice's password requirements.

✔️ **You have completed Exercise 7.1**

Setting Up Care Providers

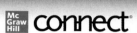 Go to https://connect.mheducation.com to complete this exercise. To see instructional notes with the steps, visit the eBook in Connect or download them from www.mhhe.com/iehr4. EXERCISE 7.2

Set Up a Care Provider

In our next scenario, there is also a new care provider starting this week, Lynette Dean, MD. The office manager will set her up in the system, assigning a user ID and user rights.

The information necessary before beginning the setup process is

Field	Value
Full name	Dean, Lynette
Sex	Female
Credentials	MD
DOB	09/04/1972
Soc. Security no.	631-55-7429
Address	12 Country Club Lane Findlay, OH 45839
Telephone number	419-555-8337
Email	ldean@sbhc.com
NPI number	9348652175
State medical license number	8215346 Expires 01/31/2023
DEA number	BD4892106
Specialty	Family Medicine
On staff at Summit Bay Health Center	Yes
Provides billable services at Summit Bay Health Center	Yes
Assigned user ID	ldean

Follow these steps to complete the exercise on your own once you have watched the demonstration and tried the steps with helpful prompts in practice mode. Use the information provided in the scenario to complete the information.

1. Click on 'Manage practice data' button.
2. Click on 'Provider information' button.

(continued)

3. Click on 'Add provider' button.
4. Click on 'First name' input field and enter 'Lynette'.
5. Click on 'Last name' input field and enter 'Dean'.
6. Click on datepicker (calendar) icon in 'Date of birth' field.
7. Click on 'Select month' and select 'September'.
8. Click on 'Select year' and select '1972'.
9. Select 'September 04 1972' date.
10. Click on 'Gender' drop-down and select 'Female'.
11. Click on 'Street' input field and enter '12 Country Club Lane'.
12. Click on 'City' input field and enter 'Findlay'.
13. Click on 'State' drop-down and select 'Ohio'.
14. Click on 'Zip' input field and enter '45839'.
15. Click on 'Primary phone' input field and enter '419-555-8337'.
16. Click on 'Primary phone type' drop-down and select 'Cell'.
17. Click on 'Email' input field and enter 'ldean@sbhc.com'.
18. Click on 'SSN' input field and enter '631-55-7429'.
19. Click on 'Credential' field and select 'M.D.'.
20. Click on 'DEA number' field and enter 'BD4892106'.
21. Click on 'Practice license number' field and enter '8215346'.
22. Click on 'License expiration date' field and enter '01/31/2023'.
23. Click on 'State issuing' drop-down and select 'Ohio'.
24. Click on 'Primary specialty' drop-down and select 'Family Medicine'.
25. Click on 'Provider NPI#' field and enter '9348652175'.
26. Click on 'Add provider' button.
27. Click on 'Tools' module.
28. Click on 'Manage access' button.
29. Click on 'Access levels' button.
30. Click on 'Lynette Dean's' access level.
31. Click on Schedules 'Select access level: Selected View and Edit' field and select 'View only'.
32. Click on Checkout 'Select access level: Selected View and Edit' field and select 'View only'.
33. Click on Claims 'Select access level: Selected View and Edit' field and select 'View only'.
34. Click on 'Save' button.

☑ **You have completed Exercise 7.2**

Setting User Rights for Staff

User rights The limitations of one's access to the functionality of the software as defined by one's job description or position within the organization.

We will take security functions a step further by adding **user rights**. Log-on rights simply mean that one is assigned a log-in and password to allow access to the computer software—in our case, EHRclinic. The user is then assigned user rights, which are privileges that limit access to only the functionality of the software needed by that individual. The position held and job description of each staff member (including care providers) dictate what privileges each person has.

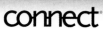
Assign User Rights to a Medical Assistant (MA)

In the scenario that follows, John Matthews is an office manager. He will be setting up the user rights for Patric Wilson, an MA who is new to the office. We will start by setting up Chart and Administrative rights by going into the Access management area located within the Tools module in EHRclinic.

Chart, or encounter, rights have to do with viewing, adding, editing, or changing documentation within patients' charts. For instance, Patric will be able to access the Patient Chart page of every patient. He will have access to a very extensive allergy module, which will include setting up a patient's allergy shot schedule, dosage calculations, and similar applications. Of course, *he will do this based only on the physician's orders.* Patric will be able to delete vital signs from a facesheet; reasons for this may be that the vitals were incorrectly typed into the facesheet or were put on the wrong patient's chart, or that the healthcare professional who entered the blood pressure, for example, did not get an accurate reading. *These privileges are very sensitive and are only given to appropriate staff members with the expertise and position within the practice to warrant such rights.* But even deleted, the original documentation is not lost forever—hidden is actually a better description for it—there is an **audit trail** that shows the original documentation and then the corrected version. The topic of data integrity and versions of documentation will be covered in more detail later in this chapter.

Custom views of the facesheet can be set up in many EHR software packages. The information displayed is consistent, but the way it looks on the screen is different. Some MAs or nurses are granted the right to sign off on lab results; *that right is determined by office policy (and may vary by care provider) as well as the level of knowledge of the individual.* An example is a standard blood test, such as a CBC, that is completely within normal limits on an established patient; the care provider may feel that an experienced MA or nurse is qualified to sign off on those results without sending them through for review by the care provider. The same applies to some prescriptions. The care provider may give a verbal order to an MA or a nurse for a prescription renewal to be called in to the patient's pharmacy or refilled by ePrescription. For example, Robyn Berkeley is a long-time patient of Dr. Rodriguez. She has a long-standing prescription for metronidazole for treatment of her rosacea, and she has run out; the MA gives Dr. Rodriguez the request, and he then authorizes her to send through a refill via ePrescribe. The MA is able to access and print (or electronically transmit) the prescription renewal with Dr. Rodriguez's digital signature.

Administrative rights, on the other hand, deal with access to scheduling, checkout procedures, patient accounts, claim completion, messages, tasks, and practice tools. Summit Bay Health Center is staffed with medical billers, medical administrative assistants, and an office manager, so administrative tasks for medical assistants are limited. For example, Patric is given access to view and edit schedules because he may make appointments for patients being seen throughout the day. He is not given access privileges for patient checkout, accounts, and claims because these administrative functions are handled by other healthcare professionals within the practice. To maintain patient privacy and security, it is important to assign access rights that are appropriate to an employee's position and job requirements.

User rights for all registration functions are also set up; if the healthcare professional works in the reception and registration areas, she would have user rights to any routine daily functions, including registering a patient for the first time, editing demographic information, scheduling an appointment, checking a patient in or out, viewing alert flags, and so on.

(continued)

Audit trail A permanent record or accounting of accesses, additions, amendments, or deletions to a health record. Also a report that shows accesses by user to each function of the software.

System rights affect just that—the overall system. The rights you will see in this exercise include importing documents that do not originate within EHRclinic and accessing patient tracking. Patric is given 'view only' access rights to the Tools module in EHRclinic, so that he can review the various databases but not make changes to them. In this case, the office manager is the only person who has access to make database changes.

Follow these steps to complete the exercise on your own once you've watched the demonstration and tried the steps with helpful prompts in practice mode. Use the information provided in the scenario to complete the information.

1. Click on 'Manage access' button.
2. Click on 'Access levels' button.
3. Click on 'Patric Wilson's' access level.
4. Click on Checkout 'Select access level' drop-down and select 'No access'.
5. Click on Accounts 'Select access level' drop-down and select 'No access'.
6. Click on Claims 'Select access level' drop-down and select 'No access'.
7. Click on Tools 'Select access level' and select 'View only'.
8. Click on 'Save' button.

✔ **You have completed Exercise 7.3**

Setting User Rights for a Manager

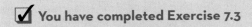   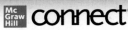

Go to https://connect.mheducation.com to complete this exercise. To see instructional notes with the steps, visit the eBook in Connect or download them from www.mhhe.com/iehr4.

Assign User Rights to an Office Manager

Office managers or administrators have increased functionality such as setting up files in accounts receivable management, chart configuration and administration, registration screens, research (clinical trial) functionality, reporting, scheduling, and overall system configuration.

As you go through this exercise, in which you will assign rights to Diane Baxter, who has just been promoted to office manager, take a look at the entire list of rights that are assigned. As office manager, Diane will have greater access than she did in her role as a medical administrative specialist.

Follow these steps to complete the exercise on your own once you have watched the demonstration and tried the steps with helpful prompts in practice mode.

1. Click on 'Manage practice data' button.
2. Click on 'Staff information' button.
3. Click on 'Search by patient first name/last name/staff member ID' field and enter 'bax'.
4. Click on 'Diane Baxter's' staff information.
5. Click on 'Position/Job title: Selected Medical administrative specialist' field and select 'Office manager'.
6. Click on 'Save changes' button.
7. Click on 'Tools' module.
8. Click on 'Manage access' button.
9. Click on 'Access levels' button.
10. Click on 'Provider name/Staff name/ID' field and enter 'bax'.
11. Click on 'Diane Baxter's' access level.

12. Click on Encounter 'Select access level' and select 'View and edit'.
13. Click on Tools 'Select access level' and select 'View and edit'.
14. Click on 'Save' button.

☑ **You have completed Exercise 7.4**

Setting Up a Group

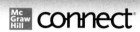 Go to https://connect.mheducation.com to complete this exercise. To see instructional notes with the steps, visit the eBook in Connect or download them from www.mhhe.com/iehr4.   **EXERCISE**   **7.5**

Create a Group

In the previous exercises, we have been working with just one staff member. In this exercise we will set up an entire group within EHRclinic. Setting up groups, such as all medical assistants, all receptionists, or all care providers, allows the office administrator to give rights by group rather than having to set up each person individually. Of course, if some of the users within the group have higher-level rights, then their profiles can be modified by adding rights individually.

Essentially, when groups are formed, the individual staff members are moved into it, and finally the group is named. Or a group may already exist and staff members are moved into it. The other advantage of groups is that if an email needs to be sent to an entire group—for instance, the health records staff—then just one email can be sent rather than a separate email to each staff member.

In Exercise 7.5 we will be working within the Task module of EHRclinic to send a message to all staff. An example is that the health records staff is required to attend an in-service meeting on HITECH regulations at 2:00 p.m. on May 5. Just one message can be sent to the entire group, notifying them of this in-service meeting.

Follow these steps to complete the exercise on your own once you've watched the demonstration and tried the steps with helpful prompts in practice mode.

1. Click on 'Tasks' module.
2. Click on 'New task' button.
3. Click on 'Task' field and enter 'HITECH in-service meeting May 5 at 2:00'.
4. Click on 'Assign to drop down' button and select 'All'.
5. Click on 'Due date' field and enter '05/05/2022'.
6. Click on 'Add task' button.

☑ **You have completed Exercise 7.5**

> **EHRclinic Tip** 〔EHRclinic〕
>
> In some EHRclinic exercises, the Path window may obstruct areas you need to click. If this happens, you can collapse the Path within the window or click to hide it in the upper left corner of the screen.

7.5   Handling Sensitive and Restricted Access

A health record contains not only pertinent clinical data but also information about a patient that may be considered embarrassing, makes a patient uncomfortable, or is just very private. Examples are personal history data such as history of abortion, having given up a child for adoption, or drug or alcohol abuse. In these instances, a record may be marked as sensitive within EHRclinic or other EHR software, so that extra care is taken when handling or releasing information.

Though all health information is confidential and is not released unless a proper authorization is on file, as required by law or for continuity of care, some health information is such that a higher level of confidentiality is vital, even from staff within an office or a hospital. Consider, for instance, a patient who is well known to the office and in the community who has a diagnosis of a sexually transmitted disease. In this case, only the care provider and staff who absolutely have a need to know in order to care for the patient, or process the record for the insurance claim, would have access to that record. Perhaps the sister-in-law of that patient is a receptionist in the office—it would not be prudent for her to handle that particular record. Or consider another patient who is on an antidepressant but does not want the record open to the entire staff because one of the medical assistants in the office is a friend of hers. In both of these examples, the record might be marked as "sensitive" within EHRclinic, and access to those records may be limited to only a select few providers and staff within the practice; this is known as "restricted access" within EHRclinic. Many practices mark records of all their staff (and often any family members) as restricted access, and only the office manager controls access to providers and other staff members who have a need to know.

Records of celebrities and other well-known individuals would also be considered sensitive and/or allow restricted access. A well-publicized case of a privacy breach involving George Clooney and his girlfriend occurred in 2007. The two were in a motorcycle accident and were taken to a New Jersey hospital. More than 20 staff members of that hospital were suspended for a month without pay due to accessing the pair's health records without a need to know and without authorization.

EXERCISE 7.6

Go to https://connect.mheducation.com to complete this exercise. To see instructional notes with the steps, visit the eBook in Connect or download them from www.mhhe.com/iehr4.

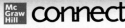

Mark a Record as Sensitive

Corinne Hess is a 17-year-old patient of Dr. Rodriguez who has been suffering from depression. The record contains information that is of a very personal nature and is going to be flagged as "sensitive."

Follow these instructions to register Corinne and input her insurance information, as well as to mark the record as sensitive. You will need the information on the registration form shown in Figure 7.1.

1. Click on 'Manage practice data' button.
2. Click on 'Patient information' button.
3. Click on 'Add new patient' button.
4. Click on 'First name' field and enter 'Corinne'.
5. Click on 'Last name' field and enter 'Hess'.
6. Click on 'Date of birth' field and enter '05/05/2005'.
7. Click on 'Gender' drop-down and select 'Female'.
8. Click on 'Marital status' dropdown and select 'Single'.
9. Click on 'Street' field and enter '904 Wrigley Road'.
10. Click on 'City' field and enter 'Carey'.
11. Click on 'Zip' field and enter '43316'.
12. Click on 'State' button and select 'Ohio'.
13. Click on 'Cell phone code' field and enter '770'.
14. Click on 'Cell phone' field and enter '555-8989'.

15. Click on 'Home phone code' field and enter '770'.
16. Click on 'Home phone' field and enter '555-3450'.
17. Click on 'Student status' drop-down and select 'Yes'.
18. Click on 'Employment status' drop-down and select 'Unemployed'.
19. Click on 'Email' field and enter 'corinnehess@patient.com'.
20. Click on 'SSN' field and enter '867-66-2489'.
21. Click on 'Preferred language' drop-down and select 'English'.
22. Click on 'Race' drop-down and select 'Caucasian'.
23. Click on 'Ethnicity' drop -down and select 'Not Hispanic or Latino'.
24. Click on 'Religion' drop-down and select 'Protestant'.
25. Click on 'Search by insurance carrier name' search field and enter 'mcg'.
26. Click on 'McGraw-Hill Healthmark'.
27. Click on 'Patient insurance id' field and enter 'GAR512374'.
28. Click on 'Add patient' button.
29. Click on 'Okay' button.
30. Click on 'Search patient' field and enter 'hes'.
31. Click on 'Corinne Hess's' patient information.
32. Click on 'Add image' field.
33. Click on 'Corrine Hess'.
34. Click on 'Choose' button.
35. Click on 'Insurance info' tab.
36. Click on 'Edit primary insurance' button.
37. Click on 'Is the plan active' drop-down and select 'Yes'.
38. Click on 'Patient responsibility' drop-down and select 'Copay'.
39. Click on 'Copay' field and enter '20'.
40. Click on 'Deductible' field and enter '0'.
41. Click on 'Deductible met' drop-down and select 'N/A'.
42. Click on 'Effective start date of coverage' field and enter '01/01/2022'.
43. Click on 'Effective end date of coverage' field and enter '12/31/2022'.
44. Click on 'Is guarantor: Selected Yes' field and select 'No'.
45. Click on 'Group insurance ID' field and enter '6501'.
46. Click on 'Add guarantor'.
47. Click on 'Search patient by first name/last name/chart no./DOB (mm/ dd/yyyy)' field and enter 'hess'.
48. Click on 'Jared Hess' patient.
49. Click on 'Guarantor' 'Relationship' drop-down and select 'Child'.
50. Click on 'Guarantor' Group insurance ID and enter '6501'.
51. Click on 'Sync Insurance Info' button.
52. Click on 'Done' button.
53. Click on 'Save changes' button.
54. Click on 'Tools' module.
55. Click on 'Manage reports' button.
56. Click on 'Patient charts and graphs' button.
57. Click on 'Search by patient first name/last name/chart number/SSN' field and enter 'hes'.
58. Click on 'Corinne Hess's' info.
59. Click on 'Sensitive' checkbox.
60. Click on 'chart and graphs' cancel button.

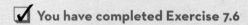 **You have completed Exercise 7.6**

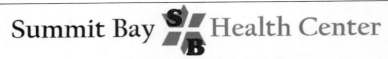

REGISTRATION FORM
(Please Print)

| **Today's date:** May 4, 2022 | | **Care Provider:** Dr. Rodriguez |

PATIENT INFORMATION

Patient's last name:	First:	Middle:	☐ Mr. ☐ Miss	Marital status (circle one)
Hess	Corinne		☐ Mrs. ☒ Ms.	(Single) / Mar / Div / Sep / Wid

Is this your legal name?	If not, what is your legal name?	(Former name):	Birth date:	Age:	Sex:
☒ Yes ☐ No			05/05/2005	17	☐ M ☒ F

Street address:	Social Security no.:	Home phone:	Cell phone:
904 Wrigley Road	867-66-2489	770-555-3450	770-555-8989

P. O. Box:	City:	State:	ZIP Code:
	Carey	OH	43316

Occupation:	Employer:	Employer phone no.:
N/A	N/A	N/A

E-mail address: corinnehess@patient.com

Race: Caucasian	Ethnicity: Not Hispanic or Latino	Primary language: English	Religion: Protestant

Other family members seen here: none

INSURANCE INFORMATION
(Presentation of Insurance Card is required at time of each visit)

Person responsible for bill:	Date of birth:	Address:	Home phone:	Cell phone:
Jared Hess	07/23/1978	904 Wrigley Road, Carey, OH 43316	770-555-3450	770-555-9172

Is this person a patient here?	☒ Yes ☐ No

Occupation:	Employer:	Employer address:	Employer phone no.:
Teacher	Carrolton Elementary	63178 Dodge Blvd, Jenera, OH 45841	770-555-5000

Is this patient covered by insurance?	☒ Yes ☐ No

Please indicate primary insurance	☒ McGraw-Hill Healthmark Insurance	☐ BlueCross/ Blue Shield	☐ [Insurance]	☐ [Insurance]	☐ [Insurance]
☐ [Insurance]	☐ Workers' Compensation	☐ Medicare	☐ Medicaid (Please provide card)	☐ Other	

Subscriber's name:	Subscriber's S.S. no.:	Date of birth:	Group no.:	Policy no.:	Co-payment:
Jared Hess	555-88-1456	07/23/1978	6501	GAR512374	$ 20.00

Patient's relationship to subscriber:	☐ Self ☐ Spouse ☒ Child ☐ Other	Effective Date: 01/01/2022

Name of secondary insurance (if applicable): None	Subscriber's name:	Group no.:	Policy no.:

Patient's relationship to subscriber:	☐ Self ☐ Spouse ☐ Child ☐ Other

IN CASE OF EMERGENCY

Name of local friend or relative (not living at same address):	Relationship to patient:	Home phone no.:	Work phone no.:
Amanda Jaxon	Aunt	(419)555-0422	(770)555-1518

The above information is true to the best of my knowledge. I authorize my insurance benefits be paid directly to the physician. I understand that I am financially responsible for any balance. I also authorize [Name of Practice] or insurance company to release any information required to process my claims.

Jared H. Hess	5/4/2022
Patient/Guardian signature	Date

Figure 7.1 Corinne Hess Registration Form

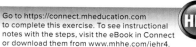

Mark a Record as Restricted Access

David Olivetti is the brother-in-law of Kaitlyn, a medical assistant at Summit Bay Health Center, and is good friends with Dr. Rodriguez. Dr. Ingram is his regular physician at Summit Bay Health Center. Because of the relationship with Kaitlyn and Dr. Rodriguez, David does not want either to have access to his EHR. In this exercise, David's record will be marked for restricted access.

1. Click on 'Manage reports' button.
2. Click on 'Patient charts and graphs' button.
3. Click on 'Search by patient first name/last name/chart number/SSN' field and enter 'oli'.
4. Click on 'David Olivetti's' info.
5. Click on 'Restricted' checkbox.
6. Click on 'Chart and graphs' cancel button.

☑ **You have completed Exercise 7.7**

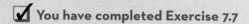

7.6 Data Integrity

Data integrity refers to the accuracy and timeliness of data collection, as well as the consistency of the definitions used to collect the data. In addition, there is an expectation that there has been no manipulation of the data once the data have been collected and reported. To maintain data integrity, the healthcare facility must have strict policies regarding who may access data, the definition of a complete record, the accuracy of data, consistent applications of data dictionary definitions, and the timeliness of data entry. Think of it this way: If a patient is seen on Wednesday but the documentation in the health record is not entered until Friday, how accurate do you think it will be? Or if one of the staff members instructs a patient to document his past surgical history but to include only surgeries done under general anesthesia in the past five years, yet the office policy shows a data dictionary definition of surgery as *any* procedure the patient has had while under local, regional, or general anesthetic at any time in the past, then how consistent are the data? What about a healthcare professional who finds a blood pressure reading of 152/80 in a patient yet enters it as 140/80 and knowingly leaves it as is, figuring it is "close enough"?If you were a care provider using the information found in your EHR database, and you knew poor documentation practices were occurring, you would not have much faith in using those data, would you? Or if you were conducting a research study and knew that the data were flawed, how valid would the study be? In other words, any data found within the health record must be accurate, complete, and documented at the time of or as close to the time of occurrence as possible.

Data integrity Maintaining the accuracy and consistency of data.

Amending a Chart Entry

Integrity also applies to the addition, amendment, or omission of documentation that has already been recorded. Any alteration in the

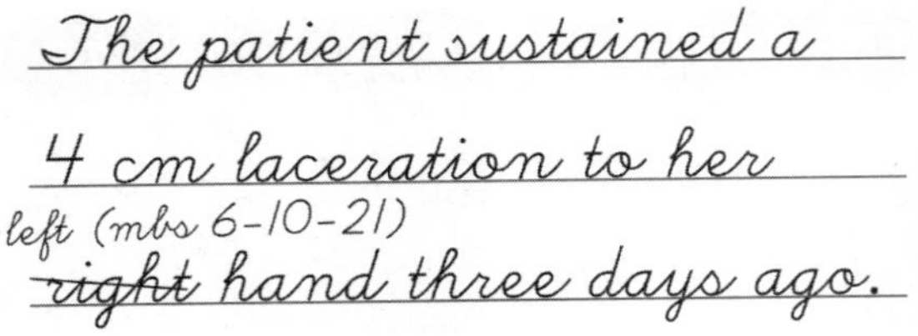

The patient sustained a

4 cm laceration to her

left (mbs 6-10-21)

~~*right hand three days ago.*~~

Figure 7.2   Example of Correction to Paper Documentation

original documentation must be recoverable. With the use of paper records, if an entry in a health record was amended or corrected, it was obvious. See Figure 7.2 for an example of a proper chart correction. You can readily see that the entry was corrected; originally, it read that the patient had sustained a laceration to her right hand, when, in fact, it was the left hand. A single line was drawn through the incorrect word, the correct word was inserted, and the correction was initialed and dated by the person who made the correction.

In an electronic record, original documentation that is found to be incorrect or incomplete may be hidden from view but is never completely "deleted." Only the corrected information is viewable to the healthcare professionals or care providers; however, that original, hidden documentation can be recovered at any time.

Standard practice dictates that only certain staff members such as those who are in lead or administrative positions have users' rights to make changes to a record in an electronic environment. This is not a procedure that is done often, nor is it done without a valid reason, such as that a note was put on the wrong patient's chart or a note pertains to that patient but not to that particular visit. Some software vendors use the term *deleting* rather than *hiding;* regardless, the deleted/hidden entry will *always* be retrievable, should the record be needed in a lawsuit, to verify some sort of inconsistency, or for insurance purposes.

7.7   Apply Policies and Procedures to Release Health Information Using EHRclinic

Another requirement of the Promoting Interoperability (formerly Meaningful Use) initiatives is to share health information with other healthcare professionals when necessary. For instance, Virginia Hill is a patient of Dr. Ingram's, and he is referring her to a specialist. It is important for the specialist to know her medical history and the reasoning behind the referral; therefore, information is released electronically. This reason is known as continuity of care.

Many releases require a written authorization from the patient or legal representative. If the specialist also has an EHR, he or she is able to access the primary care physician's health record of Virginia Hill, but let's say Dr. Ingram's office printed Mrs. Hill's record and mailed it to the specialist. Now, we will be accounting for the disclosure. Release of information in the case of this referral would not require an authorization, nor would release of information to an insurance company for purposes of payment of the claim, nor release of information to public health agencies, as required by law. Written authorization is required for all releases of information to physicians' offices or hospitals that are not a result of a direct referral. Authorization is also required to release health information to attorneys, employers (if not a Workers' Compensation claim), spouses, children, and law enforcement agencies. Also, certain records such as those related to drug and alcohol abuse, mental health, and HIV/AIDS have more stringent release of information regulations; those will be discussed in great detail in another course.

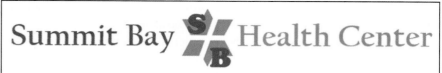

Summit Bay Health Center

Authorization to Release Medical Records

Name: _Juan Ortega_   DOB: _2/28/2001_

Address: _1710 Red Oak Lane, McComb, OH 45858_ .

I, _Juan Ortega_ , hereby grant my permission to _Summit Bay Health Center_ (name of practice) to release the following information:

physical exam, lab results, cardiac test results .

_____

to _Dr. Ingram_ of Summit Bay Health Center.

Reason for Request:

Continuity of care and second opinion .

_____

_____

Signature of Patient or Legal Guardian: _Juan Ortega_

Printed Name: _Juan Ortega_

Relationship to Patient: _Self_

Date: _5/4/2022_   Date Authorization Expires: _8/1/2022_

This authorization can be revoked at anytime by notifying Summit Bay Health Center. You have the right to refuse to grant authorization to release medical information.

9741 Madison Ave ● Findlay, OH 45840 ● (419) 555-3079 ● fax (419) 555-0017

Figure 7.3   **Authorization to Release Records**

In addition to providing releases of information for records to be sent to other entities, it is often necessary for patients to have records sent to the healthcare practice. Figure 7.3 shows an authorization for other providers to release records to Summit Bay Health Center. If a patient is new to the practice or has seen another provider, such as a specialist, obtaining relevant health records is important for continuity of care.

Releasing information without a required authorization is known as a **breach of confidentiality**. Offices and healthcare facilities are required to report breaches, as was discussed earlier in this chapter, as part of the

Breach of confidentiality Releasing information without a required, properly executed authorization or as restricted by law.

HITECH regulations. Not only is the office or facility held liable for any breaches, but individual staff members may be as well.

As previously discussed, healthcare practices are obligated to provide a Notice of Privacy Practices (NPP) to their patients. This document explains patient rights, as described by HIPAA, related to the practice's use and disclosure of protected health information. New patients are provided with an NPP and asked to sign an acknowledgment that they received it, which is then placed in their charts. A new acknowledgment should be signed each time the NPP is updated by the practice.

 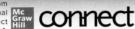

EXERCISE   7.8

Go to https://connect.mheducation.com to complete this exercise. To see instructional notes with the steps, visit the eBook in Connect or download them from www.mhhe.com/iehr4.

Post an Acknowledgment of Notice of Privacy Practices to a Patient's Chart

Corinne Hess has just registered as a new patient to Summit Bay Health Center and is waiting for her appointment to see Dr. Rodriguez. Her father, Jared, has been given a Notice of Privacy Practices and just signed a statement acknowledging that he received the NPP, which needs to be documented in Corinne's electronic health record.

Follow these steps to complete the exercise on your own once you've watched the demonstration and tried the steps with helpful prompts in practice mode. Use the information provided in the scenario to complete the information.

1. Click on 'Manage reports' button.
2. Click on 'Patient charts and graphs' button.
3. Click on 'Search by patient first name/last name/chart number/SSN' field and enter 'hes'.
4. Click on 'Corinne Hess's' info.
5. Click on 'Add form' button.
6. Click on 'Form name' input field and enter 'NPP'.
7. Click on 'Description' input field and enter 'Acknowledgment of receipt'.
8. Click on Attachment 'Browse' button.
9. Click on 'Choose' button.
10. Click on 'List of forms done' button.

✓ **You have completed Exercise 7.8**

7.8   Accounting of Information Disclosures

An accounting of the releases is also necessary to comply with regulations. As noted earlier, most releases require a written authorization, but to comply with HITECH, *all* releases must be accounted for, whether the disclosure is to internal staff members or to external requestors.

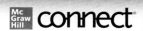
Document Disclosure of a Patient's Information

In this scenario, the office manager is processing release of information requests. She received a signed authorization from Corinne Hess' father, authorizing the disclosure of Corinne's office visit summary to her pediatrician, Dr. Hanna. Once the information has been sent to Dr. Hanna, an accounting for the release of records must be documented in Corinne's chart. Use the information provided in the scenario to complete the information.

Follow these steps to complete the exercise on your own once you have watched the demonstration and tried the steps with helpful prompts in practice mode. Use the information provided in the scenario to complete the information.

1. Click on 'Manage reports' button.
2. Click on 'Patient charts and graphs' button.
3. Click on 'Search by patient first name/last name/chart number/SSN' field and enter 'hes'.
4. Click on 'Corinne Hess's' info.
5. Click on 'Add new note' button.
6. Click on 'Note title' button and enter 'Disclosure of records'.
7. Enter 'Office visit summary sent to Dr. Hanna, as authorized by patient's legal guardian (father).' in 'Note' button.
8. Click on 'Done' button.

✔️ **You have completed Exercise 7.9**

7.9 Information Exchange

Communicating with other healthcare providers is another requirement of promoting interoperability. It is known as health information exchange (HIE). An advantage of utilizing an EHR is that patient care improves through the sharing of patient information at the point of care. With this functionality, care providers can access the findings of other physicians or test results immediately. Of course, this sharing is done through a secure environment, and there are regulations that address telecommunications and networking security as well. Secure email is one way that information can be shared between providers, the National Health Information Network (NHIN) Exchange is another, and there are state and private HIE programs as well. The State HIE Cooperative Agreement Program operates through the use of ONC funding, and its purpose is to coordinate local HIEs or serve as the HIE for a given area.

for your information fyi

Using a search engine, take the time to find your state's HIE on the Internet; each HIE has its own site and includes valuable information for care providers and staff.

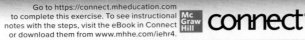
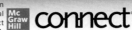
Exchange of Information for Continuity of Care

In this scenario, Ian Mikeals is a pediatric asthma patient of Dr. Ingram. Dr. Ingram is referring Ian to a pediatric asthma specialist. Before Ian's referral can be sent, the provider must be added to the referring provider database in EHRclinic.

Follow these steps to complete the exercise on your own once you've watched the demonstration and tried the steps with helpful prompts in practice mode.

1. Click on 'Manage practice data' button.
2. Click on 'Referring provider' button.
3. Click on 'Add new referring provider' button.
4. Click on 'First' name field and enter 'Jack'.
5. Click on 'Last' name field and enter 'Williams'.
6. Click on 'Street' input field and enter '900 Farmore Ave'.
7. Click on 'City' input field and enter 'Carey'.
8. Click on 'Zip' input field and enter '43380'.
9. Click on 'State' drop-down and select 'Ohio'.
10. Click on 'Phone number' input field and enter '419-555-0286'.
11. Click on 'Fax' input field and enter '419-555-3711'.
12. Click on 'Credentials' drop-down and select 'M.D.'.
13. Click on 'Primary specialty' drop-down and select 'Pulmonary'.
14. Click on 'NPI #' input field and enter '9618753220'.
15. Click on 'Add referring provider' button.

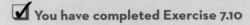 You have completed Exercise 7.10

Exchange of Information outside the Organization

There is another type of information exchange that has nothing to do with continuity of care, business purposes, or insurance purposes. It involves communicating *about* care via **social media**. Social media includes Facebook, YouTube, Twitter, **blogs** (ongoing conversations about a topic that take place online), and the like. These outlets are used by patients to share their experience with a healthcare organization or to recount their journey through an illness; they can also be used by the organizations themselves as a means of marketing or public relations. Take a look at the Facebook page of Children's Hospital, Boston, for example, by going to http://www.facebook.com/ and searching for the hospital. There you will find videos, testimonials, facts and figures about its patient population; links to related sites; support groups and blogs; awards the organization has won; and a link to its social media policy, which is short and to the point and, in summary, states that although all comments are welcome, they should not be offensive, should be on-topic, and should not violate the privacy of patients or their families.

There is some risk in allowing patients to provide comments, since not all of them will be positive, but by the same token, patient feedback is a vehicle to promote the institution, its accomplishments, and its services. The

Social media Interactive communication sites via the Internet. Examples are Facebook, YouTube, Instagram, Snapchat, and Twitter.

Blog Ongoing conversations about a topic that take place online via the Internet.

appropriate use of social media also provides a service to the community by including needed information about the organization as well as links to related sites such as public health sites, educational sites, and support groups.

Employees of an organization also use social media (Facebook, Twitter, and LinkedIn, for example) and may contribute to blogs about their organization. Since what they say and how they say it can sometimes be misconstrued, it is imperative that healthcare organizations develop a policy to address the use of social media, and such a policy should include the following information:

- The circumstances under which an employee may access any social media site during work hours
- Penalties or potential disciplinary action for failure to comply with the organization's social media policy
- Requirements:
  - Employees should maintain a positive tone in their posts and be respectful of the organization and its staff when posting on an organization-sponsored site.
  - The PHI of patients should *never* be posted (directly or implied).
  - The identity of any patients (directly or implied) should *never* be posted.
  - No copyrighted materials should be posted.
  - No information about the organization may be posted, as this is the responsibility of the marketing or public relations department.

The use of social media to share information about a particular person is gaining popularity. Use is set up and maintained by someone authorized by the patient, with the objective of keeping family and friends updated on the patient's condition. One such site is Caring Bridge (to locate Caring Bridge's home page, type "CaringBridge" into a search engine). What the patient or family cares to share on this site is under their control, but healthcare professionals who are or were involved in the patient's care need to be careful. A posting that you intend to be caring and helpful may be misinterpreted and perceived as intrusive by the family, so before posting, you should think twice about what you want to say and how you say it!

7.10 Compliance Plans

Think of all the regulations that affect healthcare—HIPAA, ARRA, and HITECH, not to mention Medicare, Medicaid, and managed care plan requirements; it is a daunting task to ensure compliance with all of them. Having a formal compliance plan is key to surviving the regulatory maze. Think of a compliance plan as your practice's or facility's policies that ensure regulations are followed and use it as a check-sheet to ensure that staff and care providers in your office or facility are following your own policies, which in turn ensure the following of rules and regulations. A compliance plan should include

- A named compliance officer—a staff member who monitors new regulations, monitors existing ones, and is the "go-to" person, should an incident occur that is not in compliance with the plan
- Written policies that cover, at a minimum,
  - Routine daily operations (registration, scheduling, human resources, etc.)
  - File backup

- Computer access (both physical access and access to software and databases)
- Release of patient information
- Breach of confidentiality, including unauthorized disclosure
- Security breaches, internal and external
- Coding and billing (including anti-fraud and anti-abuse practices)

Policies should be kept in a location accessible to all office staff. All policies should also include the disciplinary process, should policies not be followed, intentionally or unintentionally.

An example of a policy statement regarding computer access and the use of passwords may read

Access to computer software, databases, and equipment shall be restricted to employees (including care providers) of Summit Bay Health Center. The extent to which access and rights are given is based on position description in order to carry out their job duties. Employees (including care providers) are required to keep their log-in user ID and password confidential; sharing with others is grounds for immediate disciplinary action, up to and including dismissal.

Reporting of compliance with promoting interoperability is also required; specific compliance strategies to conform with promoting interoperability will be covered later in this text.

The use of formal internal audits, which should be performed on every staff member (including care providers) on a periodic basis, not only allows the administrative staff to be proactive in finding and correcting problems but also serves as a reminder and an educational tool for staff.

7.11 Safeguarding Your System and Disaster Recovery Planning

Protecting computer hardware and software is as important as protecting the information within the systems. Computer crime, unauthorized access to information, and natural disasters are all security concerns that must be addressed in any healthcare organization that processes or stores digital data.

Written policies, as noted in Section 7.10, are deterrents at a very basic level—in particular, regarding controlling access. Restricting access in offices or areas where computers are present to employees only, turning computer screens away from public view, and shredding printed documents that include patient information are all examples. Encryption of data is necessary to deter unauthorized access to what is documented. Tracking the computer accesses of all employees on a periodic basis helps ensure that access is only on a need-to-know basis. Carefully screening job applicants and verifying previous employment are additional important screening mechanisms since people are the greatest threat to computer security.

Backing up data on a daily basis is crucial. Backup can be made to online secondary storage, hard disk, optical disk, magnetic tape, and/or flash memory. A key component of backup is that the backed-up files should be stored at an off-site location. Should a fire or flood occur in your office, and the backup files also become damaged by the flood, they will do little good.

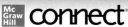
Perform a Backup of Data in EHRclinic

At the end of each day, Summit Bay Health Center's office manager performs a backup of data. Doing so protects the clinical, financial, and administrative records in the event of a problem with the system or a disaster occurs.

Follow these steps to complete the exercise on your own once you have watched the demonstration and tried the steps with helpful prompts in practice mode. Use the information provided in the scenario to complete the information.

1. Click on 'Take backup' button.
2. Click on 'Backup my data' button.
3. Click on 'Proceed' button.

✓ **You have completed Exercise 7.11**

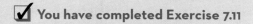

Over the past few years, worldwide disasters have shown the need for having a **disaster recovery plan**. The plan must be written, and staff must know what to do in the event of a disaster that affects the computer systems within the facility (Williams and Sawyer).

At a minimum, the plan should include

- An accounting of all functions that are performed electronically within the office
- A listing of all computer hardware, software, and data related to each of those functions
- The specific location of the backup files and the format used for the backup
- Step-by-step procedures for restoring the backed-up data
- An alert system to notify personnel of the disaster
- Required security training for all personnel

Unfortunately, many facilities lack a disaster recovery plan and may not realize its importance until a data loss, security breach, or other disaster occurs. Not only should facilities have a plan, but they should actually carry out the plan periodically as any other disaster plan would be practiced.

The importance of keeping *all* computerized functions safe, confidential, and secure cannot be overstated.

disaster recovery plan A written document that details an inventory of hardware and software, backup procedure, including location of backup files, the system used to alert users of the disaster, required security training for personnel, and procure for restoring backup files.

APPLYING YOUR SKILLS

Write a timeline and summary of the regulations that govern the collection, storage, and release of health information kept in an electronic format. Keeping in mind paper records versus electronic records, why was there a need for more stringent rules?

chapter 7 **Summary**

LEARNING OUTCOME	CONCEPTS FOR REVIEW

7.1 Identify the HIPAA privacy and security standards.	– HIPAA passed in 1996
	– Contains Privacy and Security Rules, among others
	– HITECH made HIPAA rules more stringent and gave government authorities the power to enforce the privacy and security rules
	– Omnibus Final Rule to HITECH went into effect March 2013 with compliance required in September 2013
	– Enhancements were made to patient privacy and patient rights, strengthened enforcement of the law, and allowed more control over business associates
	– Fines for privacy breaches were increased
	– Providers using an EHR must provide patients with electronic copies of their records when requested
	– Patients paying by cash may instruct the provider not to bill their insurance and not to divulge any information regarding the treatment to the insurance company
	– The intent is to ensure that protected health information (PHI) is private and secure
	– Covered entities include any healthcare facilities, health plans, clearinghouses, and other businesses that handle PHI
	– Only the minimum necessary information may be released
	– Standards include
	  • Define directory information
	  • Use of authorization to release PHI
	  • Enforce minimum necessary information release
	– Password configuration and protection
	– Appointment of a privacy and/or security officer
	– System configured to minimize the number of log-in attempts
	– Protection from viruses and malware
	– Use of security audits to monitor access
	– Policy to address remote access to the system
	– Policy on use and protection of hardware, particularly wireless devices
	– Written policy and procedures on breach notification
	– Staff education

7.2 Evaluate an EHR system for HIPAA compliance.	– Password protection – Use of unique identifier for each user – Access to PHI only for those who have a need to know – Accounting of all disclosures (internal and external) – Security policy that addresses backup of data, storage, and restoration of backed-up data – Ability to audit by user or by patient who has accessed a record, and which areas of the record were viewed, edited, or deleted – Use of code sets—ICD-10-CM/PCS, CPT®, and HCPCS—to store and transmit information

LEARNING OUTCOME	CONCEPTS FOR REVIEW
7.3 Describe the role of certification in EHR implementation.	– HIMSS—Health Information and Management Systems Society – AHIMA—American Health Information Management Association – CMS and the Office of the National Coordinator for Health Information Technology (ONC) – Independent agencies
7.4 Apply procedures to set up security measures in EHRclinic.	– Add new clinical users – Assign password to new clinical users – Set up a care provider's user rights – Assign user rights to a healthcare professional (medical assistant for example) – Assign user rights to an office manager – Create a group – Set general system-wide security requirements – Run an audit trail report
7.5 Follow proper procedures to access sensitive or restricted-access records.	– Sensitive information may or may not be clinical in nature but is embarrassing in nature; therefore, the record is flagged – Restricted-access records are marked as such, so that only select providers or staff may access them
7.6 Apply procedures to ensure data integrity.	– Integrity of data can be ensured only if it is complete, accurate, consistent, and timely and has not been altered, destroyed, or accessed by unauthorized individuals – Strict organization-wide policies that are adhered to must be in place – Amendments and deletions to entries must be obvious, and the original format must remain – Amend a chart entry – Hide a chart entry – Recover a hidden chart entry
7.7 Apply procedures to release health information using EHRclinic.	– Release of information is necessary for a multitude of reasons, including continuity of care – Authorization to release information may be required and must be addressed in written organization policies – Must account for all disclosures to comply with HITECH
7.8 Account for data disclosures using EHRclinic.	– Internal and external disclosures of PHI must be accounted for – Run a report of information disclosures from a patient's chart

(continued)

LEARNING OUTCOME	CONCEPTS FOR REVIEW
7.9 Exchange information with outside healthcare providers for continuity of care using EHRclinic.	- Promoting interoperability (meaningful use) standards require exchange of information between providers for smooth continuation of care - Sharing of electronic information must be through secure means - Exchange information for continuity of care using EHRclinic
7.10 Outline the content of compliance plans.	- Healthcare organizations must have written compliance plans that address how the organization ensures compliance with all regulations governing operation of the organization as well as privacy, security, meaningful use, and general health information regulations - Written policies must be kept and available to all staff at all times
7.11 Appraise the importance of disaster recovery planning.	- Contingency plan is equivalent to a backup plan, should the system fail or a natural or other disaster occur - All potential security concerns should be addressed with a detailed backup plan - Importance of written disaster recovery plan

MATCHING QUESTIONS

Match the terms on the left with the definitions on the right.

_____ 1. **[LO 7.7]** breach of confidentiality

_____ 2. **[LO 7.1]** confidentiality

_____ 3. **[LO 7.1]** hardware

_____ 4. **[LO 7.4]** audit trail

_____ 5. **[LO 7.1]** computer virus

_____ 6. **[LO 7.1]** covered entity

_____ 7. **[LO 7.1]** password

_____ 8. **[LO 7.11]** disaster recovery plan

_____ 9. **[LO 7.1]** directory information

_____ 10. **[LO 7.1]** encryption

a. person or group who has legal right to access protected health information by virtue of being a healthcare provider, clearinghouse, or health insurance plan

b. private, secure code that allows a user access to computer systems and software

c. security measure in which words are scrambled and can only be read if the receiving computer has the code to read the message

d. listing of patient information, such as hospital room number

e. documentation for addressing critical issues in the event of a crisis

f. permanent record of the changes made to various documents; available even after files are deleted

g. break or failure of security measures that results in information being compromised

h. devices such as laptops, PDAs, and desktop computers that are at risk for theft

i. keeping information about a patient to oneself

j. deviant program, stored on a computer floppy disk, hard drive, or CD, that can destroy or corrupt data

MULTIPLE-CHOICE QUESTIONS

Select the letter that best completes the statement or answers the question:

1. **[LO 7.7]** In the event of a breach, who may be held responsible?
   a. providers
   b. office staff
   c. the facility
   d. all of these

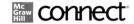

Enhance your learning by completing these exercises and more at **https://connect.mheducation.com!**

2. **[LO 7.1]** Which of the following would be considered a covered entity?
   a. healthcare provider
   b. friend
   c. significant other
   d. teacher

3. **[LO 7.4]** Of the following, which factor contributes to the user rights allowed a user?
   a. annual job performance
   b. job description
   c. level of education
   d. number of patients seen

4. **[LO 7.11]** It is critical that backup files be stored
   a. in paper form.
   b. off-site.
   c. on-site.
   d. with the originals.

5. **[LO 7.8]** HITECH regulations require that _____ information releases are accounted for.
   a. all
   b. external
   c. internal
   d. no

6. **[LO 7.2]** According to HIPAA regulations, healthcare providers must use _____, as opposed to written documentation, to store and transmit information to insurance carriers.
   a. CPT® codes
   b. ICD-10 codes
   c. HCPCS codes
   d. all of these

7. **[LO 7.3]** Promoting Interoperability standards require offices to select an EHR that is
   a. certified.
   b. comprehensive.
   c. fast.
   d. simple.

8. **[LO 7.7]** Releasing information without proper authorization is called a/an
   a. breach of confidentiality.
   b. breach of trust.
   c. information breach.
   d. security breach.

9. **[LO 7.6]** When a document is amended in an EHR, the original documentation is
   a. deleted.
   b. hidden.
   c. printed.
   d. visible.

10. **[LO 7.10]** An office's compliance manual should be kept in a/an _____ location.
    a. accessible
    b. external
    c. electronic
    d. protected

11. **[LO 7.9]** The sharing of health information must be done in a _____ environment.
    a. healthcare
    b. private
    c. public
    d. secure

12. **[LO 7.4]** Under a care provider's order, medical assistants and nurses _____ allowed to send an ePrescription or call in a refill prescription to a pharmacy.
    a. are
    b. are not
    c. might be
    d. should not be

13. **[LO 7.1]** To help guard against security breaches, emails containing protected health information should be
    a. deleted.
    b. encrypted.
    c. forbidden.
    d. sent.

14. **[LO 7.3]** The mission of HIMSS is to
    a. develop competencies for health information education programs.
    b. ensure information security.
    c. lead healthcare transformation through the use of health information technology.
    d. train facilities on HIPAA regulations.

SHORT-ANSWER QUESTIONS

1. **[LO 7.2]** According to the ONC website, how does health information technology help care providers better manage patient care?

2. **[LO 7.7]** Define continuity of care.

3. **[LO 7.5]** If all health information is confidential, explain why it may still be necessary to mark some health records as "sensitive" or "restricted."

4. **[LO 7.6]** Why must a user enter her password in order to change a chart entry in EHRclinic?

5. **[LO 7.10]** List at least six pieces of information that must be included in an office's compliance plan.

6. **[LO 7.11]** List the six pieces of information that form the minimum requirements of a disaster recovery plan.

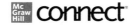 Enhance your learning by completing these exercises and more at **https://connect.mheducation.com**!

7. **[LO 7.4]** When new physicians or employees are hired in a physician's practice, the office manager or office administrator typically has the responsibility to set the physician or employee up in the PM and EHR system(s) as part of the security measures. Explain each type of security role in EHRclinic.

8. **[LO 7.3]** What does it mean if an EHR system has been certified by the Office of the National Coordinator?

9. **[LO 7.1]** Explain what a security audit is and list one example of when a security audit might need to take place.

10. **[LO 7.9]** Explain one advantage of using an EHR for communicating with other healthcare providers, as discussed in the text.

11. **[LO 7.10]** What is the best way to ensure that your office staff are following all the different regulatory bodies governing healthcare?

12. **[LO 7.8]** Why must an office manager account for all information released, including that released internally?

13. **[LO 7.4]** Would a care provider and a medical assistant be assigned the same rights in EHRclinic? Why or why not?

14. **[LO 7.2]** List six things that an office's EHR team should keep in mind when rolling out a new system.

15. **[LO 7.11]** List three methods to safeguard computer hardware and software systems.

16. **[LO 7.1]** Give an example of when directory information would be needed.

APPLYING YOUR KNOWLEDGE

1. **[LOs 7.1, 7.9]** Discuss two advantages and two disadvantages of using email to send information between providers.

2. **[LOs 7.1, 7.2, 7.4, 7.10, 7.11]** Discuss why many practices require users to change their passwords after a specified period and why they do not allow users to reuse the same passwords over and over again.

3. **[LO 7.3]** Imagine that you are working in a small healthcare practice. Your supervisor has asked you to spearhead the adoption of an EHR program. Follow the link provided in the text to find the website listing certified EHRs. After browsing the site and looking at the sheer number of products listed, discuss some methods your healthcare office could use to choose the best EHR option.

4. **[LOs 7.6, 7.7]** Provide one example each of an internal and an external breach of confidentiality that might occur in a healthcare setting and list a possible consequence of each breach. (For example, letting a temporary employee access a patient's chart with your username would be an internal breach; a consequence could be that a patient's health information is compromised when a temp accidentally sends the patient's chart information out in an accidental "reply all" email.)

5. **[LOs 7.1, 7.4, 7.6, 7.10, 7.11]** You are in the office lounge getting some water. One of your colleagues is at her desk, working on a laptop. She gets up to join you at the water cooler. As the two of you are talking, another staff member sits down in your colleague's chair and begins using the laptop to check her email. What is wrong with this scenario?

6. **[LOs 7.1, 7.2, 7.4, 7.6, 7.7, 7.9]** Paul Davies presents to County Hospital's ER with an arm injury. He refuses to talk about how he sustained the injury and says he wants his medical records released to his sister, who will be coming to take him home. How would the objectives of an EHR make handling Mr. Davies' case easier?

7. **[LO 7.4]** Stephanie Byrd is a coder at Summit Bay Health Center. Her user ID is sbyrd. She recently got married and wants her user ID changed to slopez, to reflect her married name. Stephanie is told by the office administrator that once a user ID is assigned, it cannot be changed. Why can't the user ID be changed?

8. **[LO 7.1]** A local TV celebrity has been admitted to the local hospital. She states that she wants her admission to remain private and does not want her room number or the fact that she is there at all released to anyone but her sister, Mary Ann Green. The registration specialist in the ER tells her that is not possible and that if anyone goes to the information desk, he or she will be given her room number. If she does not wish to see the visitor, she will have to ask the nurses on the unit to put a "do not disturb" sign on the door of her room. Is this correct? Explain your answer.

chapter references

Abdelhak, M., Grostick, S., Hanken, M.A., and Jacobs, E. (2007). *Health Information: Management of a Strategic Resource* (3rd ed.). Philadelphia: Elsevier.

American Medical Association. (1995–2019). *HIPAA Violations and Enforcement.* Retrieved from https://www.ama-assn.org/practice-management/hipaa-violations-enforcement.

Centers for Medicare & Medicaid Services, Office for Civil Rights. *Collection Use and Disclosure Limitation. The HIPAA Privacy Rule in Electronic Health Information Exchange in a Networked Environment.* Retrieved from www.hhs.gov.

Certification Commission for Health Information Technology. (2011). Retrieved from http://www.cchit.org/.

CNN.com Entertainment. 27 Suspended for Clooney File Peek. Retrieved from http://www.cnn.com/2007/SHOWBIZ/10/10/clooney.records/.

Cox, J.W., Turner, K., and Zapotsky, M.C. "Virus Infects MedStar Health System's Computers, Forcing an Online Shutdown." *The Washington Post*, March 28, 2016.

Department of Health and Human Services. (2010, March 10). Proposed Establishment of Certification Programs for Health Information Technology; Proposed Rule. *Federal Register*, *75*(46): 11327–11373. Retrieved from http://edocket.access.gpo.gov/2010/2010-4991.htm.

Dimick, Chris. (2010, February). Empowered Patient: Preparing for a New Patient Interaction. *Journal of AHIMA*, *81*(2): 26–31.

HIPAA Journal. What Is the Civil Penalty for Knowingly Violating HIPAA? (2018). Retrieved from https://www.hipaajournal.com/civil-penalty-for-knowingly-violating-hipaa/.

Heubusch, Kevin. (2011, July). Access Report: OCR Tries Subtraction through Addition in Accounting of Disclosure Rule. *Journal of AHIMA*, *82*(7): 38–39.

HIMSS. (2016). *About HIMSS.* Retrieved from http://www.himss.org/ASP/aboutHimssHome.asp.

McGuireWoods. (2013). *HIPAA Final Omnibus Rule Implements Tiered Penalty Structure for HIPAA Violations.*

Miaoulis, William M. (2010, March). Access, Use, and Disclosure: HITECH's Impact on the HIPAA Touchstones. *Journal of AHIMA*, *81*(3): 38–39, 64.

Williams, B.K., and Sawyer, S.C. (2010). *Using Information Technology: A Practical Introduction to Computers & Communications* (9th ed.). New York: McGraw-Hill Companies.

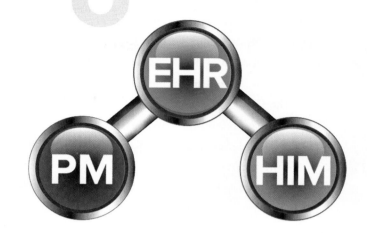

chapter **eight**

Management of Information and Communication

Learning Outcomes

At the end of this chapter, the student should be able to

8.1 Use software as an internal communication tool.

8.2 Differentiate the steps used to import documents using scanning technology.

8.3 Build master files and templates using EHRclinic.

8.4 Create custom screens within EHRclinic.

8.5 Develop a Task List within EHRclinic.

8.6 Set up system flags within EHRclinic.

Key Terms

Flags
Internet
Intranet
Live
Master file

Optical character recognition (OCR)
Resolution
Scanner
Templates

What You Need to Know and Why You Need to Know It

So far in this text, we have mainly looked at the collection of data, which in turn becomes information about a patient. In this chapter, we will look at communicating that information. The information collected in a healthcare environment is shared with external sources such as other healthcare providers, public health agencies, Medicare, Medicaid, insurance companies, and professional organizations. The information included may be in the form of a summary of a patient's record; a report that answers a question, such as the local public health office asking how many cases of flu-related illnesses were seen during a given time period; or a piece of correspondence from one care provider to another. Additionally, the communication may be internal—within the facility. With PM and EHR software, communicating internally through the use of an internal email system is efficient. Information is key to almost everything we do, personally and professionally, so having the information we need at our fingertips and communicating that information accurately and in a timely fashion are key to a well-run organization. Taking it a step further, patients who receive timely, accurate information and who experience good communication within the practice will have more confidence in the practice as a whole.

Internet A series of networks that allow instant access to information from around the world.

Intranet A secure environment or private internal network that is available only to a select group (e.g., the staff within an organization).

8.1 | Internal Communications

The **Internet** is a series of networks that allow instant access to information from around the world. Some Internet sites are private, requiring a user ID and password to gain access, and some are public sites that can be viewed by anyone. Within an organization, however, an **intranet** exists. An intranet is a secure environment or private internal network that is available only to a select group, such as the staff within the organization. The following table lists examples of what might be shared on an intranet site.

Facility's mission and value statements	Directory of staff and care providers	Compliance officer's name and contact information
Policies and procedures	FAQs	Forms, publications, and newsletters
Organization charts	Office meeting minutes	Calendar of events
Link to the IT department		Internal webmail links

The intranet is a one-stop-shop for staff and providers of a practice or other healthcare organizations to gain access to all the information they need to stay informed, as well as a way to send and receive messages among colleagues. Of course, someone (usually a webmaster) has to keep the information up to date; outdated information is not information at all. There is no benefit to having an intranet that contains outdated information. When staff starts noticing that the site is not being kept current, they will stop accessing it and sharing information. If your current employer has an intranet, take some time to navigate it—look there for the information listed in this section as well as other useful information.

The use of internal messaging improves communication within an office. It is particularly helpful for avoiding the "no one ever told me" syndrome. When internal email is used to communicate work-related information, and is not cluttered with personal communications, it is even more valuable. Many organizations have policies regarding use of the office email account; though they may not mandate that it cannot be used as a personal means of communication, such use is most likely frowned upon and may lead to more stringent policies. Some offices use a priority rating on their work-related emails. This is particularly helpful to care providers in sifting out what needs to be done immediately versus what can wait for a later time. High-priority messages include patient care matters, those of medium priority include changes in meeting dates or time-sensitive information, and low-priority messages might be information such as that lunch is ready in the lounge. When establishing rules for the priority system, everyone should at least be clear on what *is* or *is not* considered high priority. Remember that if everything is marked as urgent, or high priority, then there is no way to differentiate an item that should truly take priority.

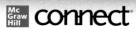

Go to https://connect.mheducation.com to complete this exercise. To see instructional notes with the steps, visit the eBook in Connect or download them from www.mhhe.com/iehr4.

EXERCISE 8.1

Send an Electronic Message Using EHRclinic Messaging

In this exercise, we will look at carrying out an internal communication using EHRclinic. In this exercise, Dr. Ingram is to attend an EMR meeting, but the date and time have been changed to Thursday at 3:30 p.m. In this instance, the message would be sent only to Dr. Ingram; if the message were for all the care providers, it would be sent using a group rather than typing in one name.

Follow these steps to complete the exercise on your own once you have watched the demonstration and tried the steps with helpful prompts in practice mode. Use the information provided in the scenario to complete the information.

1. Click on 'Messages' module.
2. Click on 'Compose mail' button.
3. Click on 'To' field and enter 'ing'.
4. Select 'jingram@sbhc.com'.
5. Click on 'Subject' field and enter 'EMR Meeting'.
6. Click on 'Text area' and enter 'Just as a reminder, the EMR meeting this week has been moved to Thursday at 3:30 p.m.'.
7. Click on 'Send' button.

for your information

The terms *electronic medical record (EMR)* and *electronic health record (EHR)* are often used interchangeably. At Summit Bay Health Center, EMR is the preferred terminology.

✓ **You have completed Exercise 8.1**

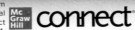
Send an Urgent Patient Message Using EHRclinic Messaging

Jason Peterson called the office asking for a call back from Dr. Ingram as soon as possible. His wife, Amy Peterson, fell in the kitchen this morning and is now complaining of a headache. Mr. Peterson is concerned that she may have hit her head.

This is an example of a message that should be given higher priority over most other messages. Dr. Ingram may want to have Mr. Peterson bring her to the office today, or he may advise that she go to the emergency department for evaluation.

Follow these steps to complete the exercise on your own once you have watched the demonstration and tried the steps with helpful prompts in practice mode. Use the information provided in the scenario to complete the information.

1. Click on 'Messages' module.
2. Click on 'Compose mail' button.
3. Click on 'To' field and enter 'ing'.
4. Select 'jingram@sbhc.com'.
5. Click on 'Subject' field and enter 'Amy Peterson'.
6. Click on 'Add patient chart' button.
7. Click on 'Search patient by first name/last name/chart no./ DOB (mm/dd/yyyy)' field and enter 'pet'.
8. Click on 'Amy Peterson' patient.
9. Click on 'Add' button.
10. Click on 'Choose template' button.
11. Click on 'Cancel' button.
12. Click on 'Text area' and enter the following details:
    - Patient:Amy Peterson
    - DOB:07/15/1950
    - Chart #:AA007
    - Caller:Jason Peterson (husband)
    - Contact Number:(567)555-0082
    - Message:Mr. Peterson states that his wife fell in the kitchen this morning and is now complaining of a headache.
13. Click on 'Mark as urgent' checkbox.
14. Click on 'Send' button.

☑ **You have completed Exercise 8.2**

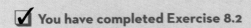

8.2   **Importing Documents to the EHR**

Communication involves many forms other than email messages. Reports, test results, and verifications of insurance coverage, just to name a few, are communicated many times throughout the day. These reports may be sent to the practice in digital or hard-copy format but, in the end, must be merged with the appropriate patient's electronic medical record.

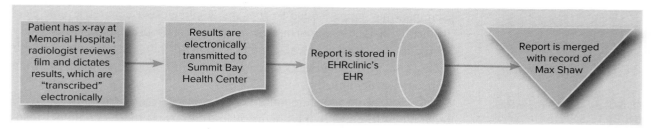

Figure 8.1   Flow of Report from Hospital to Merging with Appropriate Record in EHRclinic

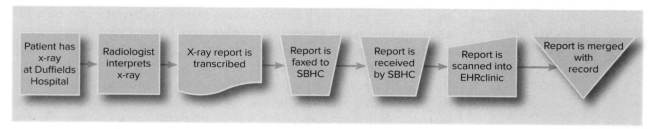

Figure 8.2   Flow of Faxed Report from Hospital to EHRclinic

For example, Dr. Ingram sent Max Shaw to Memorial Hospital for a chest x-ray. The x-ray is completed and the report of the radiologist's findings is sent electronically to Summit Bay Health Center. It then needs to be merged with (attached to) the patient's chart; the flow of this is depicted in Figure 8.1.

Not all documents can be sent electronically, however. Let's say a patient, David Malone, had his chest x-ray at Duffields Hospital, which does not yet have electronic capability. Instead, the report of the x-ray findings is in hard-copy form only. It can be faxed, mailed, or picked up from the hospital by a staff member. Since the goal of Summit Bay Health Center is a paperless office with a unit record for all patients, a hard-copy image needs to be manually scanned into the EHR once it arrives at the office (Figure 8.2).

When a hard-copy document needs to be sent electronically the healthcare professional uses a **scanner** to save the image. This is done by feeding the paper copy through a document scanner such as the one seen in Figure 8.3 or uses a flat-bed scanner, where the document is laid flat on the screen, similar to a photocopier. The image is digitized into a format that is readable by a computer. Various prompts that appear on the computer screen are followed, and finally, the electronic version of the document is merged with the correct patient's electronic record within EHRclinic. Care must be taken in this process because just as a hard-copy document can be misfiled, so can a scanned image. Before a scanned image is attached to a patient's health record, the healthcare professional verifies that the correct patient and correct visit are selected. Also, the type of document (correspondence, authorization, history, or physical exam, for

Scanner A piece of equipment that digitizes documents into a format that is readable by a computer.

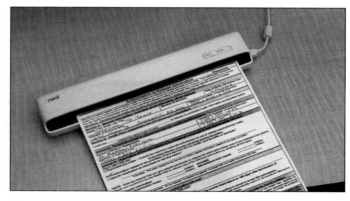

Figure 8.3   Scanner Used to Import a Document
Image: McGraw Hill Education

example) may be bar-coded so that the document is easily retrievable electronically. It is also important to remember that, although it is necessary to include relevant medical documentation in patients' electronic health records, scanned documents take up "space," or memory, so avoid scanning unnecessary documents.

The scanning of documents utilizes **optical character recognition (OCR)** technology to convert the document into a format that is computer-readable. It is important to ensure that scanned images are as good as the originals. This is known as **resolution**, in which the higher the resolution, the better the quality of the image. There are other scanning functions that you may be aware of and not even realize it—in a grocery store, for instance, the cashier passes the bar code from a can of green beans across a small light source, scanning the bar code, so that the computer reads it as a 15.5-ounce can of green beans with a price of $1.25. In that case, the optical reader reads a bar code rather than words. This process not only results in a price for the item but is also part of an inventory control system—the persons responsible for re-order now know that there is one fewer can of beans on the shelf.

8.3 Master Files and Templates

Care providers and all other healthcare professionals are extremely busy. Their first concern is the patient, not documentation, but documentation is essential to patient care. So to make documenting easier and faster, **master files** (datasets that provide structure and are the building blocks for parts of the chart notes) and **templates** (preformatted documents built into practice management [PM] and electronic health record [EHR] systems) are used. Master files and templates are used often in an electronic health record system, for instance, when documenting a history and physical exam. Figure 8.4 is an example of a master file for selecting conditions in a patient's past medical history.

At Summit Bay Health Center, before the EHR went **live**, staff members built these master files with input from care providers. Master files list common conditions and diagnoses that patients at Summit Bay Health Center have had. Diagnoses can be added to an individual's record, or to the master file itself. Other master files in EHRclinic include PE (physical exam), ROS (review of systems), orders, diagnosis favorites, and HPI (history of present illness).

Building templates within the system is an administrative task that is done prior to going live, but templates can be edited as necessary. These preformatted documents allow screenshots to be built, letters to be written, and progress notes to appear out of individual selections from master files. Care providers may prefer their documentation to look a certain way, so a practice that has five care providers may have five templates for written progress notes. Templates can also be used to facilitate return-to-work or school notes, draft letters to patients, document lab results, and assist with a number of other functions.

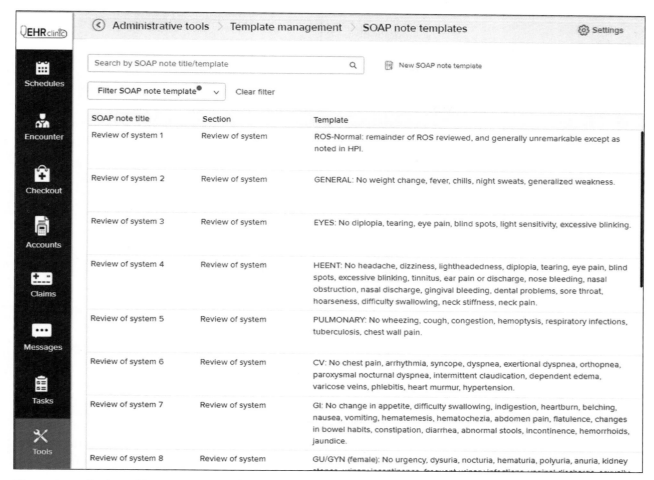

Figure 8.4   Review of System Master File

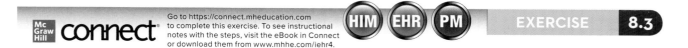

Go to https://connect.mheducation.com to complete this exercise. To see instructional notes with the steps, visit the eBook in Connect or download them from www.mhhe.com/iehr4.

HIM   EHR   PM

EXERCISE   8.3

Build a Master File in EHRclinic

To build or revise a master file in EHRclinic, the Tools module will be accessed and then Review of Systems will be selected from the SOAP note templates menu. In this exercise, we will build the master file for Review of Systems (ROS). The end product will indicate what this care provider wants as the default values (the values that automatically appear in a field on the ROS screen and appear each time he sees a patient). For instance, the care provider wants the default value for weight loss to be a negative response; in other words, if a patient is asked if she has experienced unexplained weight loss, most of the time the answer will be no; therefore, this response will show as (-) weight loss on the ROS screen.

Setting up these default values is done from the Tools module within the Template management menu.

Follow these steps to complete the exercise on your own once you have watched the demonstration and tried the steps with helpful prompts in practice mode.

1. Click on 'Manage templates' button.
2. Click on 'SOAP note templates' button.

(continued)

3. Click on 'Filter SOAP note template' drop-down and select 'Review of system' option.
4. Click on 'Close' button.
5. Click on 'New SOAP notes template' button.
6. Click on 'SOAP note field' drop-down and select 'SOAP notes: Review of system'.
7. Click on 'Title' field and enter 'Patient symptoms'.
8. Click on 'Template' field and enter 'Patient is c/o the following symptoms:'.
9. Click on 'Add template' button.
10. Click on 'New SOAP notes template' button.
11. Click on 'SOAP note field' drop-down and select 'SOAP notes: Review of system'.
12. Click on 'Title' field and enter 'Past medical history'.
13. Click on 'Template' field and enter 'Patient's past medical history includes:'.
14. Click on 'Add template' button.
15. Click on 'Template management' button.

☑ **You have completed Exercise 8.3**

8.4 Customization

Care providers, registration staff, medical assistants, nurses, therapists, billers, and coders all use the information in the PM and EHR software. But not all of the users "see" things the same way. The way subsets of information display in relation to one another on a computer screen is often most effective when the user is satisfied with how the information appears. Many PM and EHR software packages include the flexibility to allow the customization of screen configurations, and EHRclinic is no exception. Care providers, and healthcare professionals in general, will be more accepting of an EHR if they know they have some say in the appearance of the information and can customize it to meet the needs of the facility.

EXERCISE 8.4

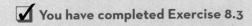

Go to https://connect.mheducation.com to complete this exercise. To see instructional notes with the steps, visit the eBook in Connect or download them from www.mhhe.com/iehr4.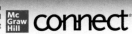

Customize a Facesheet Screen

We will now look at a couple of exercises in which customization is possible. The first task is to customize a Facesheet screen. In this scenario, the healthcare professional is going to customize a facesheet. He starts by entering the User Settings Admin within the System Set-up module that is in the Chart menu. Watch as he chooses the elements that will show on the facesheet and then how he changes the order in which they appear.

Follow these steps to complete the exercise on your own once you have watched the demonstration and tried the steps with helpful prompts in practice mode.

1. Click on 'Tools' module.
2. Click on 'Manage reports' button.

198

3. Click on 'Patient charts and graphs' button.

4. Click on 'Alexis Shaw's' info.

5. Click on 'Collapse all' button.

6. Click on 'Expand patient info' header (+).

7. Click on 'Expand patient medical history' header (+).

8. Click on 'Expand surgical history' header (+).

9. Click on 'Expand social history' header (+).

10. Click on 'Expand medication list' header (+).

11. Click on 'Expand list of notes' header (+).

12. Click on 'Add new note' button.

13. Click on 'Note title' button and enter 'Facesheet'.

14. Click on 'Note' button and enter 'Customized facesheet'.

15. Click on 'Done' button.

16. Click on 'Chart and graphs' cancel button.

☑ **You have completed Exercise 8.4**

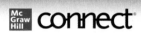 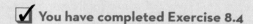

Go to https://connect.mheducation.com to complete this exercise. To see instructional notes with the steps, visit the eBook in Connect or download them from www.mhhe.com/iehr4.

EXERCISE **8.5**

Customize User Preferences in EHRclinic

In addition to the facesheet, user preferences can also be customized to desired font size and preferred units of measurement (US customary or Metric units).

In this exercise, you will change the font to large and choose Metric units to change your user preferences.

Follow these steps to complete the exercise on your own once you have watched the demonstration and tried the steps with helpful prompts in practice mode.

1. Click on 'Settings' button.

2. Click on 'Increase font size button' to Large.

3. Click on 'Metric unit' radio button.

4. Click on 'Save' button.

☑ **You have completed Exercise 8.5**

8.5 Using Software to Organize Your Work—Task Lists

With all the requirements we deal with in healthcare, having help with organizational skills is certainly an advantage! In EHRclinic, there is a functionality called Task List or Tasks, whereby a care provider or other healthcare professional assigns tasks to another staff member or to an entire group. For instance, Dianna Pike, a care provider, wants a particular report to be run by the office administrator, Jon Daniels. The request is simply put into Jon's Task List, so that he is aware that he has a task to complete. Or a task—for instance, the completion of a computerized in-service—that needs to be completed by an entire group such as the health information department staff can be assigned to the group rather than to each individual, saving the office administrator much time and ensuring that everyone gets the *same* message.

Some examples of tasks include

- Calling patients to change appointments due to the change in a provider's vacation dates
- Registering for an upcoming seminar
- Calling a patient regarding the need for a follow-up laboratory test
- Making reservations for the office holiday party
- Ordering supplies or equipment

As you can see, the tasks may not be clinical; they can be anything that needs to be done by an individual or individuals in the practice.

EXERCISE 8.6   Go to https://connect.mheducation.com to complete this exercise. To see instructional notes with the steps, visit the eBook in Connect or download them from www.mhhe.com/iehr4.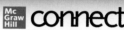

Create a Task for the Receptionist

In the scenario that follows, Dr. Ingram left the following message on your workstation:

Will you please ask Diane to contact EHRclinic and arrange a training session covering ePrescribe? I would like to have this done between June 1 and July 31. Thanks!

In this exercise, you will assign Dr. Ingram's request to the medical receptionist, Diane Baxter, for completion by April 15, 2022. While you are assigning this task, you notice that the task to send referral thank-you notes is still open from last week and needs to be marked as complete.

This function also allows the user to select the priority of the task—high, medium, or low. Practice policy may dictate what circumstances dictate each, and whether prioritization is used at all.

Follow these steps to complete the exercise on your own once you have watched the demonstration and tried the steps with helpful prompts in practice mode. Use the information provided in the scenario to complete the information.

1. Click on 'Tasks' module.
2. Click on 'New task' button.
3. Click on 'Task' field and enter 'Contact EHRclinic and arrange ePrescribe training between June 1 and July 31'.
4. Click on 'Assign to drop down' button and select 'Diane Baxter'.
5. Click on datepicker (calendar) icon in 'Due date' field and select 'April 15, 2022'.
6. Click on 'Add task' button.
7. Click on 'Send February referral thank you notes due on 03/25/2022' checkbox to mark it as completed.

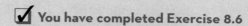 You have completed Exercise 8.6

8.6 Using Software as a Reminder

If you work in healthcare, you have a lot to remember, as you have already seen. It would be next to impossible to remember every situation about every patient. However, using the functionality of PM or EHR software, including EHRclinic, makes keeping on top of everything easier by including alerts, or reminders, in a patient's chart through a series of flag alerts (reminders) or icons, each of which has a particular meaning.

Flags can be added in the system in the Notes area of the patient's Facesheet and be used for all patients. Examples of common flags include these:

Flag A message that appears on a screen in written form or as an icon to serve as a reminder to staff and care providers.

- Patient frequently cancels appointments
- Phone number on file is no longer in service
- Confidentiality messages (such as do not leave message on home phone)
- Co-pay is required (and can include amount)
- Patient is noncompliant
- Account in collections
- Do not charge late fee
- Payment plan set up
- Allergic to penicillin (can have several different medications)
- Environmental allergy to _____
- Sensitive information contained in chart
- Clinical alerts
  - Bone density scan due
  - Diabetic patient
  - Requires patient education
  - Pap smear due

A flag can be set up in the system for just about anything the office sees a need for. A word of caution, though: Do not set up so many flags that it is difficult to remember their meaning or that the alert becomes the rule rather than the exception and therefore is ignored.

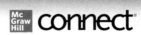 Go to https://connect.mheducation.com to complete this exercise. To see instructional notes with the steps, visit the eBook in Connect or download them from www.mhhe.com/iehr4.

EXERCISE 8.7

Assign a Note (Flag) to a Patient's Chart

In this exercise, you will set up a system flag for a patient. In this case, Mark Shaw is allergic to latex, so the healthcare professional will add that flag to Mark's chart.

Follow these steps to complete the exercise on your own once you have watched the demonstration and tried the steps with helpful prompts in practice mode. Use the information provided in the scenario to complete the information.

1. Click on 'Manage reports' button.
2. Click on 'Patient charts and graphs' button.

(continued)

3. Click on 'Search by patient first name/last name/chart number/SSN' field and enter 'sha'.
4. Click on 'Mark Shaw's' info.
5. Click on 'Add new note' button.
6. Click on 'Note title' button and enter 'Flag'.
7. Click on 'Note' button and enter 'Allergic to latex'.
8. Click on 'Done' button.

As you can see, computerization of the practice management and health record functions has many other benefits to care providers and staff than just maintenance of the information they collect. The use of software streamlines the processes and increases efficiency.

✓ **You have completed Exercise 8.7**

APPLYING YOUR SKILLS

Virginia Park called Dr. Hilliard today. He was looking at her medical history in her EHR, then sent an email to his nurse from within the history section of EHRclinic. The body of the email read "Jane, Ms. Park has called five times with the same questions. I'm tired of her calling me. Please take care of this—I have better things to do than to deal with a hypochondriac."

Could this become an issue for Dr. Hilliard? Defend your answer.

chapter 8 **summary**

LEARNING OUTCOME	CONCEPTS FOR REVIEW
8.1 Use software as an internal communication tool.	– Difference between Internet and intranet – Examples of information commonly shared on an intranet – Send a message using EHRclinic
8.2 Differentiate the steps used to import documents using scanning technology.	– Reports within a chart are a type of communication – Documents may be imported from within EHRclinic or from an external source – Scanning a document involves a process of feeding (or laying flat) the document in the scanner, then attaching the document to the appropriate patient's chart – Scanning digitizes documentation into readable format – Optical character recognition (OCR) allows scanned images to be edited
8.3 Build master files and templates using EHRclinic.	– Master file—list of possible choices such as a list of allergies, list of conditions, or list of surgeries – Templates allow for building an end product such as a progress note, a piece of correspondence, or a screen view – Build a master file for an ROS
8.4 Create custom screens within EHRclinic.	– Allow flexibility and personalization for individual users – Design a Facesheet view for a user
8.5 Develop a Task List within EHRclinic.	– Tasks are reminders that a job has been assigned – Can be made by any user – Can be a task set for a single user or a group – Assign a task to a user in EHRclinic
8.6 Set up system flags within EHRclinic.	– Flags are alerts, or reminders – Use them sparingly; otherwise, they no longer point out the exception to the rule but rather become the rule – Set up a flag on a patient's record in EHRclinic

MATCHING QUESTIONS

Match the terms on the left with the definitions on the right.

_____ 1. **[LO 8.6]** flag

_____ 2. **[LO 8.3]** default value

_____ 3. **[LO 8.3]** master file

_____ 4. **[LO 8.3]** templates

_____ 5. **[LO 8.1]** intranet

_____ 6. **[LO 8.3]** live

_____ 7. **[LO 8.2]** scanner

_____ 8. **[LO 8.2]** optical character recognition (OCR)

a. secure internal environment available only to a select group

b. device that digitizes documents into a format readable by computers

c. alert, or reminder, that appears in a patient's chart

d. dataset that provides structure and is the building block for parts of the chart notes

e. technology that converts a document into a computer-readable format

f. using something in real time

g. preassigned value that automatically appears in a field

h. preformatted documents built into an EHR or PM system

MULTIPLE-CHOICE QUESTIONS

Select the letter that best completes the statement or answers the question:

1. **[LO 8.1]** The Internet is _____ and an intranet is _____.
   a. public; private
   b. private; public
   c. private; private
   d. public; public

2. **[LO 8.2]** A hard-copy document is attached to a patient's electronic chart by
   a. copying.
   b. emailing.
   c. scanning.
   d. shredding.

3. **[LO 8.3]** Using templates makes it easier for care providers to focus on their first priority, which is
   a. documentation.
   b. patient care.
   c. office staff.
   d. training.

4. **[LO 8.4]** EHRclinic allows each user to _____ certain features to their liking.
   a. access
   b. customize
   c. delete
   d. revise

5. **[LO 8.1]** A facility needs to make sure that the information on its intranet does not become
   a. outdated.
   b. overused.
   c. private.
   d. secure.

6. **[LO 8.6]** It is _____ to have too many flags set up in EHRclinic.
   a. impossible
   b. possible
   c. necessary
   d. recommended

7. **[LO 8.3]** The Review of Systems menu choices in EHRclinic are an example of a/an
   a. index.
   b. master file.
   c. real-time menu.
   d. template.

8. **[LO 8.5]** A healthcare professional may assign work to another user with EHRclinic's _____ functionality.
   a. Assignment
   b. Groups
   c. Tasks
   d. Workload

9. **[LO 8.6]** Jane Howard often misses appointments; an alert is set to appear on her record; this alert is known as a/an _____ in EHRclinic.
   a. flag
   b. avatar
   c. decal
   d. symbol

10. **[LO 8.4]** Which of the following EHRclinic functions may be customized by a user?
    a. Access Rights
    b. Insurance Policies
    c. Patient Information
    d. Screen Layout

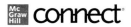

Enhance your learning by completing these exercises and more at https://connect.mheducation.com!

SHORT-ANSWER QUESTIONS

1. **[LO 8.1]** List four topics that might be found on an organization's intranet.

2. **[LO 8.3]** Can a medical office have more than one template for a referral letter? Explain.

3. **[LO 8.1]** What will happen if an office's intranet is not kept current? Be specific.

4. **[LO 8.3]** List four advantages of using master files and templates in a healthcare office.

5. **[LO 8.6]** List at least eight common flags used in EHRclinic.

6. **[LO 8.6]** Why might it be good to have a "Sensitive information contained in chart" alert pop up when users access specific patient charts?

7. **[LO 8.5]** Explain how using the Task List function in EHRclinic helps organize work.

8. **[LO 8.4]** Why might healthcare professionals be more accepting of an EHR if they are able to customize it in some way?

APPLYING YOUR KNOWLEDGE

1. **[LO 8.4]** How might a care provider "see" the information display in EHRclinic in the same way a patient registration staff member does?

2. **[LOs 8.1, 8.2, 8.6]** As office manager, what are some ways for you to ensure that staff members remember to attach hard-copy documents to the patient charts they are working on?

3. **[LO 8.3]** Discuss two advantages and any potential disadvantages to using templates for communication documents.

4. **[LOs 8.5, 8.6]** You are the office manager for a small practice. Since your office recently implemented an EHR system, you would like to have a staff training session to set forth guidelines and best practices for using system flags. Explain how you would use EHRclinic to assist you in your task and come up with four talking points about the proper use of flags and alerts.

5. **[LOs 8.3, 8.4]** Dr. Stewart hired a new associate, Dr. Reynolds, about six months ago. Dr. Reynolds has been trying without success to use EHRclinic efficiently. Though he likes the template method of documenting, he has found that much of what he prefers to document is not part of the existing templates, and he has to type freehand a lot of that data. He feels he is not paying as much attention to his patients as he should during visits because he is typing, and he is concerned that his E&M code levels are lower than they should be. He comes to you, the office manager, to vent his frustrations. What, if anything, can be done to make his use of EHRclinic more effective and efficient? Would any of this have an impact on Dr. Reynolds' E&M code levels?

chapter references

Williams, B.K., and Sawyer, S.C. (2015). *Using Information Technology: A Practical Introduction to Computers & Communications* (11th ed.). New York: McGraw-Hill Companies.

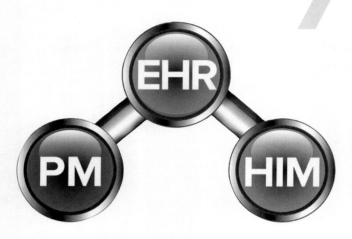

Promoting Interoperability and Compliance Support

Learning | Outcomes

At the end of this chapter, the student should be able to

9.1   Describe the uses of the dashboard in EHRclinic to meet Interoperability standards.

9.2   Explain how data and information are used in decision support.

9.3   Set up system reports using EHRclinic.

9.4   Set up custom reports using EHRclinic.

9.5   Illustrate uses for an index.

9.6   Describe uses for a registry.

9.7   Explain how data gathered in EHRclinic are used in the credentialing process.

Key | Terms

Aggregate

Benchmarking

Centers for Medicare and Medicaid Services (CMS)

Core objectives

Credentialing

Custom report

Dashboard

Detail report

Drug formulary

Drug Enforcement Agency (DEA) Number

Healthcare Integrity and Protection Data Bank (HIPDB)

Index

In-network

Menu objectives

Merit-based Incentive Payment System (MIPS)

National Practitioner Data Bank (NPDB)

Physician Quality Reporting System (PQRS)

Query

Registry

Summary report

Value-based payment modifier program

Variable

What You Need to Know and Why You Need to Know It

Running reports, supplying information to government agencies, and ensuring compliance with Meaningful Use, now known as the Promoting Interoperability Program, licensing agencies, Medicare/Medicaid rules, managed care plans, and accrediting agencies are all responsibilities of administrative personnel. This person may be an MA who is an office manager, a health information management (HIM) professional, or a healthcare administrator. Participation in the Promoting Interoperability Program will require the submission of data that show compliance with specific standards in order to receive incentive payments and avoid penalties based on the Merit-based Incentive Payment System (MIPS). In this chapter, we will cover EHRclinic functionality that proves compliance with the requirements of interoperability, the Medicare Quality Payment Program, licensing agencies, insurance providers, and state and federal regulation reporting requirements.

9.1 Using the Dashboard in EHRclinic to Meet Regulations and Standards

In order for eligible professionals and hospitals to receive stimulus money, as part of HITECH legislation, they have been required to successfully show meaningful use and interoperability of electronic health data. In other words, eligible professionals and hospitals that implemented (or upgraded) certified electronic health record systems and complied with the core and menu objectives (covered in this section) have been eligible for monetary grants and avoided penalties for noncompliance.

Promoting Interoperability (formerly Meaningful Use) was developed to ensure that the use of EHRs by healthcare providers would improve quality, safety, and efficiency, as well as reduce health disparities within healthcare. Specifically, Meaningful Use legislation was developed with the following health outcomes policy priorities in mind:

- Improving quality, safety, and efficiency, as well as reducing health disparities
- Engaging patients and families in their own health
- Improving the coordination of care
- Improving population and public health
- Ensuring adequate privacy and security protection for personal health information

The **Centers for Medicare & Medicaid Services (CMS)** administered the Meaningful Use program and developed a plan for implementing three stages within five years. Stage 1 of the evolution of Meaningful Use focused on data capturing and sharing and was effective with fiscal year (FY) 2011. The 15 Stage 1 **core objectives** that were required to show Meaningful Use of electronic health records are listed in Table 9.1. Stage 2 of Meaningful Use began in FY2013 for eligible hospitals and FY2014 for eligible providers. Its focus was meeting a certain number of core and menu objectives as outlined in Table 9.3 and Table 9.4, done in two stages. Starting in 2019, all eligible professionals, eligible hospitals, dual-eligible hospitals, and critical access hospitals are required to use the 2015 edition of **Certified Electronic Health Record Technology (CEHRT)** to meet the

Centers for Medicare & Medicaid Services (CMS) An agency of the Department of Health and Human Services, and it is responsible for developing and enforcing regulations that govern Medicare- and Medicaid-related issues.

Core objectives Basic functions or collection of data that should be completed on a patient's visit or hospitalization.

Certified Electronic Health Record Technology (CEHRT) A complement to Meaningful Use Stage 2; certification by the Office of the National Coordinator (ONC) of EHR software that meets certain standards.

requirements of the Promoting Interoperability Program (CMS Program Requirements).

Eligible professionals (EPs) and hospitals (including critical access hospitals, or CAHs) had to meet Stage 1 Meaningful Use of electronic health data before progressing to Stage 2. Though the final rule for Stage 2 was effective on September 4, 2012, implementation of Stage 2 requirements were extended through 2016, and Stage 3 began in 2018 for providers who completed at least two years in Stage 2.

TABLE 9.1	Medicare Core Objectives, 2011, Stage 1
Core Objective	**Explanation**
Use of computerized physician order entry (CPOE)	Medication orders made by care providers are done electronically rather than in writing in a paper record.
Drug–drug and drug–allergy checks	An alert system exists, based on the medications and allergies entered for a patient, for potential drug-to-drug or drug-to-allergy effects.
ePrescribing	Care providers place prescriptions electronically rather than by paper.
Recording of patient demographic information	The following demographics must be collected on all records: – Preferred language – Gender – Race – Ethnicity – Date of birth
Recording of a problem list	A list of all current and active diagnoses for which the patient is being treated
Recording of a medication list	A list of all current and active medications being taken by the patient—if the patient is on no medications, the record must reflect that as well
Recording of a medication allergy list	A list of medication(s) to which the patient is allergic
Recording of vital signs and patient measurements	On each visit, the following must be recorded: – Height – Weight – Blood pressure – Body Mass Index (BMI) – Maintenance of a growth chart (for children 2–20 years, including BMI)

Core Objective	Explanation
Recording of smoking status	For patients 13 years of age and older, smoking status must be recorded.
Clinical decision support functionality	At least one clinical decision support rule must be implemented. Example: A patient with a fasting blood sugar above 120 mg/dL may trigger an alert for diabetes mellitus, type 2.
Reporting clinical quality measures	Each provider must specify the Reporting Numerators, Denominators, and Exclusions for each quality measure reported.
Ability to exchange key clinical information between/among care providers	The capability to share among care providers such information as a problem list, medication list, allergies, and diagnostic test results
Ability to provide an electronic copy of health information	Patients must be provided with electronic health information upon request, including test results, problem list, medication list, and medication allergies.
Ability to provide clinical summaries	For each office visit, a clinical summary should be provided to each patient.
Privacy and security provisions	The software in use meets or exceeds standards set forth by the ONC Meaningful Use standards and includes technical specifications that ensure the privacy and confidentiality of information found in the database.

Source: Centers for Medicare & Medicaid Services. Medicare & Medicaid EHR Incentive Program: Meaningful Use Stage 1 Requirements. Retrieved from https://www.cms.gov/EHRIncentivePrograms /Downloads/MU_Stage1_ReqOverview.pdf.

For hospitals, the core objectives include all of those listed in the table *except* ePrescribing.

The 2011 **menu objectives** for Medicare included those listed in Table 9.2. Of the 10 listed, 5 needed to be met, 1 of which had to include a population/ public health measure.

Hospitals had to incorporate 5 of the 10 menu objectives listed in Table 9.2 to be eligible for incentive grants in 2011.

Menu objectives are additional functions that allow for greater use of EHR functionality—for instance, running statistical reports, registries, or lists; checking for drug interactions; and providing patients with educational materials about their illness. See Figure 9.1 for a Clinical Visit Summary given to a patient at the conclusion of a visit, satisfying the Summary of Care objective.

Menu objectives Additional functions that allow for greater use of EHR functionality.

TABLE 9.2   **Medicare Menu Objectives, 2011, Stage 1**

Drug formulary A list of provider-preferred generic and brand-name drugs covered under various insurance plans.

Menu Objective	Explanation
Drug-formulary checks	The office or hospital has access to at least one internal or external **drug formulary**.
Lab test results documented in the EHR	Results of laboratory tests ordered must be entered into the patient's EHR rather than being filed in paper format; results may be entered electronically through electronic data interchange, scanned into the record via manual scanning methods, or manually keyed into the record from the paper results.
Keeping of patient lists	The ability to generate a list of patients with a specific condition in order to satisfy quality improvement initiatives, reduce disparities, for research, or for outreach to patients with that diagnosis
Patient reminders generated	The ability to send reminder letters (or electronic reminders) for preventive and/or follow-up care
Timely electronic access	The ability to provide patients with their electronic record within four business days of the information being available in electronic form
Patient education	Access to educational resources using EHR technology and providing the resources to patients, if appropriate
Medication reconciliation	Documentation of medications the patient is taking as prescribed by other care providers
Summary of care	The care provider submits a summary of care to physicians or another healthcare facility that is assessing the patient or taking over the care of the patient.
Immunization registries	The capability to submit electronic data to immunization registries or other immunization information systems in accordance with applicable law
Syndromatic surveillance	The capability to submit electronic data to public health agencies in accordance with applicable law

Source: Centers for Medicare & Medicaid Services. Medicare & Medicaid EHR Incentive Program: Meaningful Use Stage 1 Requirements. Retrieved from https://www.cms.gov/EHRIncentivePrograms /Downloads/MU_Stage1_ReqOverview.pdf.

Medicaid-eligible providers (physicians, dentists, nurse midwives, nurse practitioners, and physicians' assistants in rural health clinics), with some restrictions based on percentage of patients who are covered by Medicaid, qualify for the full stimulus amount in the first year if a practice shows it has adopted, upgraded, or implemented EHR.

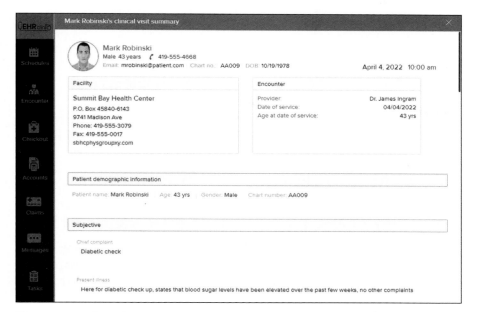

Figure 9.1   Clinical Visit Summary

Go to https://connect.mheducation.com to complete this exercise. To see instructional notes with the steps, visit the eBook in Connect or download them from www.mhhe.com/iehr4.

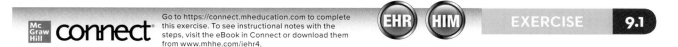

EXERCISE 9.1

Print a Clinical Visit Summary for a Patient

After his office visit on March 31, 2022, Mark Robinski asks for a copy of the details from his encounter. In this exercise, the healthcare professional will print Mr. Robinski's clinical visit summary.

Follow these steps to complete the exercise on your own once you have watched the demonstration and tried the steps with helpful prompts in practice mode. Use the information provided in the scenario to complete the information.

1. Click on 'Tools' module.
2. Click on 'Manage reports' button.
3. Click on 'Patient charts and graphs' button.
4. Click on 'Search by patient first name/last name/chart number/SSN' field and enter 'rob'.
5. Click on 'Mark Robinski's' info.
6. Click on 'Patient office visits 1' view button.
7. Click on 'Patient office visits' print button.
8. Click on 'Okay' button.
9. Click on 'Patient office visits' cancel button.
10. Click on 'Add new note' button.
11. Click on 'Note title' button and enter 'Clinical visit summary'.
12. Click on 'Note' button and enter 'Printed'.
13. Click on 'Done' button.
14. Click on 'chart and graphs' cancel button.

✓ **You have completed Exercise 9.1**

EHRclinic Tip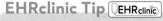

In some EHRclinic exercises, the Path window may obstruct areas you need to click. If this happens, you can collapse the Path within the window or click to hide it in the upper left corner of the screen.

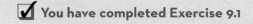

Table 9.3 lists the EP Core Objectives for Stage 2 as excerpted from the CMS Stage 1 vs. Stage 2 Comparison Table. All 17 were required to meet Stage 2 Meaningful Use.

TABLE 9.3	Eligible Professional (EP) Core Objectives: Stage 2 Meaningful Use
Stage 2 Explanation	**Comparison to Stage 1**
CPOE to be used for medication, laboratory, and radiology orders directly entered by any licensed healthcare professional who can enter orders into the medical record per state, local, and professional guidelines	Stage 1 addressed medications only, and at least 30% of unique patients had to have medication(s) ordered using CPOE. Stage 2 requires more than 60% of medication, 30% of laboratory, and 30% of radiology orders created by the EP during the EHR reporting period be recorded using CPOE.
Generate and transmit permissible prescriptions electronically (eRx)	Stage 1 required that more than 40% of permissible prescriptions written by an EP were transmitted electronically. Stage 2 requires more than 50% of all permissible prescriptions written by the EP to be compared to at least one drug formulary and transmitted electronically using Certified EHR Technology.
EHR must show evidence that the following demographics are included in the EHR of each patient: • Gender • Preferred language • Race • Ethnicity • Date of birth	Stage 1 required more than 50% of unique patients' EHR to show evidence of collection of the demographics collected in structured format. Stage 2 requires more than 80% of unique patients to have the demographics collected in structured format.
The following vital signs must be recorded: • Height • Weight • Blood pressure • Calculate and display BMI • Plot and display growth charts for children 2–20 years, including BMI	Stage 1 required more than 50% of all unique patients age 2 and over to show evidence of blood pressure, height, and weight recorded as structured data. Stage 2 requires more than 80% of unique patients to have blood pressure (for patients age 3 and over only) and height and weight (for all ages) recorded as structured data.
The smoking status of patients 13 years of age and older must be recorded as structured data.	Stage 1 required more than 50% of patients 13 years old or older to have smoking status recorded as structured data. Stage 2 requires more than 80% of patients 13 years old or older to have smoking status recorded as structured data.

Stage 2 Explanation	Comparison to Stage 1

Use clinical decision support to improve performance on high-priority health conditions.	Stage 1 required the EP to implement one clinical decision support rule.
	Stage 2 requires the following:
	  1. Five clinical decision support interventions related to four or more clinical quality measures, if applicable, be implemented at a relevant point in patient care for the entire EHR reporting period
	  2. The EP or hospital EHR has functionality for drug–drug and drug–allergy interaction checks be in place for the entire EHR reporting period

Provide patients the ability to view online, download, and transmit their health information within four business days of the information being available to the provider.	Stage 1 required that more than 50% of all patients who request an electronic copy of their health information be provided it within three business days. Stage 2 requires more than 50% of patients seen during the EHR reporting period be provided timely (available to the patient within four business days after the information is available to the provider) online access to their health information. And more than 5% of all patients seen during the EHR reporting period (or their authorized representative) be able to view, download, or transmit to a third party their health information.
Provide clinical summaries for patients for each office visit.	Stage 1 required that clinical summaries be provided to patients for more than 50% of all office visits within three business days. Stage 2 requires that clinical summaries be provided to patients within one business day for more than 50% of office visits.
Protect electronic health information created or maintained by the Certified EHR Technology through the implementation of appropriate technical capabilities.	Stage 1 required EPs to conduct or review a security risk analysis and implement security updates as necessary and correct identified security deficiencies as part of their risk management process. Stage 2 requires an EP to conduct or review a security risk analysis, including addressing the encryption/security of data at rest, and implement security updates as necessary and correct identified security deficiencies as part of its risk management process.
Incorporate clinical lab test results into Certified EHR Technology as structured data.	Stage 1 required more than 40% of all clinical lab test results ordered by the EP during the EHR reporting period whose results were either in a positive/negative or numeric format be included in the EHR as structured data. Stage 2 requires more than 55% of all clinical lab test results ordered during the EHR reporting period whose results are either in a positive/negative or numeric format be included in the EHR as structured data.

(continued)

Stage 2 Explanation	Comparison to Stage 1
Generate lists of patients by specific conditions to use for quality improvement, reduction of disparities, research, or outreach.	Stage 1 required an EP to generate at least one report listing patients of the provider with a specific condition. The Stage 1 requirement remained the same in Stage 2.
Use clinically relevant information to identify patients who should receive reminders for preventive/follow-up care.	Stage 1 required more than 20% of all unique patients 65 years or older or 5 years old or younger to be sent an appropriate reminder during the EHR reporting period. Stage 2 requires the use of EHR technology to identify and provide reminders for preventive/follow-up care for more than 10% of patients with two or more office visits in the last 2 years.
Use Certified EHR Technology to identify patient-specific education resources and provide those resources to the patient if appropriate.	Stage 1 required more than 10% of all patients seen by the EP be provided patient-specific education resources. Stage 2 requires patient-specific education resources identified by Certified Electronic Health Record Technology (CEHRT) be provided to patients for more than 10% of all unique patients with office visits seen by the EP during the EHR reporting period.
The EP who receives a patient from another setting of care or provider of care or believes an encounter is relevant should perform medication reconciliation.	Stage 1 required that the EP perform medication reconciliation for more than 50% of transitions of care in which the patient is transitioned into the care of the EP. The Stage 1 requirement remained the same in Stage 2.
The EP who transitions a patient to another setting of care or provider of care or refers a patient to another provider of care should provide a summary of care record for each transition of care or referral.	Stage 1 required that the EP who transitioned or referred the patient to another setting of care or provider of care provide a summary of care record for more than 50% of transitions of care and referrals. Stage 2 requires the following: 1. The EP who transitions or refers a patient to another setting of care or provider of care to provide a summary of care record for more than 50% of transitions of care and referrals 2. The EP who transitions or refers a patient to another setting of care or provider of care to provide a summary of care record either (a) electronically transmitted to a recipient using CEHRT or (b) where the recipient receives the summary of care record via exchange facilitated by an organization that is a NwHIN Exchange participant or is validated through an ONC-established governance mechanism to facilitate exchange for 10% of transitions and referrals

Stage 2 Explanation	Comparison to Stage 1
	3. The EP who transitions or refers a patient to another setting of care or provider of care to either (a) conduct one or more successful electronic exchanges of a summary of care record with a recipient using technology that was designed by a different EHR developer than the sender's or (b) conduct one or more successful tests with the CMS-designated test EHR during the EHR reporting period
Capability to submit electronic data to immunization registries or immunization information systems and actual submission except where prohibited and in accordance with applicable law and practice	Stage 1 required the performance of at least one test of Certified EHR Technology's capacity to submit electronic data to immunization registries. Stage 2 requires successful ongoing submission of electronic immunization data from Certified EHR Technology to an immunization registry or immunization information system for the entire EHR reporting period.
Use secure electronic messaging to communicate with patients on relevant health information.	This objective did not exist in Stage 1. Stage 2 requires the capability for a secure message to be sent using the electronic messaging function of CEHRT by more than 5% of unique patients seen during the EHR reporting period.

Source: Centers for Medicare and Medicaid Services. (2012, August). *Stage 1 vs. Stage 2 Comparison Table for Eligible Professionals.* Retrieved from http://www.cms.gov/Regulations-and-Guidance /Legislation/EHRIncentivePrograms/Downloads/Stage1vsStage2CompTablesforEP.pdf.

The following Stage 1 core objectives were incorporated elsewhere in Stage 2, or they were eliminated from Stage 1 and they are no longer an objective for Stage 2, and therefore there was no need to list them:

- Implement drug–drug and drug–allergy interaction checks.
- Maintain an up-to-date problem list of current and active diagnoses.
- Maintain an active medication list.
- Maintain an active medication allergy list.
- Report clinical quality measures (CQMs) to CMS or the states.
- Have the capability to exchange key clinical information (e.g., problem list, medication list, medication allergies, diagnostic test results) among providers of care and patient-authorized entities electronically.
- Implement drug-formulary checks.
- Provide patients with timely electronic access to their health information (including lab results, problem list, medication lists, medication allergies) within four business days of the information being available to the EP.

Hospitals (including CAHs) have similar core objectives to those listed here for eligible professionals. The requirement to generate and transmit permissible prescriptions electronically is a menu objective rather than a core objective in hospitals. Also, the requirement to receive reminders for preventive/follow-up care does not apply to hospitals, since hospitals care for patients during acute illnesses, rather than provide the ongoing care of a patient's medical issues as is done by primary care providers and specialists. The demographics objectives for hospitals include those listed for eligible professionals and include date and preliminary cause of death in the event of mortality in the eligible hospital or critical access hospital. Eligible hospitals are required to submit electronic syndromic (diagnostic) surveillance data to public health agencies. Also in core objectives, eligible hospitals must have the capability to electronically transmit and track medications from order to administration using assistive technologies in conjunction with an electronic medication administration record (eMAR). In the paper system, that was known as the medication administration record (MAR).

Table 9.4 recaps the menu objectives for Stage 2 as they applied to eligible professionals. EPs were required to comply with three of the six menu objectives to qualify for Meaningful Use.

TABLE 9.4	Eligible Professional (EP) Menu Objectives: Stage 2 Meaningful Use
Stage 2 Explanation	**Comparison to Stage 1**
Have the capability to submit electronic syndromic surveillance data to public health agencies and actual submission except where prohibited and in accordance with applicable law and practice.	Stage 1 required at least one test of Certified EHR Technology's capacity to provide electronic syndromic surveillance data to public health agencies. Stage 2 requires successful ongoing submission of electronic syndromic surveillance data from Certified EHR Technology to a public health agency for the entire EHR reporting period.
Record electronic notes in patient records.	Stage 1 did not include this menu objective. Stage 2 requires an EP to enter at least one electronic progress note created, edited, and signed for more than 30% of unique patients.
Imaging results consisting of the image itself and any explanation or other accompanying information are accessible through CEHRT.	Stage 1 did not include this menu objective. Stage 2 requires more than 10% of all scans and tests whose result is an image ordered by the EP for patients seen during the EHR reporting period be incorporated into or accessible through Certified EHR Technology.
Record patient family health history as structured data.	Stage 1 did not include this menu objective. Stage 2 requires more than 20% of all unique patients seen by the EP during the EHR reporting period to have a structured data entry for one or more first-degree relatives or an indication that family health history has been reviewed.
Have the capability to identify and report cancer cases to a state cancer registry, except where prohibited, and in accordance with applicable law and practice.	Stage 1 did not include this menu objective. Stage 2 requires successful ongoing submission of cancer case information from Certified EHR Technology to a cancer registry for the entire EHR reporting period.
Have the capability to identify and report specific cases to a specialized registry (other than a cancer registry), except where prohibited, and in accordance with applicable law and practice.	Stage 1 did not include this menu objective. Stage 2 requires successful ongoing submission of specific case information from Certified EHR Technology to a specialized registry for the entire EHR reporting period.

Source: Centers for Medicare & Medicaid Services. (2012, August). *Stage 1 vs. Stage 2 Comparison Table for Eligible Professionals.* Retrieved from https://www.cms.gov/Regulations-and-Guidance/Legislation/EHRIncentivePrograms/Downloads/Stage1vsStage2CompTablesforEP.pdf.

Eligible hospitals (including CAHs) attempting to meet Stage 2 menu objectives were required to meet three of six possible objectives, which included the following:

- Record whether a patient 65 years old or older has an advance directive.
- Record electronic notes in patient records.

- Imaging results consisting of the image itself and any explanation or other accompanying information are accessible through CEHRT.
- Record patient family health history as structured data.
- Generate and transmit permissible discharge prescriptions electronically (eRx).
- Provide structured electronic lab results to ambulatory providers.

As you read through the core and menu objectives, notice how often "structured data" is mentioned. These data elements must be chosen from libraries within the EHR system rather than in free-text within the EHR notes.

Not only was more functionality added in Stage 2, but the measure thresholds were increased as well.

In Stage 2, the ability to share patient information with other providers and healthcare facilities is a major emphasis; after all, a prime goal of using electronic health records is the improvement of patient care and outcomes by sharing patient information between and among providers, hospitals, and other healthcare facilities. A 2012 study conducted by CapSite, a healthcare technology research firm, revealed that 71% of hospitals in the United States planned to join a health information exchange (HIE) (CapSite, September 2012), and a 2013 study conducted by the same research firm found that 46% of U.S. physician groups planned to join an (HIE) (CapSite, June 2013).

Having the ability to view Meaningful Use **dashboards** has been an important component of all EHR programs, as it allows a practice or an organization to compare actual performance to the required performance level in order to ensure compliance. An example of a dashboard is depicted in Figure 9.2. Note that the dashboard's color-coding helps users identify areas of strength or weakness.

Dashboards A visual comparison of actual performance to required performance.

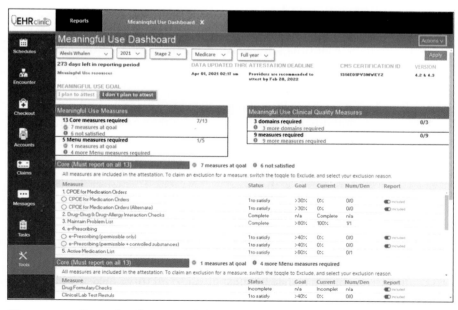

Figure 9.2   **Example of Meaningful Use Dashboard**

Meaningful Use Stage 3 "paused" in the summer of 2016, after the Final Rule was published in the *Federal Register* on October 6, 2015. Part

Physician Quality Reporting System (PQRS) A voluntary pay-for-performance incentive program. Participating care providers submit data on any of the 100 designated quality measures and receive monetary incentives for doing so.

Value-based payment modifier program Part of the Merit-based Incentive Program, payment to solo practitioners (physicians who do not practice as part of a group) and medical practice groups per the Medicare Physician Fee Schedule (PFS) but based on the quality of care furnished compared to the cost of care during a performance period. The Value Modifier was an adjustment made to Medicare payments for items and services.

Merit-based Incentive Payment System (MIPS) A reimbursement system that replaces the Sustainable Growth Rate formula previously used by Medicare Part B with a value-based system. The value-based system is called the Quality Payment Program (QPP).

of the program's scoring is tied to EPs using Certified EHR Technology and attaining Meaningful Use. The Medicare Access and CHIP (Children's Health Insurance Program) Reauthorization Act (MACRA) was passed, and the result was a combination of Meaningful Use, the **Physicians' Quality Reporting System (PQRS)**, and the **value-based payment modifier program**, or MIPS—the **Merit-based Incentive Payment System (MIPS)**.

Effective with FY2018, all eligible hospitals and healthcare professionals are required to show proof that a certified electronic health record (EHR) system is in use, which

1. Protects health information. Providers must conduct security audits and conduct a security risk analysis.

2. Uses ePrescribing. More than 60% of a provider's permissible prescriptions must be queried for drug formulary interactions and transmitted to pharmacies electronically.

3. Implements five clinical decision support (CDS) measures or the active use of drug–drug and drug–allergy interaction checks, which are available within the certified EHR platform used in the practice.

4. Uses computerized provider order entry (CPOE) functionality for medication, lab, and diagnostic imaging orders.

5. Provides patient access to their own EHR for more than 80% of the practice's patients, with the option to both view and download their own records. Additionally, eligible physicians must offer the option to view educational data regarding the condition(s) the patient is being treated for, to more than 35% of their patients.

6. Provides coordination of care through patient engagement. Physicians encourage patients to actively engage in their care by educating them and offering them the ability to view their own health data. In addition, at least 25% of patients in a practice interact with their EHR, at least 35% of patients receive a secure digital message from a care provider, and providers encourage the collection of patient-generated health data from fitness trackers or wearable devices from more than 15% of patients. Eligible providers must attest to all three measures; however, the thresholds for two of the three must be met.

7. Provides for health information exchange. This is better known as interoperability and requires that more than 50% of care transition and referrals include the exchange of medical records, such as continuity of care documents electronically. The second measure of HIE requires providers who are seeing a patient for the first time to receive care documents electronically from other caregivers (providers, hospitals) more than 40% of the time. The third measure is that the provider will use e-prescribing functionality to reconcile medication lists from online sources with their own EHR for more than 80% of new patients they treat. As with the coordination of care incentive, eligible providers must attest to all three measures but meet the thresholds for two of the three.

8. Allows reporting to public health and clinical data registries. Eligible providers periodically report to three out of five available EHR reporting destinations. Reporting options include an immunization registry, syndromic surveillance, cases, a public health registry, and a clinical data registry.

According to the Healthcare Information Management and Systems Society (HIMSS), "Clinical Decision Support (CDS) is defined broadly as a clinical system, application, or process that helps health professionals make clinical decisions to enhance patient care. Clinical knowledge of interest could range from simple facts and relationships to best practices for managing patients with specific disease states, new medical knowledge from clinical research, and other types of information" (HIMSS, 2013).

CDS includes reminders and alerts, diagnostic and therapeutic guidance, links to expert resources (the Centers for Disease Control and Prevention (CDC), the Mayo Clinic, and clinical trials, for example), and results of best practices. Many EHR vendors link directly to one of these expert sites. The trigger that a clinical alert or support should be displayed comes from the data that has already been captured in the patient's record. This is where the data dictionary and structured data that we covered in an earlier chapter apply. Typically, there is a piece or combination of pieces of data (or lack thereof) within the patient's record that "triggers" or "flags" a record when a particular test or treatment may be needed for that patient. For example, a 50-year-old patient without a CPT® code for any of the recommended screening tests for colon cancer on the patient's current or past records may be flagged for "colon cancer screening," since the CDC's U.S. Preventive Services Task Force recommends colon cancer screening between the ages of 50 and 75. This is an example of clinical decision support and is a functionality of an EHR, the value of which cannot be overexaggerated. The use of CDS tools improves patient safety, decreases duplication of procedures, reduces the performance of unnecessary testing, and as a result reduces the cost of healthcare while improving patient outcomes, efficiency of care, and the provision of clinically relevant, evidence-based care. Clinical decision support tools are built into most EHRs, and they are instrumental in improving patient compliance and assisting physicians in providing quality care.

It was noted earlier that Meaningful Use required that at least five clinical decision support interventions related to four or more clinical quality measures be implemented during the entire reporting period. An alert that pops up to ask a patient if he or she has had a colonoscopy does not meet the requirement unless that alert appears based on certain information found in the EHR about *that* patient compared to evidence-based criteria that have been embedded in the EHR software. For instance, an alert for colonoscopy would appear when a patient was 50 years of age or older and/or there was an entry in the patient's problem list showing a history of rectal bleeding or a family history of colon cancer was documented in the history section of his chart and no CPT® procedure codes for colonoscopy have appeared in the patient's visit history in the past five years.

By setting parameters (age, diagnosis, length of time since the last procedure was performed, etc.) for specific objectives and wellness initiatives, such as with a colonoscopy, a mammogram, or cholesterol testing, EHR systems have the ability to audit patients' charts to identify if they are due or overdue for screening or testing. This ensures that providers can order tests, procedures, immunizations, and screenings when they are needed. Doing so provides opportunities for patients to remain proactive in their own healthcare and can even lead to early detection of disease, which will result in improved patient outcomes and a lower overall cost of healthcare.

Of course, if a care provider has this functionality available through the practice's EHR software and does not use it, then it is not beneficial to the patient, to the care provider, or to the practice, nor does it satisfy Meaningful Use standards. There are still care providers who view CDS systems as "cookbook medicine"—those who find it too time consuming or who are annoyed by the pop-up reminders. One incentive to encourage the use of a CDS is pay-for-performance programs available in certain managed care plans. In other words, if the practice's fiscal position is improved by using CDS technology, then the care providers are more accepting of CDS systems.

Conversely, there are times when the office staff may need to search the database for particular cases rather than have the cases flagged one at a time. These are called "filters," which will select (or exclude) patients from the database who do (or do not) meet certain criteria. For example, a provider can **query** the database for patients who are 50 years of age or older and who have not had any of the colonoscopy CPT® codes attached to any of their visits for the past five years; once this alert is set up, their electronic record will then have a visual alert of some kind (for instance, a red ribbon icon) attached to show that a screening colonoscopy is needed. To query means to search, or "ask," the database for records that meet (or do not meet, depending on how the query is written) the criteria noted in the filters. In our example, we are querying the database for patients who are 50 years of age or older and who *do not* have one of the colonoscopy codes we've specified on any of their visits over the past five years.

Query Searching a database for patients who meet certain criteria.

9.3 Use of Report-Writer for System Reports

EHRclinic and other PM/EMR software offer a multitude of standard reports that are set to run at certain times (end of the month, for example) or on demand as the information is needed. This type of report is known as an "ad hoc" report, meaning the data are needed as soon as possible and for one-time use. Some of the standard reports available in EHRclinic are

- Patient day sheet
- Practice analysis
- Billing/payment status
- Patient ledger
- Patient collections
- Collection letter
- Patient remainder aging (the length of time the portion of the bill for which the patient is responsible remains unpaid)
- Insurance aging
- Patient remainder statement

Other common reports that may be seen include:

- Payment analysis
- Procedure code analysis
- Provider revenue summary
- Patient balances
- Referring provider
- Appointment analysis report

These standard reports and others in the reports library are necessary for the efficient running of the office. Not keeping a close watch over revenue or balances and constantly battling scheduling conflicts are not good business practices. Surprises in any of these areas can negatively impact the bottom line and cause unhappy staff, providers, and patients.

Running standard reports is as easy as a click of a button. It is always important to know the date ranges you want to include. If they are reports you run on a routine basis, you should always use the same parameters for consistency. In other words, if you run a report routinely that includes all of the care providers, do not make the mistake of running it next time with just a few of the providers; otherwise, you are not comparing apples to apples! Figure 9.3 shows the A/R Management Report Selection screen. For example, this is the screen from which you would choose to run a procedure code analysis report, which shows all procedures performed by the providers (or specific provider(s)), during a specific time period, and the volume of each. The procedures are listed by CPT® code. If you work for a dermatologist, the CPT® code 42400, biopsy of salivary gland, should not appear on your procedure code analysis report, for example, because dermatologists typically do not excise salivary glands. If it does, then someone has made a coding error. If this does happen, then the affected account should be found and the code corrected. Another use for this type of report is cost justification. If one of the providers in your practice wants to purchase a newer model of a particular piece of equipment, and it will cost approximately $200,000, the managing partners in the practice most likely will not approve the purchase if only a small number of the procedures for which it will be used are performed each year. When making large purchasing decisions, all practices should consider the return on investment (ROI) of the item(s), meaning when they can expect to make their money back. A $200,000 piece of equipment is not likely to turn a profit, or even pay for itself, if not enough procedures are performed using it. Running the practice analysis report shown in Figure 9.3, then setting parameters of

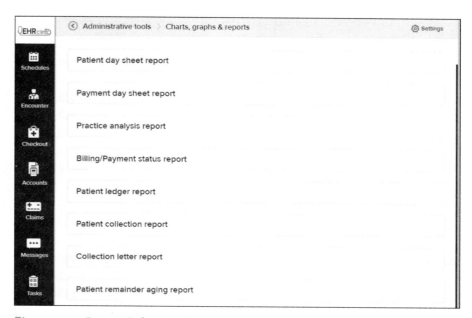

Figure 9.3 **Report Selection Screen**

what procedures, diagnoses, time frame to be included, etc. will provide the data needed for an informed decision-making process.

Major decisions, especially those that involve funding, should always be analyzed, and standard reports are a good starting point for the analysis. The findings from these reports give information—either baseline findings or changes over time. If information in these reports is not analyzed, decisions will be made arbitrarily rather than based on facts. Additionally, reports can be used to identify trends, which help practices forecast for the future.

Standard clinical reports are used as well. Examples include a listing of all active patients in the practice with a particular diagnosis and a listing of all patients with an alert flag of smoker. You may want to run this type of report to answer a survey, where just the number of active smokers is requested. In this case, a **summary report** that includes only the **aggregate** number of active smokers for a specific time period is included rather than their name, address, and so on. Reports that do include patient identifying information and list each case individually are known as **detail reports**.

Figure 9.4 depicts a provider revenue summary report in EHRclinic.

Summit Bay Health Center	
Practice Analysis	
Show all data where the procedure code range is between 00000 - 99999	
March 1, 2022 - March 31, 2022 for ALL PROVIDERS	
Total procedure charges	$ 12013.75
Total global surgical charges	$ 2075.97
Total product charges	$ 1621.82
Total inside lab charges	$ 3067.21
Total outside lab charges	$ 710.99
Total billing charges	$ 1607.85
Total charges	$ 21097.59
Total insurance payments	$ 9493.92
Total cash payments	$ 385.00
Total check copayments	$ 860.00
Toal credit card copayments	$ 1025.00
Total patient cash payments	$ 210.00
Total patient check payments	$ 640.00
Total credit card payments	$ 815.82
Total receipts	$ 13429.74
Total credit adjustments	$ 497.51
Total debit adjustments	$ 612.05
Total insurance debit adjustments	$ 1708.74
Total insurance withholds	$ 296.3
Total adjustments	$ 3114.6

Figure 9.4   Provider Revenue Summary Report

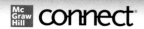
Create a Patient Collections Summary Report

The first report we will run is a detail report of all patients with outstanding collection balances between November 1, 2021, and March 31, 2022. You may need to run this report to determine which patients are due for collection letters, for example.

Follow these steps to complete the exercise on your own once you have watched the demonstration and tried the steps with helpful prompts in practice mode.

1. Click on 'Manage reports' button.
2. Click on 'Patient collection report' button.
3. Click on 'Chart number range from' field and enter 'aa001'.
4. Click on 'Chart number range to' field and enter 'aa025'.
5. Click on 'Initial billing date range from' field and enter '11/01/2021'.
6. Click on 'Initial billing date range to' field and enter '03/31/2022'.
7. Click on 'Status' drop-down and select 'Open'.
8. Click on 'Close' button.
9. Click on 'Generate report' button.
10. Click on 'Print' button.
11. Click on 'Okay' button.

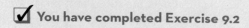
You have completed Exercise 9.2

9.4 Custom Report Writing

A **custom report** can be built to include **variables**. We select the variables in these reports that we want our patients to meet or not meet. In Exercise 9.2 there was only one variable—the date range of the collections report—which had to be between November 1, 2021, and March 31, 2022. If we had wanted to narrow our search to patients who have outstanding balances who live in ZIP code 44804, then we would have had to run a custom report with two variables in order to capture only those patients who live in the locality with a ZIP code of 44804 and have statements due between November 1, 2021, and March 31, 2022.

The custom reports are often run to answer inquiries from managed care agencies, federal or state departments of health, public health agencies, and accrediting agencies. We may even do so for a newspaper reporter or a student who just wants aggregate data about a particular diagnosis in order to write an article or a research paper. A cardiology practice may take part in a study with other cardiology practices in town and run a custom report to compare its patient demographics to those of the other practices. When statistics concerning one practice or hospital are compared to the statistics of other practices or hospitals, this is referred to as **benchmarking**, which is the comparison of one set of statistics to the overall statistics (using the same variables). As always, remember HIPAA! While we can run reports and share generic information, we are not able to share specific or identifiable

Custom report Report that is designed by the office or hospital rather than coming as part of a software package (standard report).

Variable In relation to a statistical report, the factor that varies from one patient to the next. Examples include age, ZIP code, and diagnoses.

Benchmarking Comparison of one set of statistics to the overall statistics when the same variables are used for each.

personal information, such as linking patients' names with the data about them, without their consent.

Other custom reports include

- The number of patients treated in the practice with a particular diagnosis—for example, congestive heart failure sorted by care provider
- The number of patients treated in the practice who live in a particular ZIP code, are smokers, and have diabetes
- The number of patients in a practice who have Medicaid as their primary source of payment and are between the ages of 30 and 64 years
- The number of patients in a practice who have not had a specific screening test, such as all female patients over the age of 40 who have not had a mammogram within one year, which would allow the provider to send letters, so that these patients will know they are overdue for testing
- The number of patients who have allergies to penicillin, are Hispanic, and live in ZIP code 12345

EXERCISE 9.3   Go to https://connect.mheducation.com to complete this exercise. To see instructional notes with the steps, visit the eBook in Connect or download them from www.mhhe.com/iehr4.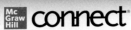

Build a Custom Report of Referring Providers

We are going to create a custom report that will show us which providers that patients are referred from, as well as which providers Summit Bay Health Center providers are referring to. The terms *referring* and *referral* are both used and mean the same thing, but it is important to understand your relationship with other medical practices in the area, both on the receiving and the sending ends of a referral. One reason a patient may be referred to another provider is that the patient needs to see a specialist, such as a cardiologist or dermatologist. If your office is family practice, then you would be referring *to* the specialist. The specialist's office would be accepting the referral. Another reason for referral may be a patient who was seen in an urgent care or emergency department; the patient would most likely be referred for follow-up to a family practitioner, an internist, or a specialist, depending on the reason for the visit. An organization may want to see where patients are being referred from so that it can do some marketing in that area, or even to see about creating a partnership with the referring organization to ensure continuity of care for patients; thus, the organization would need to run a referral report to locate the names of physicians or practices that are referring to your practice.

Follow these steps to complete the exercise on your own once you have watched the demonstration and tried the steps with helpful prompts in practice mode.

1. Click on 'Tools' module.
2. Click on 'Manage practice data' button.
3. Click on 'Referring provider' button.
4. Click on 'Amyra Sanchez's provider' information.
5. Click on 'Secondary specialty' drop-down and select 'Family Medicine'.
6. Click on 'Save changes' button.

☑ **You have completed Exercise 9.3**

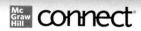
Build a Custom Report of Insurance Payments

The Summit Bay Health Center billing manager notices that the insurance payments have not been received for several McGraw-Hill Healthmark patients for March 1, 2022. Before reaching out to the insurance company, she runs a custom report to determine if any payments have been made at all for that date of service by McGraw-Hill Healthmark.

In this exercise, we will see how easy it is to use various filters, such as dates of service, chart numbers, and insurance companies, to create a custom report detailing payments.

Follow these steps to complete the exercise on your own once you have watched the demonstration and tried the steps with helpful prompts in practice mode.

1. Click on 'Manage reports' button.
2. Click on 'Billing/Payment status report' button.
3. Click on 'Date created range from' field and enter '03/01/2022'.
4. Click on 'Date created range to' field and enter '03/01/2022'.
5. Click on 'Chart number range from' field and enter 'aa001'.
6. Click on 'Chart number range to' field and enter 'aa025'.
7. Click on 'Patient insurance carrier' drop-down and select the McGraw-Hill Healthmark option.
8. Click on 'Close' button.
9. Click on 'Generate report' button.
10. Click on 'Close' button.

The custom report that was created states that 'no data' is available. This information tells the office manager that McGraw-Hill Healthmark did not remit any insurance payments for patients AA001 through AA025 on March 1, 2022. Now that she has this information, she will be able to contact the insurance company to determine why the payments have not yet been sent.

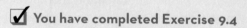 You have completed Exercise 9.4

9.5 Uses of Indexes

An **index** is a listing. Indexes, also known as indices, are generally used to find basic information; a Disease Index is run and is sorted by ICD-10-CM diagnosis code, and under each code is a list of patients by name and/or health record number (dates of admission/discharge, attending physician, and discharge disposition may also be included). Hospitals run the Disease Index to get a grasp of the types of patients being seen in the facility. This is also a good way to check for inaccuracies in coding. Another example of an index is a listing of all patients who are assigned to each care provider individually. In inpatient and outpatient settings, the Disease, Operation (procedure), and Physicians' Indexes are commonly run reports.

Managed care insurance plans often want to see a Physicians' Index or Disease Index to get a profile of the type of patients treated by a practice before considering it for **in-network** status (meaning that there is a contract

Index A listing—for instance, a Diagnosis Index is a report that is sorted by diagnosis code and includes the total number of patients seen with that disease for a given period of time, and a Master Patient Index (MPI) is a listing of all patients who have ever been seen in a hospital or a practice.

In-network Care providers who contract with a managed care plan to offer services to members of the managed care plan at a prenegotiated rate.

between a managed care plan and the provider to offer services to members of the managed care plan at a pre-negotiated, lower rate, called capitation). Another reason to see any of these indexes is to provide proof that a physician has cared for a certain number of patients or type of patients when he or she is seeking board certification, as in the case of a board-certified urologist or obstetrician. Disease Indexes are also used for case finding for the cancer registry, trauma registry, birth defect registry, and so on. Registries will be discussed in the next section.

A common index in a hospital setting is the Master Patient Index (MPI) (the listing of all patients seen in a hospital), which includes basic identifying information. The entire MPI may be run to look for missing information, duplicate patients, or names entered outside the practice's defined specifications (making sure that names are formatted according to data dictionary specifications).

| 9.6 | **Uses of Registries** |

Registry A listing that is filed in chronological order based on when something occurred. Examples include a birth registry, a death registry, a cancer registry, and a trauma registry.

Whereas an index is a listing of information, a **registry** is also a listing, but it is in chronological order. Examples in a hospital are admission and discharge registries, which are run on a daily basis and include the names of all patients admitted and all patients discharged on a certain date. Another example is a birth registry—it is kept by date and time of birth, but it is sorted by the name of the newborn and includes the name of the mother, the time of birth, and the name of the attending physician. And death registries, which are kept by date and time of death, include the patient's name, the cause of death, and the signature of the person pronouncing the death, among other data elements.

Cancer registries are registries of all patients diagnosed or treated for cancer and are required by law. These registries are sent to state cancer registries, where statewide statistics are compiled on the incidence of each type of cancer, as well as survival rates by type of cancer in each state. Each state registry is responsible for reporting to the CDC. Hospitals, physicians' offices, outpatient radiation therapy facilities, and ambulatory care centers may keep and report a registry of cancer patients on a yearly basis. Take the time to look for the most commonly diagnosed cancers in the United States, found at http://www.cdc.gov/cancer/dcpc/data/types.htm.

Trauma registries are one of the newer registries, created in the early 1990s; as the name implies, they are registries of all patients diagnosed or treated with traumatic injuries, such as fractures, burns, and open wounds. The 2016 Annual Report of the American College of Surgeons' National Trauma Databank can be found at https://www.facs.org/quality-programs /trauma/ntdb/docpub. It is interesting to page through the report and see the enormous amount of data reported by hospitals throughout the country. In Table 15 on page 39 of the report, you will see a breakdown by the mechanism of injury (fall, fire/flame, suffocation, transport vehicles, motor vehicle accidents, etc.). From there, the data gets more specific—for instance, the incidence of falls by age or incidents by region of the country (Table 41, page 99). As you can see, the southern part of the country has the highest incidence of traumatic incidents, at 39.09%. The Northeast has the lowest, at 17.65%. State and local health and safety officials can use this information to analyze reasons for a higher-than-average incidence (in the case of the South) or a lower-than-average incidence (as in the Northeast).

Immunization registries are of particular importance to public health. Some private physicians' offices keep a registry of immunizations by patient; however, not all medical practices do; it may just be a public health department that does so. Some states require reporting of immunizations by law. For instance, a West Virginia state law requires all providers to report all immunizations they administer to children under age 18 within two weeks of administering the immunization.

Other registries include those listing birth defects, diabetes, implants (any material implanted into the body), transplants, and HIV/AIDS patients. The requirements for them vary from state to state, as well as by managed care plan or other third-party requirements, and for quality reporting purposes.

EHR systems make the process of running an index or a registry very fast, but its accuracy depends on whether entry of the data was correct in the first place! This is another reason accuracy and attention to detail are so important. Remember that data obtained from any software program is only as good and accurate as the accuracy of the person who inputs it.

The Medicare Quality Payment Program, through its Merit-based Incentive Payment System, is the quality payment incentive program that rewards value and outcomes. Providers are scored on four performance indicators: quality, promoting interoperability, improvement activities, and cost. Prior to 2018, the pay-for-performance incentive program was known as the Physician Quality Reporting System (PQRS).

The first indicator, quality, directly relates to the quality of care delivered to a provider's patients based on performance measures that have been created by CMS and certain medical professional and stakeholder groups. The provider then selects six measures of performance that are most related to his or her practice.

The focus of the interoperability indicator is patient engagement as well as the electronic exchange of health information through the use of Certified Electronic Health Record Technology. The Promoting Interoperability Programs replaced the Medicare and Medicaid EHR Incentive Programs. The goal is for eligible providers and hospitals (including CAHs) to share health information with other providers, clinicians, and hospitals as necessary and appropriate. This includes test results, visit summaries, and treatment plans to coordinate care and demonstrate meaningful use of CEHRT.

The newest category, Improvement activities, includes choices of activities that assess how the provider might improve processes, enhance patient engagement, and increase the patients' access to care.

The system used now to address the cost of healthcare is value-based medicine (VBM). The cost of the care provided is calculated by CMS and is based on the provider's Medicare claims. MIPS uses cost measures as a guideline of the total cost of care during the year or during a particular hospital stay. Beginning in 2018, this performance category counted toward the provider's MIPS final score.

There are times when hospitals, medical practices, or other healthcare entities contribute to outside registries. Of note is the **National Practitioner Data Bank (NPDB)**, which came about as part of the Health Care Quality Improvement Act of 1986. This is a database of malpractice payments, revocation of privileges, licensure denial or suspension, denial of medical staff privileges, and the like. Reporting any of these adverse actions to the NPDB is required by law. Hospitals and offices

National Practitioner Data Bank (NPDB) Required by law, a database of malpractice payouts, revocation of privileges, licensure denial or suspension, denial of medical staff privileges, and similar actions.

considering granting privileges to or hiring care providers, state boards of medical examiners or licensing boards, state boards of medicine, or the care providers themselves can query the data bank when necessary. Healthcare entities that are considering granting privileges to a physician must query the NPDB during the hiring/privileging process.

Hospitals, care providers, and all other healthcare organizations must report adverse actions related to fraud and abuse to the **Healthcare Integrity and Protection Data Bank (HIPDB)**. The HIPDB is part of the National Practitioner Data Bank; more information about both of these can be found at http://www.npdb-hipdb.com/.

Healthcare Integrity and Protection Data Bank (HIPDB) A database of adverse actions related to fraud and abuse; part of the National Practitioner Data Bank (NPDB).

| 9.7 | **The Credentialing Process** |

Credentialing is the process of ensuring that a care provider has the proper qualifications to practice medicine. In other words, if a physician claims to be a cardiac surgeon, then the practice or hospital must establish that he/she has the educational background and experience (medical residency) necessary to perform surgeries typically carried out by a cardiac surgeon. It must verify that he or she has shown verification that he or she is a qualified medical professional in that specialty.

Credentialing The process of ensuring a care provider has the proper qualifications (education, experience, malpractice coverage) to practice medicine.

Credentialing does not involve a database. It is mentioned here because the information is captured and maintained for reporting purposes when a healthcare professional files for renewal of a medical license, applies for board certification (and continuing board certification), applies for hospital privileges (or maintaining such privileges), and reports to managed care entities.

Credentialing also means that a care provider is in compliance with specific policies (called bylaws) for that organization and that he has purchased sufficient malpractice insurance coverage. Some insurance carriers will not reimburse providers who perform medical care for which they are not qualified. Further, some will not invite physicians to be participating providers in an insurance plan unless they are board-certified. Board certification involves successfully completing a test that is directly related to the specialty area and that goes above and beyond state medical licensure.

Drug Enforcement Agency number A numeric identifier assigned to a health care provider, for instance a physician, optometrist, dentist, or veterinarian, by the United States Drug Enforcement Administration, which allows him/her to write prescriptions for controlled substances.

Physicians must be Medicare-credentialed in order to submit claims to Medicare for payment. When a medical practice hires a new care provider, information regarding education, experience, state license number, **Drug Enforcement Agency (DEA) number**, National Provider Identifier (NPI) number, proof of malpractice insurance, and documentation of any pending or settled claims against the care provider are all on file, usually within the PM software. And as noted earlier, the NPDB and HIPDB must also be queried prior to granting privileges, hiring care providers, or including them as participating providers by insurance carriers.

APPLYING YOUR SKILLS

In the chapter on reimbursement, we discussed the outcome-based pay-for-performance reimbursement method, the Accountable Care Organization (ACO). How do the concepts in this chapter apply to care professionals and hospitals who are part of an ACO?

chapter 9 summary

LEARNING OUTCOME	CONCEPTS FOR REVIEW
9.1 Describe the uses of the dashboard in EHRclinic to meet Interoperability standards.	– List Meaningful Use Stage 1 and 2 core objectives for providers and hospitals – List Meaningful Use Stage 1 and 2 menu objectives for providers and hospitals – View a dashboard in EHRclinic to assess performance
9.2 Explain how data and information are used in decision support.	– Define clinical decision support – Use improves patient safety, decreases duplication, reduces unnecessary testing, and reduces cost of healthcare – Use improves patient outcomes and improves efficiency – Some care providers are not accepting of CDS technology
9.3 Set up system reports using EHRclinic.	– Standard reports are commonly used by most medical practices – Standard reports are system built – Administrative as well as clinical standard reports are available – Differentiate between summary and detail reports
9.4 Set up custom reports using EHRclinic.	– Custom reports are run based on specific parameters or variables – Custom reports are used when standard reports do not provide the level of detail necessary
9.5 Illustrate uses for an index.	– An index is a list – Typically used to find all patients who meet certain criteria – Examples: Master Patient Index, Disease Index, Procedure Index, Physicians' Index
9.6 Describe uses for a registry.	– A listing of information in chronological order – Examples: birth registry, cancer registry, trauma registry, PQRS Measures registry – Submissions required by National Practitioner Data Bank (NPDB)

9.7 Explain how data gathered in EHRclinic are used in the credentialing process.	– Verification that care provider holds certain credentials
	– Included in the credentials are
	  • Education (undergrad as well as medical school)
	  • Residency(ies) dates and institution(s)
	  • Pending or settled malpractice cases
	  • Proof of purchase of malpractice insurance

chapter **review**

MATCHING QUESTIONS

Match the terms on the left with the definitions on the right.

_____ 1. **[LO 9.1]** dashboard

_____ 2. **[LO 9.5]** in-network

_____ 3. **[LO 9.1]** Meaningful Use

_____ 4. **[LO 9.1]** Centers for Medicare & Medicaid Services (CMS)

_____ 5. **[LO 9.6]** registry

_____ 6. **[LO 9.5]** index

_____ 7. **[LO 9.2]** clinical decision support

_____ 8. **[LO 9.1]** Certified Electronic Health Record Technology (CEHRT)

_____ 9. **[LO 9.3]** summary report

_____ 10. **[LO 9.1]** core objectives

_____ 11. **[LO 9.1]** Merit-based Incentive Payment System

_____ 12. **[LO 9.1]** drug formulary

_____ 13. **[LO 9.7]** credentialing

_____ 14. **[LO 9.1]** The Medicare Access and CHIP Reauthorization Act (MACRA)

_____ 15. **[LO 9.3]** detail report

a. the law that introduced value-based reimbursement

b. consolidated clinical data that removes any patient information in the printout

c. tool built into most EHRs that provides staff with results of research and best practices to enhance patient care

d. software used to capture health information that meets standards set by the Office of the National Coordinator

e. incentive program that rewards value and outcomes

f. consolidated clinical data that includes specific, demographic, or patient identifying information in the printout

g. verification process that ensures that a care provider is legally authorized through education and experience to practice medicine

h. care provider or practice that contracts with insurance companies to provide care to its subscribers at a reduced rate

i. feature of EHRclinic that allows a provider to visually track its fulfillment of core objectives

j. requirements that must be met for a professional to receive Medicare stimulus money to purchase or upgrade an EHR

k. benchmark tasks that demonstrate Meaningful Use of electronic health information

l. agency to which quality reporting measures are reported

m. list of specified information, such as all patients covered by one care provider

n. list of provider-preferred generic and brand-name drugs covered under various insurance plans

o. chronological list used in calculating statistics and record-keeping

MULTIPLE-CHOICE QUESTIONS

Select the letter that best completes the statement or answers the question:

1. **[LO 9.7]** In order to be a credentialed provider (for instance, a physician) within a healthcare facility, one requirement is
   a. being hired by a professional organization.
   b. gaining additional medical degrees.
   c. being covered by malpractice insurance.
   d. knowing procedures outside one's specialty.

2. **[LO 9.1]** In what year did Stage 2 of Meaningful Use begin for eligible providers?
   a. 2011
   b. 2012
   c. 2013
   d. 2014

3. **[LO 9.2]** When an alert is created, specifying a detail such as "search for patients 30 years or older" is an example of using a/an
   a. decision.
   b. filter.
   c. outlier.
   d. trend.

4. **[LO 9.5]** A healthcare professional typically uses an index to run a report of _____ information—for instance, all patients with gastroesophageal reflux disease, without esophagitis, ICD-10-CM code K21.9.
   a. basic
   b. encrypted
   c. statistical
   d. virtual

5. **[LO 9.1]** Healthcare facilities had _____ year[s] after the adoption of an EHR to prove Meaningful Use.
   a. one
   b. two
   c. three
   d. four

6. **[LO 9.3]** EHRclinic's reports can be used to
   a. justify the cost of new equipment.
   b. perform quality checks.
   c. track care provider data.
   d. all of these.

7. **[LO 9.2]** Meaningful Use requires that a practice not only implement at least one clinical support rule but also
   a. reduce alerts.
   b. reduce costs.

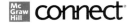

Enhance your learning by completing these exercises and more at **https://connect.mheducation.com**!

    c. track compliance.

    d. use evidence.

8. **[LO 9.4]** Custom reports have at least _____ variable(s) that is/are not available through a standard report.

    a. one

    b. two

    c. three

    d. four

9. **[LO 9.6]** You are reviewing a report that shows the patients born at Memorial Hospital from January 1, 2018, through December 31, 2018. The report is sorted by date and includes patient name, name of mother, time of birth, and name of obstetrician. Which type of report are you reviewing?

    a. dashboard

    b. index

    c. registry

    d. summary

10. **[LO 9.3]** EHRclinic's referring provider report is an example of a _____ report.

    a. clinical

    b. custom

    c. special

    d. standard

11. **[LO 9.5]** Care providers who contract with insurance carriers are known as being "in-network" and typically agree to a _____ rate of reimbursement for those services.

    a. higher

    b. lower

    c. special

    d. standard

12. **[LO 9.7]** Dr. Howard has just been hired by Memorial Orthopedic Associates. She must provide proof of her medical school education, experience, her state medical license number, her DEA number, and her _____.

    a. national provider identifier number

    b. driver's license number

    c. birth certificate

    d. proof of citizenship

SHORT-ANSWER QUESTIONS

1. **[LO 9.1]** What does it mean for a healthcare setting to report clinical quality measures?

2. **[LO 9.5]** Why might a hospital need to periodically print its entire Master Patient Index?

3. **[LO 9.3]** Contrast a summary report and a detail report.

4. **[LO 9.1]** Discuss the consequences (if any) if a provider does not achieve her core menu/objective percentages.

5. **[LO 9.2]** Explain the purpose of using filters when running a report.

6. **[LO 9.7]** What information is included in a provider's credentials?

7. **[LO 9.4]** If you needed to run a report of all the patients in your practice who were diagnosed with asthma, were African American, and were under the age of 15, what type of report would you be running? Explain your answer.

8. **[LO 9.3]** What is a procedure code analysis report?

9. **[LO 9.2]** List the benefits of clinical decision support.

10. **[LO 9.6]** List three things a registry might be used for.

11. **[LO 9.1]** Discuss the difference between the Stage 1 and Stage 2 Meaningful Use requirements for providing patients the ability to view or transmit their health information.

APPLYING YOUR KNOWLEDGE

1. **[LO 9.1]** Why might hospitals be exempt from the e-Prescribing core objective?

2. **[LOs 9.1, 9.3, 9.4, 9.5, 9.6]** As a healthcare professional, part of your job is answering patient questions. One day, a patient comes in, very concerned. When you ask what's wrong, she says, "I read about this term called *syndromatic surveillance*, and it really worries me! I don't want the government keeping tabs on me when I'm sick!" What would you say to her to alleviate her fears?

3. **[LO 9.6]** Why are registries kept in chronological order?

4. **[LO 9.2]** How can EHRclinic assist a practice in the fight against cancer?

5. **[LOs 9.2, 9.3, 9.4, 9.6]** Imagine that the state you reside in recently passed a measure requiring that a report of all immunizations administered at your practice be submitted to the state office of public health. How would you go about fulfilling this request while maintaining patient confidentiality? How can your office use the data to improve patient care?

6. **[LO 9.7]** Dr. Smith is a new provider in your office. Currently, he does not have board certification. Is it imperative that he obtain this credential? Why or why not?

7. **[LO 9.7]** Explain the DEA number and its use.

8. **[LO 9.1]** Discuss why the Stage 2 Meaningful Use requirements are more stringent than those for Stage 1.

9. **[LO 9.4]** Why are variables necessary in a custom report?

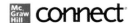

Enhance your learning by completing these exercises and more at **https://connect.mheducation.com**!

chapter references

Capsite: *2012 Ambulatory EHR & PM Study.* (2012, September). Retrieved from http://capsite.com/assets /Uploads/2012-Ambulatory-EHR-PM-StudyTOC.pdf.

Capsite: *2012 Health Information Exchange Study.* (2012, September). Retrieved from http://capsite.com /assets/Uploads/2012-Health-Information-Exchange-StudyTOC2.pdf.

Capsite: *Fifth Annual Ambulatory PM and EHR Study.* (2013, June). Retrieved from http://capsite.com /assets/Uploads/2013-Ambulatory-EHR-Study-TOC6.pdf.

Centers for Medicare & Medicaid Services. (2012, August). *Stage 1 vs. Stage 2 Comparison Table for Eligible Hospitals and CAHs.* Retrieved from https://www.cms.gov/regulations-and-guidance/legislation /ehrincentiveprograms/downloads/stage1vsstage2comptablesforhospitals.pdf.

Centers for Medicare & Medicaid Services. (2017). *Eligible Professional Medicaid EHR Incentive Program Stage 3 Objectives and Measures Objective Objectives 2 of 8* Guidance/Legislation/EHRIncentive Programs/Downloads/MedicaidEPStage3_Obj2.pdf

Centers for Medicare & Medicaid Services. (2018). *Stage 3 Program Requirements for Eligible Hospitals, CAH and Dual-Eligible Hospitals Attesting to CMS.* https://www.cms.gov/Regulations-and-Guidance /Legislation/EHRIncentivePrograms/Stage3_RequieEH.html.

Centers for Medicare & Medicaid Services. (2019, February). *2019 Program Requirements.* Retrieved from https://www.cms.gov/Regulations-and-Guidance/Legislation/EHRIncentivePrograms/2019Program RequirementsMedicare.html.

Centers for Medicare & Medicaid Services. (2019, April). *Value-Based Payment Modifier.* Retrieved from https://www.cms.gov/medicare/medicare-fee-for-service-payment/physicianfeedbackprogram /valuebasedpaymentmodifier.html.

HIMSS. (2016). *Clinical Decision Support.* Retrieved from http://www.himss.org/ASP/topics_clinicalDecision .asp.

U.S. Department of Health and Human Services. (2016). *The DataBank.* Retrieved from http://www.npdb-hipdb .hrsa.gov/.

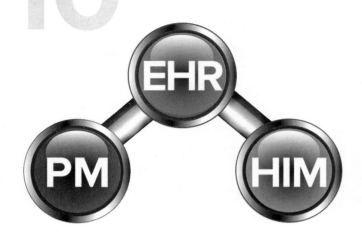

chapter ten

Looking Ahead— The Future of Health Information and Informatics

The Big Picture

What You Need to Know and Why You Need to Know It

Technology is part of the healthcare world, whether you are a clinician or an administrator. It was mentioned earlier that healthcare as a whole has been reluctant to embrace the digital age. However, that is not so when it comes to the computerization of medical technology such as diagnostic and treatment procedures. Newer technologies are less invasive, require shorter recovery time, require less (or no) hospitalization, and are safer overall than previous procedures. Though we are far ahead in the use of medical technology for diagnostic and treatment purposes, healthcare has lagged far behind other industries where computerization of *information* is concerned. In this chapter we will explore some of the more common methods to access electronic records and will discuss newer (at least to healthcare) technologies that have increased in use in the past few years, and how they have improved aspects of healthcare. As a healthcare professional, it is imperative that you stay abreast of emerging technologies. Even if you do not initially hold a position where you are involved in selection or implementation, you will definitely use technology in all the positions you will hold throughout your career. And since you have chosen healthcare as a profession, you have also chosen to become a lifelong learner—do not get too comfortable with how something is done today, as it will surely change in the blink of an eye!

Health information management (HIM) A profession that encompasses services in planning, collecting, aggregating, analyzing, and disseminating individual patient and aggregate clinical data (in paper or electronic format).

Health informatics The management of automated health information; the technological side of managing health information—the design, development, structure, implementation, integration, and management of the technical aspects of electronic (automated) health record-keeping.

10.1 Health Information versus Health Informatics

The American Health Information Management Association (AHIMA) Committee on Professional Development states the vision of **health information management (HIM)** as follows:

> *Health information management is the body of knowledge and practice that ensures the availability of health information to facilitate real-time healthcare delivery and critical health related decision-making for multiple purposes across diverse organizations, settings, and disciplines.* (AHIMA)

The health information management professional's role in the provision of quality healthcare is to ensure the availability of complete, accurate, timely health information and the collection of data necessary to make healthcare decisions, whether related to a particular patient or to the population as a whole.

Whereas health information management pertains to both paper and automated capture, retrieval, storage, and use of health information, **health informatics** is the management of automated health information in particular. Health information professionals whose work is geared more toward informatics focus on the structure of data, interoperability, the design of input and output tools, security controls, the development of data dictionaries, workflow configuration in an automated environment, and the classification systems and terminologies used in a computerized healthcare system.

In short, health informatics is managing the technology that houses health information—the design, development, structure, implementation, integration, and management of the technical aspects of electronic record-keeping. HIM professionals have historically ensured accurate, complete, readily available health information for use by care providers, administrators, researchers, public health officials, and insurers. Their focus is the content of the record, the integration of systems, and the ability to share electronic information. They manage health information regardless of the media on which it is kept. The HIM professionals and the IT professionals within a facility have always worked very closely to ensure that standards are met and information is available while maintaining the privacy and security of the information. In health informatics, there is a melding of the two disciplines—IT expertise with HIM expertise—and both may be embodied in the same person.

For years, health information management programs at all levels have included coursework in information-related software, as well as electronic record-keeping, in their curricula. Colleges and universities include in-depth coverage of the electronic health record in their medical assisting, medical billing and coding, medical office management, and healthcare administration programs. Providing instruction in these core concepts is instrumental in preparing students in these allied health disciplines for their careers in healthcare.

In a physician's office as well as other outpatient or even long-term care facilities, there may not be degreed health information professionals per se, but there is an individual in the facility who should know the requirements of a legal electronic health record, documentation requirements, and privacy and security regulations. Software service providers also have support staff who actively participate in the installation and training of a PM or EHR system, as well as know the most up-to-date IT security requirements for the storage, retrieval, and sharing of sensitive patient data. They advise practices and facilities on using the software efficiently and effectively to ensure the security and privacy of the information collected, as well as to ensure that documentation requirements are being met. If the practice does not have a full- or part-time technology position staffed, the office will contract with either a consultant or the software service provider's team.

Check Your Understanding

1. Between health information management and health informatics, which discipline is most closely associated with IT and which with information itself?
2. How can a practice management software service provider assist an office or a facility that does not have a degreed HIM professional on staff?

10.2 Initial Adoptions of Electronic Health Records

In the early years of transitioning from paper health records to electronic health records, there was resistance to giving up paper. No doubt there are still healthcare workers who have been a part of the transition to EHRs yet continue to prefer the paper record.

For years, care providers have been documenting the health records of patients by writing orders, progress notes, and chart notes or by dictating history & physicals (H&Ps), discharge summaries, operative reports, consultation reports, and correspondence. They were used to it, as that was how it had always been done. Providers would have known that if a laboratory test result was needed during a patient's visit, they needed only to flip to the laboratory tab of the patient's folder and it would be there (well, hopefully, it would be). Additionally, paper and folders are inexpensive, relatively speaking, so this was perceived as the ideal way to create, maintain, and store patient records. If it was impossible to complete the record at the time the patient was seen, the record was sent to the health information department for completion at a later time, or if a patient was seen in the office and the provider needed to dictate the chart note, it was easy enough to take the record back to her private office to complete later. Many care providers saw this paper system as being easier, and it may have seemed more efficient; however, the quality of the documentation that was written or dictated days (or even weeks) after the care was provided could be considered questionable. Handwritten paper records were often illegible, and if dictation and transcription were used, there was a lag time before the typed report could be filed in the record. Additionally, from a security perspective, a paper record could easily be picked up by someone with no need to have the record or see its contents, and if a paper record was lost, hours of staff time would have been spent searching for it.

Implementing and maintaining an electronic record is expensive, that is true. But the argument for patient safety, higher-quality medical care, point of care documentation, faster access to results of diagnostic tests, and the ability to both share information with other care providers when necessary and access a patient's health information from any location (not to mention access clinical decision support) should outweigh the "high cost" argument. Financial incentives through HITECH were the initial driving forces for many practices that had decided to convert to a paperless (or almost paperless) system. Beginning in 2011, hospitals and physicians' practices that adopted and proved meaningful use of EHRs started receiving an incentive payment. Shortly afterward, physicians were expected to begin the transition of compliance, and there was neither an incentive nor a penalty. In 2015, facilities and eligible providers who had held out and had not implemented an EHR, likely thinking that it would go away, began to receive penalties and fines for noncompliance.

Converting from a paper system to an electronic system was considered a lengthy, sometimes chaotic process. It no doubt caused a loss of productivity for both staff and care providers. When office procedures that seemed efficient in the manual form became computerized, errors in conversion were expected, some steps in the process may have been overlooked, and many of those involved became frustrated. However, planning, heeding the advice of the software service provider's installation team, and accepting the fact that the conversion, training of staff, and use of the system were expected to be a difficult and lengthy transition made the process more tolerable. In any healthcare facility or practice using an EHR, it took a great deal of time and effort to convert to and use the electronic systems, but the same can be said for any change in procedure in any profession. The use of EHRs is now an industry expectation, and it has proven to provide better functionality, an increase in patient safety, and improved continuity of care.

A study published by the American Medical Association in 2016 reported provider comments ranging from a preference for communicating with patients virtually (to answer patients' follow-up questions) and touting the benefits of ePrescribing to the detrimental effects of multiple clicks on a computer screen and slow response time, causing a clinician to feel more like clerical staff than a clinician.

Check Your Understanding

1. Healthcare facilities and eligible providers that do not adopt electronic record technology began facing penalties in what year?
2. What was the initial driving force behind facilities adopting EHRs?

10.3 Ancillary Technologies

Patient Portals

Patients today are more interested and involved in their own healthcare than ever before. They are taking a more active role and, thanks to the Internet, arrive at their appointments knowing what their care provider may ask and why, as well as what treatment options exist. They have a list of questions ready for the care provider, which allows for a more productive visit. **Patient portals** are another means for better, more meaningful communication with a care provider, and these portals are a functionality of EHRs that satisfies Meaningful Use. A patient portal is a method of accessing portions of one's own office health record. These portals are secure and can be accessed only with a user ID and password. Through it, patients can

> **Patient portal** A method of accessing portions of one's own health information from the care provider's or hospital's electronic health record.

- Email the practice with questions or concerns regarding care
- Make appointments
- Complete history forms and authorizations online
- Request prescription refills
- See the results of diagnostic tests
- Access the contents of one's own health record

By using the secure portal, the office staff spends less time answering phone calls, calling patients back (or playing phone tag), and entering data in the record; patients are more satisfied because their questions are answered more promptly, and they feel that they are more in control of their care. You may not realize that your care provider offers a patient portal; if the office is automated, and an EHR is in use, ask about it!

Many insurance plans have similar options for their subscribers, including communicating with a nurse or care provider to answer questions about symptoms, treatment options, coverage, and the like. Take a few moments to look at the website for your own health insurance—does it have patient portal capability? If so, what functionalities are provided? How can you use this to engage in your own healthcare?

Personal Health Records (PHRs)

A **personal health record (PHR)**, which is maintained and kept by the patient, is a record of his or her past and current health information, including drug allergies or reactions, immunization dates, past, and present medical conditions, surgical procedures, family history, list of current medications, and insurance information. The PHR is not a legal record because it is just that—personal; there are no safeguards to ensure that it is complete, it is not written by a medical professional, much of it may have been compiled from memory, and it does not meet the legal requirement of "being compiled during the normal course of business."

> **Personal health record (PHR)** A record, kept by the patient, that contains a person's health history, immunization status, current and past medications, allergies, and instructions given by a care provider; it often includes patient education materials as well.

However, it is a valuable tool when a patient seeks medical care, particularly if emergency care is required or if there has been a change in care providers. The PHR is only as good as the information in it—*all* of the information should be up-to-date and accurate. It also needs to be available when needed. If patients expect their PHR to be a useful document, family members should know where it is kept, and it should be taken to office visits or to the emergency department when such visits occur and updated with any new or changed information. Patients may keep the PHR in a paper format or online (or may print it from the online portal). There are many options for doing so, including the PHR websites of many major insurance carriers. Or patients may choose free online sites such as HealthVault at https://www.healthvault.com/ and Healthspek at https://www.healthspek.com/. Both are easy tools to keep up-to-date records of health history, medication history, immunizations, hospitalizations, and so on. PHRs are not new, but their use is becoming increasingly widespread.

Telemedicine

Telehealth Associated with preventive care, telehealth is the use of audiovisual equipment through which the patient and the care provider or healthcare professional can connect remotely.

Telemedicine The use of technology to remotely monitor a patient's vital signs and perform tests such as an EKG or to forward radiologic images.

Telehealth and **telemedicine** are of great benefit to patients who do not have the means to travel to a doctor's appointment or who live in remote, medically under-served areas. Telehealth, also referred to as eHealth, would typically be used in preventive or counseling visits which used to be done over the phone. Often it is a nurse who conducts these telehealth sessions, but can be other healthcare providers as well. Through telemedicine technology, a patient's blood pressure, heart rate, respiratory rate, EKG tracing, or medical imaging can be monitored remotely. Should the care provider find something that is not within normal limits, the patient would then need to seek on-site care or have emergency care dispatched. The imaging technology of Picture Archiving and Communications Systems (PACS), whereby radiologic images are viewed remotely, is one of the original uses of telemedicine.

Using telemedicine offers cost savings to both the insurance carrier and the patient; patients who would not otherwise be able to make visits to their care providers now have better access to care, which in turn improves outcomes and generally is more convenient for patients, particularly those who do not have transportation or who live a distance away from their care provider.

The Institute of Medicine's report *Telemedicine: A Guide to Assessing Telecommunications for Health Care* can be downloaded online by searching by the title.

Many Veterans Affairs Medical Centers provide telemedicine or telehealth to assist in the care of veterans. The Department of Veterans Affairs telehealth website can be found at http://www.telehealth.va.gov/index.asp.

Patient-Centered Medical Home (PCMH)

Patient-Centered Medical Home (PCMH) A model that was developed by the American Academy of Family Practitioners to care for patients with chronic conditions, to encourage and facilitate a patient's (and family's) involvement in his or her own care.

Patient-Centered Medical Home (PCMH) is a model that was developed by the American Academy of Family Practitioners to care for patients with chronic conditions. The premise encourages and facilitates the patient's (and family's) involvement in his or her own care. It is mentioned in this chapter because it ties in with the concept of a patient-centric health model. The PCMH also encourages a primary care physician approach to patient care. This is also the premise of many managed care insurance plans that require a "gatekeeper" to reduce redundancy and overutilization of testing and services and to provide overall more efficient and effective healthcare.

The use of health information technology is paramount to the PCMH model because the use of quality measures, including registries, referral tracking, results tracking, medication alerts, performance measures, evidence-based medicine, updated problem lists, and current medication lists, is part of the PCMH model—all of the elements that are requirements of Meaningful Use as well.

Evidence-Based Medicine

Meaningful use of data requires decision support capability as part of the EHR. This is also known as **evidence-based medicine (EBM)** because physicians have the ability to quickly access medical journals and academic sites that provide them with the most current diagnostic and treatment protocols that are relevant to that particular patient's condition. The patient's current and past health information is right in front of the physician, in the patient's EHR; from within that EHR, one click will take the physician to those protocols and best practices to treat the patient's condition. Through evidence-based medicine, a patient's plan of care is based on current, proven practice. Alerts, or reminders, automatically appear in a patient's chart based on data captured about that patient. An example is a female patient who has just passed her fortieth birthday. The FDA Office of Women's Health recommends that a screening mammogram be performed at the age of 40 and every one to two years thereafter (FDA). Current EHR software makes it possible for physicians to be alerted to the latest diagnostic and treatment recommendations and modalities, which in turn improves efficiency, patient care, and clinical outcomes. An office, for example, can set parameters within the EHR software that meet the industry standards for wellness screening, such as that all female patients over the age of 40 have an annual mammogram. Once these parameters are set, the EHR can perform wellness screening searches to determine which patients are overdue for testing and screening, which gives the practice an opportunity to send out reminders to patients that it is time to make an appointment because a screening test is due. Better compliance with these initiatives results in earlier diagnosis and treatment of diseases and conditions. It is clear why the use of evidence-based medicine is part of the Meaningful Use regulations.

Evidence-based medicine (EBM)
Diagnostic and treatment protocols that are based on proven research and documented best practices.

Check Your Understanding

1. What are the diagnostic and treatment protocols of evidence-based medicine based on?
2. Is a patient's personal health record a legal document? Explain your answer.
3. For a patient being monitored using telemedicine, what would happen if an abnormal reading were found?
4. How might a PCMH make a patient's experience more positive?

10.4 Making the World of Health Informatics User Friendly and Convenient

In order for an electronic health record system to be successful, the care providers need to be satisfied with the product. They typically look for portability, mobility, flexibility, and convenience—all the qualities of the products used in the 21st century and all requirements available to the healthcare team if they are to work efficiently.

Local area network (LAN) A network linking computers and related devices that are physically close to one another such as within a building.

Wide area network (WAN) Connects computer networks together that are not physically close.

Personal digital assistant (PDA) A mobile device that is small enough to fit in one's hand yet allows access to local area networks (LANs), wide area networks (WANs), and the Internet; may also have telephone capability.

Smartphone Telephone that allows Internet browsing, audio, video, and camera functionality.

Tablet computer Computer that is larger than a PDA or smartphone yet smaller than a laptop computer; allows access to local area networks (LANs), wide area networks (WANs), and the Internet.

Portable devices allow for flexibility and mobility. They are advantageous because they are convenient (the provider does not have to find a computer to use); they are cost-effective (the provider can use an inexpensive device and there is no need to rework because notes and procedure codes are entered at the point of care, which reduces the number of lost or missing charges); they improve accuracy (the care provider does not have to jot down notes that must be transferred into the record later); and, in general, they create overall satisfaction, since the information needed to care for patients is available at any time from any location. A connection to the EHR may be through a **local area network (LAN)** or a **wide area network (WAN)**. LANs link computers and related devices that are in close proximity to one another. WANs connect computer networks together that unlike LANs, are not in close proximity. (Figure 10.1). And, of course, access can be via the Internet. One type of portable device is a **personal digital assistant (PDA)**; PDAs, though not seen often, are still in use, and are compact devices that not only allow access to LANs, WANs, and the Internet, but also may double as a phone. **Smartphones** are telephones that also allow Internet browsing, as well as audio, video, and camera functionality; and **tablet computers** are larger than PDAs and smartphones yet smaller than laptop computers—they, too, provide access to LANs, WANs, and the Internet. Though PDAs and tablets are used, smartphones have much of the same functionality, and many users prefer carrying one device rather than two or more. As with all healthcare technology, HIPAA requirements should be considered to ensure the privacy and safety of protected health information (PHI) accessed via devices such as these.

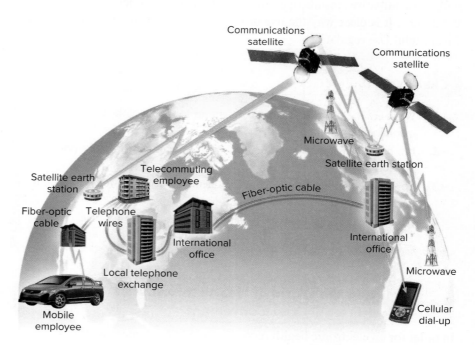

Figure 10.1 Depiction of a Wide Area Network (WAN)

Source: Williams, B.K., and Sawyer, S.C. (2011). *Using Information Technology: A Practical Introduction to Computers & Communications* (9th ed.). New York: McGraw-Hill Companies.

1. What are smartphones?
2. Describe three instances when access to an EHR on a mobile device would improve a care provider's efficiency or save time.

10.5 Advancing the Use of EHRs Remotely Yet Securely

EHRs have advanced medicine and certainly have brought documentation into the 21st century. But they have also brought challenges as well.

Can you imagine going back to "wired" technology in your personal use of electronic devices? Probably not, so at this point, most healthcare professionals would find that nearly impossible. To use mobile functionality, a wireless, high radio frequency connection is necessary, known as Wi-Fi. This is known as **Wi-Fi**, which sends data via high radio frequency. Of course, using mobile technology does require high levels of security. The use of a **virtual private network (VPN)** is one way to ensure the security of the information flowing between the mobile device and the EHR. The data being sent through mobile technology is "coded," known as encryption, as it is sent over the Internet. This encryption takes place within the software of the virtual private network. On the receiving end the data is decrypted, known as **decryption**, meaning that it is translated into meaningful form. A VPN also verifies the identity of the user through his or her user ID and password, and it allows access only to users who have been granted permission to sign on to the network. A VPN is also used for employees who telecommute (work from home) and are dialing into the facility's computer system from a home computer or laptop. A VPN provides a secure environment for users to share information with other users at remote locations. In addition to the VPN, a firewall is another security method (Figure 10.2).

Wi-Fi Data exchange via high radio frequency.

Virtual private network (VPN) Software that encrypts (codes) the data being sent as well as interprets the data being received.

Decryption Interpretation of data being received in encrypted (scrambled) form.

Virtual Private Networks (VPNs)

Firewalls prevent unauthorized access into or out of the network through the use of both hardware and software devices that filter activity over the network. Based on predefined rules, the firewall acts as a barrier; activity that passes the rules may continue into or out of the network, but an activity that does not pass the rules may not.

These security measures are necessary to exchange information on a small scale within or among related medical practices or hospitals, as well as between the health information exchanges (HIEs) that are the vision of the Office of the National Coordinator (ONC).

Cloud Computing

In recent years, there has been a rise in the number of systems that do not reside on a physical server owned, maintained, and operated by a hospital or medical practice. Rather, the data is housed "in the cloud." In **cloud computing**, the cloud service provider, rather than an Internet service provider, is in control, and a cloud environment has unlimited processing and storage capacity. In a private cloud configuration, the storage space is solely for a single organization. It is scalable—the facility or office uses just

Cloud computing The housing of data in a cloud environment, which is a commercially maintained site on the Internet.

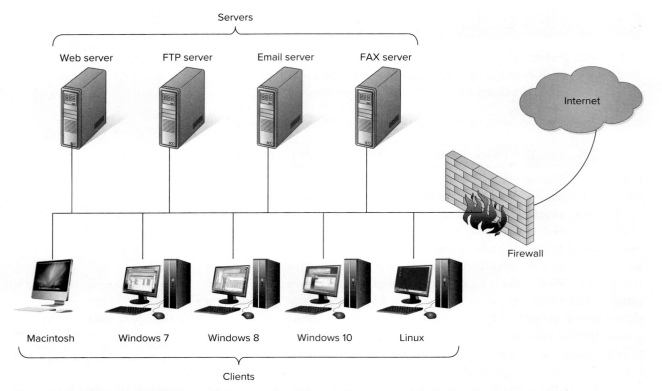

Figure 10.2 **Placement of a Firewall between Computers, Servers, and the Internet**

Source: C. Holcombe and J. Holcombe (2012). *Survey of Operating Systems* (3rd ed.). New York: McGraw-Hill Companies.

the amount of storage space it needs and then expands its storage space as needed, thus paying only for space it is using (Dinh). If there should be an equipment failure or damage of some sort, the database is not affected. Think of email services such as Gmail® (Google) or Yahoo!® or document storage services such as Google Docs, Evernote, or Dropbox; if a person loses his or her laptop or if a desktop computer is destroyed in a fire, emails and documents are not lost, since the data is stored on Google's or Yahoo!'s server. The security of the data is ensured. There is no hardware cost (for servers) associated with data stored in the cloud, and the system is mobile, allowing care providers to utilize mobile devices to access records and receive important, time-sensitive notifications at any time.

Cloud computing means that data is still Internet-centric, so privacy and security of the data is a concern. Compliance with HIPAA regulations must be considered before choosing a cloud service provider.

Data Analytics

Throughout this worktext, we've discussed data—collecting it, ensuring its accuracy, maintaining it, securing it, and keeping its privacy. It is being kept for a purpose—future healthcare of the patient and analysis of it to improve healthcare for generations to come. To do so effectively and efficiently, it is necessary to use **artificial intelligence (AI)**.

Artificial intelligence goes a step further because, with so much data available to them, researchers are learning more than they had ever imagined. There is knowledge within what is learned from the data collected. For instance, a study may be done to answer a question about Alzheimer's disease, which leads researchers to answers about a completely different disease process that they weren't even looking for in the first place.

artificial intelligence (AI) The use of computer systems that are able to perform tasks that had typically required the use of human intelligence. Examples include the use of robotics to fill prescriptions in pharmacies, the use of natural language processing in speech recognition technology, and facial recognition technology.

But all of this data needs to be managed and governed properly. The data also must be analyzed and reported responsibly. Regulatory oversight is necessary to ensure compliance.

Cybersecurity Threats

As with any electronic system, healthcare data is also prone to risk and threats of data hacking and breaches. It is the responsibility of healthcare organizations to ensure that their systems are properly protected to reduce their risk of either. In a hospital setting, this is often a combined effort between the IT and the HIM departments.

What Is on the Horizon?

Interoperability has not been an easy nut to crack in the healthcare technology journey, at least not where sharing health information is concerned. In addition, the introduction of electronic records has made health information more fragmented and is kept under close control, often being difficult to access when needed to make critical clinical decisions.

Since the third edition of this worktext was written, the idea of using blockchain technology has become a potential solution to one of the major roadblocks to acceptance of the electronic health record. What is **blockchain**? It is a distributed database that is stored on multiple computers that may or may not be in the same location. The recordings or data are known as blocks, and new blocks are constantly being added. Each is time-stamped and linked to the previous block, thus forming a chain. Everyone within the organization or the system, as in a healthcare system, gets a copy of the chain; thus, they all have access to the entire database.

Blockchain A distributed database that is stored on multiple computers that may or may not be in the same location.

All blocks remain part of the record forever, documents cannot be manipulated, and all transactions are time- and date-stamped. All blocks are encrypted, so anyone with a need to know has access to needed information, but only users having a special cryptographic key can add a new record to a chain. The chains can only be added to; nothing can be taken away or changed once a transaction is part of the chain.

The core concepts of blockchain are

1. Private key cryptography—only a person who has a cryptographic key, a coded message—i.e., a series of numbers, letters, and symbols that equate to a person's identity but keeps that person's identity private, used to access network housing information, for instance, electronic health information

2. Distributed network—a system whereby the programming, software, and data are spread across multiple computers but communicate through nodes (computers) and are dependent upon each other

3. Transaction ledger—the health record, paper records scanned into the EHR, and claims documents (billing information), which are encrypted, digitally signed, and stored in the blockchain; once stored, they cannot be changed or erased

A cryptographic key is similar to a password, but only the person who has that cryptographic key can alter a particular transaction (for instance, a history & physical report). As long as the author of the report remains the only person who knows the key, no one can manipulate his or her transactions. In addition, cryptography is used to guarantee the synchronization of copies of the blockchain on each computer (or node) in the network. This method makes the data both accessible and secure.

Pulling It All Together

The intent of this worktext has been to introduce students to the automation of health information, with emphasis on those who have chosen to study health information management, medical assisting, and medical billing and coding. Having chosen one of these professions, you will work closely with automated systems. Many of you will be lucky enough to be involved in choosing a system from the very first steps, others will use the systems on a daily basis, and yet others will climb the ladder into the implementation, training, and development of computer programs and systems that will enhance the automated exchange of information.

Medicine and healthcare are not static; changes occur daily. Those changes must be communicated, implemented, and tracked to determine their impact on patient care. As a healthcare professional, you will not be observing from the sidelines; instead, you will be an active participant in improving quality healthcare through the availability of complete, accurate, and secure health information.

Check Your Understanding

1. How does a VPN verify a user's identity?
2. What role does encryption play in using VPNs?
3. Explain what is meant by the *scalability* of cloud computing.
4. Explain how blockchain can be used in health information.

APPLYING YOUR SKILLS

As a healthcare consumer, name 5 to 10 experiences you have had or have witnessed in which any aspect of healthcare was electronic rather than manual.

chapter 10 summary

LEARNING OUTCOME	CONCEPTS FOR REVIEW
10.1 Compare health information management to health informatics.	– Define health information management – Define health informatics – Role of HIM professional in each
10.2 Discuss barriers that remain to the adoption of electronic health records.	– Written records and dictation have been the norm – Paper and dictation are fairly inexpensive – Lengthy process to convert to electronic records – Extensive training time – Loss of productivity – High frustration level
10.3 Describe ancillary technologies or models that are improving the care of patients through information technology.	– Patient portals—means of communication between patients and medical practice – Personal health record—patient keeps own record of history, immunizations, allergies, surgeries, past conditions, and family history – Telemedicine allows patient to be "seen" without leaving the home – Patient-Centered Medical Home (PCMH)—primary care physician is leader of a team that cares for the patient; patient is more involved than in traditional approach; use of technology inherent in the process – Evidence-based medicine—technology "researches" best practices and decision support to assure that patient is receiving most up-to-date diagnostic and treatment options
10.4 Illustrate three mobile devices that will make the collection and sharing of health information more timely and efficient.	– Use of EHR can be more convenient by making it mobile; use of personal digital assistants (PDAs), smartphones, and tablet computers allow for portability – Wireless (Wi-Fi) connections are required to use portable devices

10.5 Describe how virtual private networks (VPNs) and cloud computing are advancing the use of EHRs.	– Though portability is necessary, so is security
	– Virtual private networks encrypt and interpret information that is sent and received via wireless networks
	– Use of firewalls as a security device
	– Cloud computing: commercially maintained storage site on the Internet
	  • Unlimited storage and processing capability
	  • Scalable (pay for as much or as little storage as used)
	  • Private cloud is for use by one organization
	  • Database not affected by equipment failure, power outages, or physical damage
	– New technology
	  • Blockchain technology

chapter review

MATCHING QUESTIONS

Match the terms on the left with the definitions on the right.

_____ 1. **[LO 10.5]** decryption

_____ 2. **[LO 10.1]** health information management (HIM)

_____ 3. **[LO 10.3]** patient portal

_____ 4. **[LO 10.3]** evidence-based medicine

_____ 5. **[LO 10.3]** personal health record (PHR)

_____ 6. **[LO 10.3]** telemedicine

_____ 7. **[LO 10.5]** virtual private network (VPN)

_____ 8. **[LO 10.5]** Wi-Fi

_____ 9. **[LO 10.1]** health informatics

_____ 10. **[LO 10.5]** cloud computing

_____ 11. **[LO 10.4]** wide area network (WAN)

_____ 12. **[LO 10.5]** blockchain

a. clinical decision support based on research and best practices

b. a distributed database that is stored on multiple computers

c. link computers within the same company that are not located in close proximity

d. uncoding coded data to make it readable

e. high radio frequency wireless connection used by smartphones, PDAs, and other electronic devices

f. unlimited storage and processing capability

g. secure method of accessing individual health records and information through an EHR

h. secure Internet environment that encrypts data and allows remote access to health information

i. medical history maintained and kept by an individual patient

j. monitoring or exchange of health information remotely

k. improving healthcare through working with data and ensuring that the best information is available for decision making

l. science that deals with health information and its structure, acquisition, and uses

MULTIPLE-CHOICE QUESTIONS

Select the letter that best completes the statement or answers the question:

1. **[LO 10.1]** Health informatics is basically the _____ part of managing health information.
   a. critical
   b. structural
   c. technological
   d. usable

2. **[LO 10.4]** One benefit of accessing the EHR through mobile devices is a reduction in
   a. cost.
   b. errors.
   c. satisfaction.
   d. both cost and errors.

3. **[LO 10.2]** Incentives are being offered to EHR adopters through _____ legislation.
   a. CCHIP
   b. HIPAA
   c. HITECH
   d. ONC

4. **[LO 10.3]** Care providers use _____ as a way to support their decisions and diagnoses.
   a. current medical trends
   b. evidence-based medicine
   c. Meaningful Use
   d. patient-centric care

5. **[LO 10.1]** Which of the following stakeholders are served by the health information management profession?
   a. patient care organizations
   b. payers
   c. research agencies
   d. all of these

6. **[LO 10.2]** Which of the following is a way to make the transition to EHRs easier?
   a. Allow staff members to be frustrated and anxious about the change.
   b. Follow the advice and suggestions of the EHR service provider's installation team.
   c. Provide immediate training, so that ramp-up is quicker.
   d. Save money for EHR costs by eliminating staff.

7. **[LO 10.3]** A PCMH focuses on _____ communication between patients and providers.
   a. decreased
   b. increased
   c. random
   d. structured

8. **[LO 10.1]** Of the following, which is an accurate statement?
   a. Eligible providers taking advantage of HITECH funds must have a credentialed or degreed health information professional on staff.
   b. In the event the eligible provider is unable to hire a credentialed or degreed health information professional on staff, he or she must use the services of a paid health information consultant.
   c. Though not required, the expertise of a health information professional on staff, as a consultant or as offered by the service provider, is helpful.
   d. The EHR software is already written to handle any health information–related issues; therefore, no additional input or services from a health information professional are necessary.

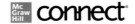 Enhance your learning by completing these exercises and more at **https://connect.mheducation.com!**

9. **[LO 10.4]** There must be a/an _____ available in order for providers to use portable devices to access health information.
   a. computer terminal
   b. Internet hookup
   c. wireless connection
   d. wireless mouse

10. **[LO 10.3]** Who is responsible for maintaining a personal health record?
    a. HIM professional
    b. patient
    c. provider
    d. medical staff

11. **[LO 10.2]** Penalties for facilities not adopting electronic health records began in
    a. 2014.
    b. 2015.
    c. 2016.
    d. 2017.

12. **[LO 10.3]** Videoconferencing and remote vital sign monitoring are part of
    a. patient-centric care.
    b. a patient portal.
    c. telemedicine.
    d. virtual health networks.

13. **[LO 10.5]** What does VPN stand for?
    a. verifying provider network
    b. verified protocol network
    c. virtual private network
    d. virtual provider network

14. **[LO 10.3]** Recent advances in healthcare rely increasingly on
    a. change.
    b. precedent.
    c. technology.
    d. tradition.

SHORT-ANSWER QUESTIONS

1. **[LO 10.1]** Explain the difference between health information and health informatics.

2. **[LO 10.3]** What are some advantages to a healthcare facility's use of the patient portal function?

3. **[LO 10.4]** What is a mobile device?

4. **[LO 10.5]** How does a VPN ensure data integrity and security?

5. **[LO 10.2]** Explain why many care providers view a paper-based system as easier than an electronic one.

6. **[LO 10.1]** What does an HIM professional do?

7. **[LO 10.2]** How can healthcare facilities make the adoption of EHRs as easy and painless as possible?

8. **[LO 10.4]** How do mobile applications reduce costs and errors?

9. **[LO 10.3]** Describe a Patient-Centered Medical Home (PCMH).

10. **[LO 10.5]** Explain what Wi-Fi is.

APPLYING YOUR KNOWLEDGE

1. **[LO 10.3]** After reading about the patient portal in your text, can you think of any potential disadvantages of patients using the patient portal system within the EHR? Justify your answer.

2. **[LO 10.2]** What is your opinion on the use of incentives to encourage healthcare facilities to adopt EHRs? Explain your answer.

3. **[LOs 10.4, 10.5]** You are a healthcare professional who has the ability to work from home on certain days. How would you go about accessing the work you needed to do on a given day from your home?

4. **[LOs 10.1, 10.2, 10.3, 10.4, 10.5]** Your healthcare office is beginning to discuss adopting an EHR system, mobile accessibility, and other new capabilities such as telemedicine. Your supervisor has asked you to come up with some brief talking points for the staff discussing the new technologies, their advantages, and ways in which each staff member will be affected by the new systems. Come up with a short outline for your presentation.

5. **[LO 10.5]** Justify why a physician's practice or hospital may choose cloud computing over on-site servers. Are there any drawbacks to using a cloud environment instead of traditional servers? Explain.

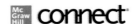

Enhance your learning by completing these exercises and more at **https://connect.mheducation.com!**

chapter references

Abdelhak, M., Grostick, S., Hanken, M.A., and Jacobs, E. (2007). *Health Information: Management of a Strategic Resource.* Philadelphia: Saunders.

American Health Information Management Association (AHIMA). (2003). Body of Knowledge, a Vision of the e-HIM Future: A Report from the AHIMA e-HIM Task Force. Supplement to the *Journal of AHIMA.*

American Telemedicine Association. Telemedicine Defined. Retrieved from www.americantelemed.org/.

Beckers Hospital Review. Things to Know about Blockchain in Healthcare. Retrieved from: https://www.beckershospitalreview.com/healthcare-information-technology/9-things-to-know-about-blockchain-in-healthcare.html March 31, 2019.

Cantrell, S. (2010). Reference and Information Services in the 21st Century: An Introduction, 2nd ed. *Journal of the Medical Library Association, 98*(3): 264–265. doi: 10.3163/1536-5050.98.3.019

Dinh, Angela K. Cloud Computing 101. *Journal of AHIMA 82*(4) (April 2011): 36–37.

FDA Office of Women's Health. (2011). *Mammograms.* Retrieved from http://www.fda.gov/.

Institute of Medicine. (1996). *Telemedicine: A Guide to Assessing Telecommunications for Health Care.* Retrieved from http://www.nap.edu/openbook.php?record_id=5296&page=R1.

LaTour, K.M., and Eichenwald-Maki, S. (2010). *Health Information Management: Concepts, Principles and Practice.* Chicago: AHIMAPress.

Menachemi, N., Powers, T.L., and Brooks, R.G. (2011). Physician and Practice Characteristics Associated with Longitudinal Increases in Electronic Health Records Adoption. *Essentials of the U.S. Health Care System, 56*(3): 183–197. Retrieved from EBSCO*host.*

Shi, L., and Sing, D.A. (2010). *Essentials of the U.S. Health Care System* (2nd ed.). Sudbury, MA: Jones and Bartlett Publishers.

Troseth, M. (2016, June 28)). Evidence-based practice: The key to advancing quality and safety in healthcare. Retrieved from http://beckershospitalreview.com/quality/evidence-based-practice-the-key-to-advancing-quality-and-safety-in-healthcare.html.

Viola, Allison. Blockchain's Role in Health IT. *Journal of AHIMA* 89, no. 9 (October 2018): 34–35, 54.

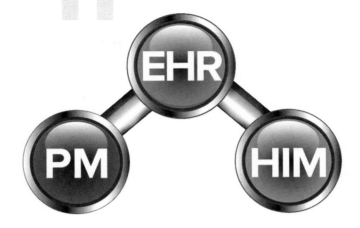

chapter eleven

Additional Practice

What You Need to Know and Why You Need to Know It

In previous chapters of the book, you had the chance to complete guided exercises using step-by-step directions. In this chapter, you will have the opportunity to apply the knowledge you have learned to a scenario that will take you through the entire medical documentation and billing process. Using source documents and references to earlier chapters, you will use your critical thinking skills to complete the simulated exercises related to the following scenario:

> *Harper Anna Jacobi has called Summit Bay Health Center to make an appointment. She says that she is a new patient and would like to see Dr. Ingram, as she has heard he is a great doctor. Harper states she would like to get in as soon as possible because she is miserable, with a sore throat, fever, and urinary symptoms.*

You will use the following source documents, located at the end of the chapter, to help you complete several of the exercises:

- Source Document A: Patient Registration Form
- Source Document B: Insurance Card
- Source Document C: Patient Intake Sheet
- Source Document D: Office Visit Notes
- Source Document E: Remittance Advice (RA)

EXERCISE 11.1

Go to https://connect.mheducation.com to complete this exercise. To see instructional notes with the steps, visit the eBook in Connect or download them from www.mhhe.com/iehr4.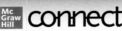

Register the Patient (Refer to Chapter 3 for assistance.)

The information the healthcare professional enters in this exercise is taken while on the initial phone call with the patient. Basic information such as full name, date of birth, address, and telephone numbers are entered into EHRclinic. The healthcare professional will email some paperwork to Harper before she arrives for her appointment. For our purposes, we will say she filled out the **Patient Registration Form** (Source Document A) and had her friend drop it off the same day she called in.

Register the patient using the information found on Source Document A. In addition, note that Harper is not a student and she works full-time. She also emailed her identification, so her image will need to be added to her new patient registration.

✔️ **You have completed Exercise 11.1**

EXERCISE 11.2

Go to https://connect.mheducation.com to complete this exercise. To see instructional notes with the steps, visit the eBook in Connect or download them from www.mhhe.com/iehr4.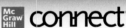

Capture Insurance Information of the Patient (Refer to Chapter 3 for assistance.)

Harper included her insurance information on the lower half of the Patient Registration Form.

Capture the insurance information from the **Patient Registration Form** (Source Document A) and enter it into EHRclinic by going into the Tools module, Manage practice data, and Patient information to access Harper's demographics. The expiration date of the insurance is 12/31/2022 and the plan is active. Harper does not have a deductible and there are no dependents.

✔️ **You have completed Exercise 11.2**

EXERCISE 11.3

Go to https://connect.mheducation.com to complete this exercise. To see instructional notes with the steps, visit the eBook in Connect or download them from www.mhhe.com/iehr4.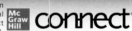

Schedule the Patient's Appointment (Refer to Chapter 3 for assistance.)

While on the initial phone call with the healthcare professional, Harper also made an appointment.

Schedule an appointment for Harper at the Summit Bay Health Center with Dr. Ingram on June 20, 2022, for a 30-minute 'new appointment' at 9:30 a.m. Enter the chief complaint using the **Office Visit Notes** (Source Document D). Do not state c/o or use the quotation marks in the visit reason.

✔️ **You have completed Exercise 11.3**

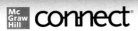
Check In the Patient Who Has Arrived (Refer to Chapter 3 for assistance.)

The scenario moves ahead and Harper has now arrived for her appointment.

Check Harper into EHRclinic. Her condition is not related to employment, auto accident, or other accident and the dates of current illness are the default dates of 6/20/2022 to 6/20/2022.

☑ **You have completed Exercise 11.4**

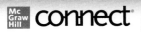

Post the Co-payment to the Account (Refer to Chapter 6 for assistance.)

Post the co-pay to Harper's account in EHRclinic. Recall that Harper has already been checked in, so payments will be accessed by going to the Accounts module. Refer to the **Insurance Card** (Source Document B) for the co-pay amount. She paid her co-pay with check number 5879. You will need to enter the check number in the appropriate field as part of the exercise.

Next, you will be adding a note to Harper's Facesheet to document the copayment. When the payment has been saved, click 'Cancel' to exit the payment details screen. Go to the Tools module, Manage reports, and Patient charts and graphs. Search for Harper Jacobi's chart; then scroll down to the Notes section in the Facesheet.

Add a new note with a title of 'Payment' and note details stating '$20 copay paid'. Click 'Done' to save the note.

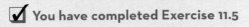 ☑ **You have completed Exercise 11.5**

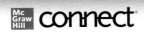

Enter the Patient's Past Medical History (Refer to Chapter 4 for assistance.)

The healthcare professional has come out to the waiting room to take Harper back to an exam room. While in the exam room, more information is gathered from the patient regarding past medical history, family and social histories, current medications, and allergies. Finally, a set of vitals is taken and entered in Harper's chart. A flag is also put on the chart to alert anyone on the healthcare team.

Enter the patient's past medical history using the **Patient Intake Sheet** (Source Document C) and the following bullet points (to provide detail not

(continued)

included in the Patient Intake Sheet and that would be gathered during the patient interview).

- Past medical history: Bronchitis details—Date onset 01/01/2004, no listed duration, and status resolved
- Surgical history: Appendectomy details—Date of surgery 04/01/2009
- Problem list: Seasonal allergies/hay fever details—ICD code edition is ICD-10-CM, ICD code is allergic rhinitis (other seasonal), no date of diagnosis or duration, and status is unresolved.
- Social history (use the Patient Intake Sheet plus this additional information):
  - Never smoked
  - Never used illicit drugs
  - Exercises frequently
  - Sleeps 8 hours per day
  - Always uses seat belt
  - Lives with parents (family)
  - Sexually active with one male partner, no history of STI diagnosis, and always uses protection
- Family medical history:
  - Mother has diabetes, type 2, and is alive.
  - Brother has asthma and is alive.

☑ **You have completed Exercise 11.6**

EXERCISE 11.7 **EHR** Go to https://connect.mheducation.com to complete this exercise. To see instructional notes with the steps, visit the eBook in Connect or download them from www.mhhe.com/iehr4. **Mc Graw Hill connect**

Enter the Patient's List of Current Medications and Known Drug Allergies (Refer to Chapter 4 for assistance.)

Enter Harper's current medications and known drug allergies into EHRclinic using the information on the **Patient Intake Sheet** (Source Document C), as well as the following additional information:

- Medications
  - The status of the OTC medication is active.
  - The dosage is 125 mg.
  - The quantity is 90.
  - The multivitamin comes in tablet form and is taken orally with a frequency of once a day (there is no dose timing, duration, or refill information).
  - The default provider is Ingram.
- Allergies
  - The type of allergy is 'drug', with allergy details of 'Codeine'.
  - The onset was childhood with a date of September 10, 2010, and no time details (default 12:00 am).
  - The allergy is severe, with an active status and an adverse reaction of "Breathing."

☑ **You have completed Exercise 11.7**

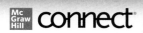 **EXERCISE** **11.8**

Go to https://connect.mheducation.com to complete this exercise. To see instructional notes with the steps, visit the eBook in Connect or download them from www.mhhe.com/iehr4.

Add Acknowledgment of NPP to the Patient's Chart (Refer to Chapter 7 for assistance.)

Harper was given Summit Bay Health Center's Notice of Privacy Practices and signed the acknowledgment that she received it. The acknowledgment of receipt of NPP must be documented in her chart.

When documenting the form, use the following information:

- The form name is *NPP*.
- The form description is *Acknowledgment of receipt*.

☑ **You have completed Exercise 11.8**

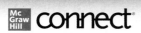 **EXERCISE** **11.9**

Go to https://connect.mheducation.com to complete this exercise. To see instructional notes with the steps, visit the eBook in Connect or download them from www.mhhe.com/iehr4.

Enter the Patient's Vital Signs (Refer to Chapter 4 for assistance.)

Enter Harper's vital signs into EHRclinic using **Office Visit Notes** (Source Document D), as well as the following information:

- Harper identifies her sore throat pain level as a 2.
- The healthcare professional performs a pulse oximetry on Harper, with a reading of 98% oxygen saturation.

☑ **You have completed Exercise 11.9**

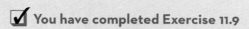   **EXERCISE** **11.10**

Go to https://connect.mheducation.com to complete this exercise. To see instructional notes with the steps, visit the eBook in Connect or download them from www.mhhe.com/iehr4.

Assign a Flag to the Patient's Chart (Refer to Chapter 8 for assistance.)

Assign the "HIPAA Form Signed" flag to Harper's chart in EHRclinic by accessing the Notes area in the facesheet and creating a new note using the following information:

- The note title is *Flag*.
- The note content is *HIPAA form signed*.

☑ **You have completed Exercise 11.10**

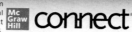
Enter Diagnosis and Procedure Codes (Refer to Chapter 6 for assistance.)

Dr. Ingram spent 20 minutes with Harper, ran a couple of lab tests (strep screen and urinalysis), and has determined she has strep throat and a UTI.

Enter Harper's office visit details, including diagnosis and procedure codes, into EHRclinic using **Office Visit Notes** (Source Document D), as well as the following information:

- For the Chief complaint, Present illness, Review of systems, and examination fields: Use the pre-formatted text on the right side of the office visit template that matches the information listed in the office visit note.
- For the prescriptions, be sure to list the additional details exactly as they are stated in the office visit note.
  - Sulfadiazine details: 500 mg, one tab by mouth twice a day until gone
  - Ibuprofen details: 200 mg, two tabs by mouth every 8 hours as needed
- Harper states that she does not know how to obtain a clean-catch midstream urine specimen, so the healthcare professional provides her with these instructions and documents it under Patient Education.
- The password to sign the note is 123456.

After Harper's office visit has been marked 'Ready for treatment', the healthcare professional must complete her plan review and document the strep test and urinalysis as complete.

After signing the note and entering the password, click on the 'Plan review' tab, and follow these steps:

- Mark both of the procedures as 'complete'.
- Click the 'Ready for checkout' button.
- Click 'Proceed'.

Harper's encounter has now been sent to the Checkout module for claim generation and submission.

☑ **You have completed Exercise 11.11**

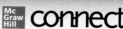
Create a Task for the Receptionist (Refer to Chapter 8 for assistance.)

Harper needs a note to return to work. Compose a return-to-work letter for her to take with her before she leaves the office. The healthcare professional sends a task to the receptionist to create the note for Harper and tells Harper to stop by the front desk to pick it up on her way out.

Send a task through EHRclinic to Alisha Acy with a message stating *Please write a note for Harper Jacobi to return to work on June 22, 2022, per Dr. Ingram.*

The due date of this task is June 20, 2022 (06/20/2022), and it should be linked to Harper Jacobi's chart.

☑ **You have completed Exercise 11.12**

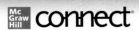
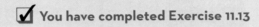
Compose a Correspondence Letter (Refer to Chapter 8 for assistance.)

Compose a correspondence letter for return to work for Harper Jacobi, entering the information for dates under care from 6/20/2022 to 6/21/2022, and returning to work on 6/22/2022 with no restrictions and no other instructions. Use the following information for assistance:

- From the Tools module, access 'Charts, graphs, and reports'.
- Click on 'Patient charts and graphs' to search for Harper Jacobi's chart.
- Scroll down to 'Letters' and click 'Add new letter' to begin the work note.
- The title of the letter is *Return to work.*
- The body of the letter should read *Patient was seen by Dr. Ingram on 6/20/2022. She is excused from work from 6/20/2022 through 6/21/2022 and will return to work on 6/22/2022 with no restrictions.*
- Print the letter; then click 'Done' to close the letter screen.

☑ **You have completed Exercise 11.13**

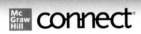

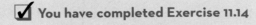
Generate the Claim and Submit It to the Insurance Company (Refer to Chapter 6 for assistance.)

At the completion of Harper's visit, the healthcare professional will generate a claim and submit it to the insurance company. First, it will be necessary to go through the checkout procedure for Harper's encounter.

As Harper is checking out, the healthcare professional realizes that her co-payment did not save to the system, so it will have to be entered again. Use the following information for assistance:

- When performing code linkage for Harper's claim, be sure that the diagnosis code for streptococcal pharyngitis is used for the strep test procedure (87880) and that the diagnosis code for the urinary tract infection is used for the urinalysis procedure (81000).
- Recall that Harper paid her $20 co-payment with check #5879. When the payment is posted, it should be applied to procedure code 81000.
- For claim generation, Harper's chart number is AA027.

☑ **You have completed Exercise 11.14**

Investigate an Unpaid Insurance Claim (Refer to Chapter 6 for assistance.)

Harper called the billing office because she received her Explanation of Benefits (EOB) and noticed the insurance company did not pay anything on her claim. The EOB has an explanation of "Not eligible for benefits."

Usually, when an EOB states "Not eligible for benefits," it means the policy is expired or that the policy or group number was entered wrong. You want to verify this with Harper, so you access her insurance information by going to 'Information management' and then 'Patient information'. Once you have retrieved her insurance information, you ask her what her policy number is on her card. She tells you it is HAJ5679045, which is not what is entered in the computer. Fix the error on her policy number in EHRclinic by clicking 'Edit' in the Insurance info screen and saving the changes.

☑ **You have completed Exercise 11.15**

  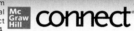
Post an Insurance Payment to an Account (Refer to Chapter 6 for assistance.)

Three weeks later, after resubmitting the claim, your office received an RA from Harper's insurance company. This includes the payments and adjustments as well as the patient responsibility for the date of service 6/20/2022.

Post the insurance payment to Harper's account in EHRclinic. Refer to **Remittance Advice (RA)** (Source Document E) for information needed for this exercise.

Recall that the total amount of the check received is found under the EFT Information on the remittance advice. Also, use the amount allowed when posting the payments to each procedure code.

☑ **You have completed Exercise 11.16**

   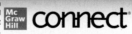
Send an Electronic Message through EHRclinic Messaging (Refer to Chapter 8 for assistance.)

Dr. Ingram is very active in the community and does many charitable fundraisers. One of the big events he does each year is to compete in the annual city triathlon, for which the proceeds go to help those in need. Dr. Ingram is sending a message to the office manager, Diane Baxter, to challenge employees to compete in this year's event. He has asked Diane to forward the message to the clinic staff. If any of them beat him in the race, he will buy everybody in the clinic lunch on Monday.

Send an electronic message using EHRclinic Messaging. Here are some details you will need:

- Send the message to the office manager, Diane Baxter, at dbaxter@sbhc.com.
- Subject should be *Up for a challenge?*
- Body of message should be *A challenge from Dr. Ingram: Beat me at the tri, and I will buy! Dr. Ingram will buy lunch for the entire clinic if any of you beat him at the triathlon this year. All money donated goes to a good cause to help those in need. Have some fun and get lunch . . . maybe!*

✓ **You have completed Exercise 11.17**

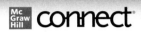 Go to https://connect.mheducation.com to complete this exercise. To see instructional notes with the steps, visit the eBook in Connect or download them from www.mhhe.com/iehr4.   **EXERCISE 11.18**

Add a New Clinical User to EHRclinic (Refer to Chapter 7 for assistance.)

The healthcare professional has been on the job for a year and a half. Her supervisor feels that she is ready for some more administrative duties, so she is shown how to add a new user to EHRclinic. A new MA and a new care provider are starting today, so the healthcare professional sets up EHRclinic user accounts for the new employees. The healthcare professional also assigns access rights to these employees.

Add the new medical assistant to EHRclinic using the following information:

- New medical assistant: Cecelia Strong
- DOB: 12/28/1989
- Gender: Female
- Address: 48209 Hollywood, Carey, OH 43316
- Primary phone: 419-555-0096 (cell)
- Email: cstrong@sbhc.com
- SSN: 819-44-0374
- Start date: 06/13/2022
- Position: Medical assistant
- Credentials: RMA (AMT)

✓ **You have completed Exercise 11.18**

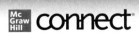 Go to https://connect.mheducation.com to complete this exercise. To see instructional notes with the steps, visit the eBook in Connect or download them from www.mhhe.com/iehr4.   **EXERCISE 11.19**

Set Up a Care Provider (Refer to Chapter 7 for assistance.)

Set up the new care provider in EHRclinic. Here is some information you will need:

- New provider: Ariana Gladstone, MD
- DOB: March 11, 1981
- Gender: Female

(continued)

- Address: 907 Harcourt Lane, Carey, OH 93316
- Primary phone: 419-555-1452 (cell)
- Email: agladstone@sbhc.com
- SSN: 987-42-1632
- Credentials: M.D.
- DEA number: BG7865147
- License number: 4875119 expires 07/01/2023 (issued by Ohio)
- Primary specialty: Cardiology
- NPI: 1039785163
- Dr. Gladstone has default 'View and Edit' access to all EHRclinic functions, with the following exceptions:
  - Schedules—View only
  - Checkout—View only
  - Accounts—No access
  - Claims—View only

✔️ **You have completed Exercise 11.19**

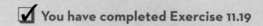   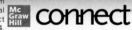

EXERCISE 11.20 **PM** **EHR** **HIM** Go to https://connect.mheducation.com to complete this exercise. To see instructional notes with the steps, visit the eBook in Connect or download them from www.mhhe.com/iehr4.

Assign User Rights to the Medical Assistant (MA) (Refer to Chapter 7 for assistance.)

The new medical assistant has been entered into the EHRclinic staff database. Before she can begin working in EHRclinic, her user rights must be assigned.

Assign the following user rights for Cecelia Strong. Here is the information you will need to set the appropriate user rights for a Summit Bay Health Center medical assistant:

- Schedules—View and Edit
- Encounter—View and Edit
- Checkout—No access
- Accounts—No access
- Claims—No access
- Messages—View and Edit
- Tasks—View and Edit
- Tools—View only

✔️ **You have completed Exercise 11.20**

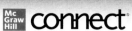   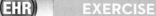
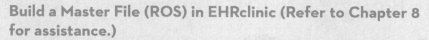

Build a Master File (ROS) in EHRclinic (Refer to Chapter 8 for assistance.)

The new provider wants specific criteria set up because her specialty is cardiology. This will allow her to enter data faster as well as spend more time examining patients.

- Enter information in the Review of Systems option.
- Title: *Cardiovascular*
- Template: - *chest pain, light-headedness, irregular heartbeats, and rapid heart rate*

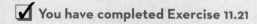 **You have completed Exercise 11.21**

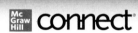
Create a Collections Summary Report (Refer to Chapter 9 for assistance.)

One part of the healthcare professional's new duties is to build a report that identifies patients who have outstanding balances and have had multiple collection attempts. The practice needs to determine if it is appropriate to refer any of these patients to a collection agency based on the length of time their oldest balance is due.

Create and print a collections summary report in EHRclinic. Here is some information you will need:

- Type of report: Patient Collection Report
- Chart number range: aa001–aa025
- Initial billing date range: 11/02/2021–03/31/2022
- Status: Open

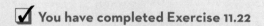 **You have completed Exercise 11.22**

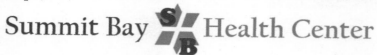

Summit Bay Health Center

REGISTRATION FORM
(Please Print)

Today's date: June 18, 2022	Care Provider: Dr. Ingram

PATIENT INFORMATION

Patient's last name:	First:	Middle:	☐ Mr. ☐ Miss	Marital status (circle one)
Jacobi	Harper	Anna	☐ Mrs. ☒ Ms.	(Single) / Mar / Div / Sep / Wid

Is this your legal name?	If not, what is your legal name?	(Former name):	Birth date:	Age:	Sex:
☒ Yes ☐ No			05/15/1995	27	☐ M ☒ F

Street address:	Social Security no.:	Home phone:	Cell phone:
7568 Catawba Lane	614-33-6849	567-555-6359	567-555-0081

P. O. Box:	City:	State:	ZIP Code:
	Jenera	OH	45841

Occupation:	Employer:	Employer phone no.:
Project Manager	Venture Corp	567-555-2378

E-mail address: hjacobi@venturecorp.com

Race: Caucasian	Ethnicity: Not Hispanic or Latino	Primary language: English	Religion: Protestant

Other family members seen here: none

INSURANCE INFORMATION
(Presentation of Insurance Card is required at time of each visit)

Person responsible for bill:	Date of birth:	Address:	Home phone:	Cell phone:
Harper Anna Jacobi	05/15/1995	7568 Catawba Lane, Jenera, OH 45841	567-555-6359	567-555-0081

Is this person a patient here?	☒ Yes ☐ No

Occupation:	Employer:	Employer address:	Employer phone no.:
Project manager	Venture Corp	4450 Cameron Blvd, Jenera, OH 45841	567-555-2378

Is this patient covered by insurance?	☒ Yes ☐ No

Please indicate primary insurance	☒ McGraw-Hill Healthmark Insurance	☐ BlueCross/ Blue Shield	☐ [Insurance]	☐ [Insurance]	☐ [Insurance]
☐ [Insurance]	☐ Workers' Compensation	☐ Medicare	☐ Medicaid (Please provide card)	☐ Other	

Subscriber's name:	Subscriber's S.S. no.:	Date of birth:	Group no.:	Policy no.:	Co-payment:
Harper Anna Jacobi	614-33-6849	05/15/1995	6500	HAJ5679015	$ 20.00

Patient's relationship to subscriber:	☒ Self	☐ Spouse	☐ Child	☐ Other	Effective Date: 01/01/2022

Name of secondary insurance (if applicable): None	Subscriber's name:	Group no.:	Policy no.:

Patient's relationship to subscriber:	☒ Self	☐ Spouse	☐ Child	☐ Other

IN CASE OF EMERGENCY

Name of local friend or relative (not living at same address):	Relationship to patient:	Home phone no.: ( )	Work phone no.: ( )

The above information is true to the best of my knowledge. I authorize my insurance benefits be paid directly to the physician. I understand that I am financially responsible for any balance. I also authorize [Name of Practice] or insurance company to release any information required to process my claims.

Harper Jacobi	*6/18/2022*
Patient/Guardian signature	Date

Source Document A   Patient Registration Form

McGraw-Hill Healthmark®

Subscriber Name:
HARPER ANNA JACOBI

Identification Number:
HAJ5679015

Group Number: 6500
Coverage Date: 01/01/2022

SINGLE

Office Copay	$20
Emergency Copay	$100
RX Generic Copay	$25
RX Brand Copay	$50
RxID: 062788	
RxNFP: 6874	

PPO℞

Source Document B   Insurance Card

Date:	6/20/2022	Provider: *Dr. Ingram*

Patient Name: *Harper Anna Jacobi* DOB: *05/15/1995*   MRN: *AA027*

Personal Health Information

Allergies (List all allergies and reactions)
Codeine, difficulty breathing and swelling of lips, tongue and throat. Reaction date 9/10/2010.

Medications (all prescription and over-the-counter)
Multivitamin once a day

Family Medical History (list age and health history)
Mother: *59 years old, diabetes Type II at 28 years*

Father: *62 years old, no medical problems*

Sister(s): *none*

Brother(s): *26 years old, asthma started at age 5*

Other:

Past Medical History	Yes	No	If yes, when?
Asthma		✓	
Bronchitis	✓		2004
Cancer		✓	
Diabetes		✓	
Gout		✓	
Heart Disease		✓	
Hernia		✓	
High Blood Pressure		✓	
High Cholesterol		✓	
HIV Positive		✓	
Kidney Disease		✓	
Liver Disease		✓	
Migraines		✓	
Pneumonia		✓	
Thyroid Problems		✓	
Other *seasonal allergies/hay fever*			
Other			
Surgeries (list below)			
Appendectomy			*2009*

Social History (Check all that apply)
Tobacco Use: (Choose one)

Current – every day? _____

Current – occasional? _____ How often? _____

Former smoker? _____

Never smoked? __✓__

Alcohol Use:

Non Drinker? _____

Social Drinker? *occasional* How often? *Monthly*

Heavy Drinker? _____ How often? _____

Caffeine Use: Yes __✓__ No___ Type? *2 cups of coffee per day*

Marital Status:

Single __✓__ Married _____

Divorced _____ Other _____

Education:

High school _____ College __✓__ Post-graduate _____

Occupation: *Project Manager (business)*

Language
Preferred language *English*

Current Medical Problems	Yes	No	Details
Unexplained weight loss		✓	
Headaches		✓	
Pain	✓		*sore throat*
Dental problems		✓	
Arthritis		✓	
Diarrhea/Constipation		✓	
Urinary problems	✓		*burning*
Menstrual problems		✓	
Fatigue		✓	
Problems with eating		✓	
Problems with memory		✓	
Chronic coughs/colds		✓	
Back problems		✓	
Other			

Source Document C   Patient Intake Sheet

Summit Bay Health Center
Office Visit Notes

Date: 6/20/2022	Provider: Dr. Ingram
Patient Name: Harper Anna Jacobi DOB: 05/15/1995	MRN: AA027

CC:	C/o sore throat and "burning with urination"
PI:	Pt states that she developed a sore throat about three days ago and has difficulty swallowing. She states that she may have had a fever, but has not taken her temperature. She has been treating her symptoms with OTC pain relievers, allergy medications, and throat spray with very little relief. Patient also states that she developed a burning sensation with urination about a week ago. She has experienced Increased frequency and urgency, slight lower abdominal pain, and pressure with urination. She has been drinking cranberry juice and has increased her water intake with no improvement in symptoms.
ROS:	ROS Normal and pt reports no signs of blood in urination, no flank or back pain, no nausea/vomiting or chills/sweats, no recent changes in weight. Abnormals: + difficulty swallowing and throat pain . + painful urination, frequency, urgency, and lower abd pain.
Vitals:	T: 99.8 °F oral R: 20 P: 84 bpm BP: 112/74 mm HG ⓇR arm, sitting Ht: 65 in Wt: 143#
Exam:	27 y/o female in no apparent acute distress, well nourished, well developed, alert, cooperative Exam: bilateral lymph nodes in the neck, throat is clear with slight tonsillar redness and swelling, abdomen soft, nontender and without distension. No notable splenic or hepatic enlargement or tenderness. Eyes: PERRLA Ears: External auditory canals and tympanic membrane clear. Nose: No nasal discharge. Lungs: Clear to auscultation and percussion. Cardiac: Regular rhythm, no peripheral edema, cyanosis, or pallor, no bruits.
Dx:	Streptococcal pharyngitis and urinary tract infection
Labs:	Strep screen; urinalysis
Rx:	Sulfadiazine 500 mg, one tab by mouth twice a day until gone
	Ibuprofen 200 mg, two tabs by mouth every 8 hours as needed
F/U	Return to clinic in one week
Signed	Dr. Ingram 6/22/22

Source Document D   Office Visit Notes

McGraw-Hill Healthmark®

Summit Bay Health Center

PAGE: 1 OF 1
DATE: 07/22/2022
ID NUMBER: HAJ5679015

PROVIDER: JAMES INGRAM, M.D.

PATIENT: JACOBI, HARPER ANNA   CLAIM: 1659AA027

FROM DATE	THROUGH DATE	PROC CODE	UNIT	AMT BILL	AMT ALLOW	AMT PAID	DED	COPAY	ADJ	COIN	PROV PAID	REASON CODE*
06/20/22	06/20/22	87880	1	22.00	18.21	18.21	0.00	0.00	3.79	0.00	0.00	PR1
06/20/22	06/20/22	81001	1	22.00	20.69	20.69	0.00	0.00	1.31	0.00	0.00	PR1
	CLAIM TOTALS			44.00	38.90	38.90	0.00	ADJ	5.10	0.00	0.00	

PAYMENT SUMMARY		TOTAL ALL CLAIMS		EFT INFORMATION	
TOTAL AMOUNT PAID	38.90	AMOUNT CHARGED	44.00	NUMBER	59715674
PRIOR CREDIT BALANCE	.00	AMOUNT ALLOWED	38.90	DATE	07/22/22
CURRENT CREDIT DEFERRED	.00	DEDUCTIBLE	0.00	AMOUNT	38.90
PRIOR CREDIT APPLIED	.00	COPAY	20.00		
NEW CREDIT BALANCE	.00	COINSURANCE	0.00		
NET DISPERSED	38.90				

*REASON CODES

PR1 - Deductible   PR3 – Co-pay   V – VOID   ADJ - Adjustment

Source Document E   Remittance Advice (RA)

CMS-1500

HEALTH INSURANCE CLAIM FORM

APPROVED BY NATIONAL UNIFORM CLAIM COMMITTEE (NUCC) 02/12

☐☐ PICA

PICA ☐☐

CARRIER →

1. MEDICARE ☐ (Medicare#)   MEDICAID ☐ (Medicaid#)   TRICARE ☐ (ID#/DoD#)   CHAMPVA ☐ (Member ID#)   GROUP HEALTH PLAN ☐ (ID#)   FECA BLK LUNG ☐ (ID#)   OTHER ☐ (ID#)

1a. INSURED 'S I.D. NUMBER (For Program in Item 1)

2. PATIENT 'S NAME (Last Name, First Name, Middle Initial)

3. PATIENT 'S BIRTH DATE MM DD YY   **SEX** M ☐ F ☐

4. INSURED 'S NAME (Last Name, First Name, Middle Initial)

5. PATIENT 'S ADDRESS (No., Street)

6. PATIENT RELATIONSHIP TO INSURED Self ☐ Spouse ☐ Child ☐ Other ☐

7. INSURED 'S ADDRESS (No., Street)

CITY   STATE

8. RESERVED FOR NUCC USE

CITY   STATE

ZIP CODE   TELEPHONE (Include Area Code) ( )

ZIP CODE   TELEPHONE (Include Area Code) ( )

9. OTHER INSURED 'S NAME (Last Name, First Name, Middle Initial)

10. IS PATIENT 'S CONDITION RELATED TO:

11. INSURED 'S POLICY GROUP OR FECA NUMBER

a. OTHER INSURED 'S POLICY OR GROUP NUMBER

a. EMPLOYMENT? (Current or Previous) ☐ YES ☐ NO

a. INSURED 'S DATE OF BIRTH MM DD YY   **SEX** M ☐ F ☐

b. RESERVED FOR NUCC USE

b. AUTO ACCIDENT? ☐ YES ☐ NO   PLACE (State)

b. OTHER CLAIM ID (Designated by NUCC)

c. RESERVED FOR NUCC USE

c. OTHER ACCIDENT? ☐ YES ☐ NO

c. INSURANCE PLAN NAME OR PROGRAM NAME

d. INSURANCE PLAN NAME OR PROGRAM NAME

10d. CLAIM CODES (Designated by NUCC)

d. IS THERE ANOTHER HEALTH BENEFIT PLAN? ☐ YES ☐ NO *If yes,* complete items 9, 9a, and 9d.

READ BACK OF FORM BEFORE COMPLETING & SIGNING THIS FORM.
12. PATIENT 'S OR AUTHORIZED PERSON 'S SIGNATURE I authorize the release of any medical or other information necessary to process this claim. I also request payment of government benefits either to myself or to the party who accepts assignment below.

SIGNED _____ DATE _____

13. INSURED 'S OR AUTHORIZED PERSON 'S SIGNATURE I authorize payment of medical benefits to the undersigned physician or supplier for services described below.

SIGNED _____

PATIENT AND INSURED INFORMATION →

14. DATE OF CURRENT ILLNESS. INJURY, or PREGNANCY (LMP) MM DD YY   QUAL.

15. OTHER DATE QUAL.   MM DD YY

16. DATES PATIENT UNABLE TO WORK IN CURRENT OCCUPATION FROM   TO

17. NAME OF REFERRING PROVIDER OR OTHER SOURCE   17a.   17b. NPI

18. HOSPITALIZATION DATES RELATED TO CURRENT SERVICES MM DD YY   MM DD YY   FROM   TO

19. ADDITIONAL CLAIM INFORMATION (Designated by NUCC)

20. OUTSIDE LAB? ☐ YES ☐ NO $ CHARGES

21. DIAGNOSIS OR NATURE OF ILLNESS OR INJURY Relate A-L to service line below (24E)   ICD Ind.

A. |_____   B. |_____   C. |_____   D. |_____
E. |_____   F. |_____   G. |_____   H. |_____
I. |_____   J. |_____   K. |_____   L. |_____

22. RESUBMISSION CODE   ORIGINAL REF. NO.

23. PRIOR AUTHORIZATION NUMBER

24. A. DATE(S) OF SERVICE From / To (MM DD YY / MM DD YY)	B. PLACE OF SERVICE	C. EMG	D. PROCEDURES, SERVICES, OR SUPPLIES (Explain Unusual Circumstances) CPT/HCPCS / MODIFIER	E. DIAGNOSIS POINTER	F. $ CHARGES	G. DAYS OR UNITS	H. EPSDT Family Plan	I. ID. QUAL.	J. RENDERING PROVIDER ID. #
1								NPI	
2								NPI	
3								NPI	
4								NPI	
5								NPI	
6								NPI	

PHYSICIAN OR SUPPLIER INFORMATION →

25. FEDERAL TAX I.D. NUMBER   SSN ☐ EIN ☐

26. PATIENT 'S ACCOUNT NO.

27. ACCEPT ASSIGNMENT? (For govt. claims, see back.) ☐ YES ☐ NO

28. TOTAL CHARGE $

29. AMOUNT PAID $

30. Rsvd for NUCC Use

31. SIGNATURE OF PHYSICIAN OR SUPPLIER INCLUDING DEGREES OR CREDENTIALS (I certify that the statements on the reverse apply to this bill and are made a part thereof.)

SIGNED _____ DATE _____

32. SERVICE FACILITY LOCATION INFORMATION

a. NPI   b.

33. BILLING PROVIDER INFO & PH # ( )

a. NPI   b.

NUCC Instruction Manual available at: www.nucc.org   *PLEASE PRINT OR TYPE*   APPROVED OMB-0938-1197 FORM 1500 (02-12)

UB-04

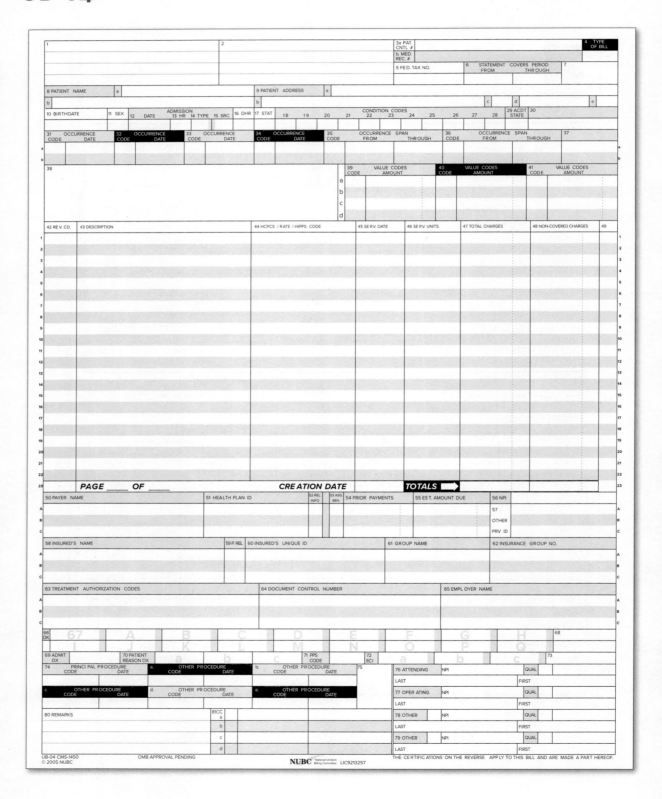

glossary

a

Abuse   Coding and billing that is inconsistent with typical coding and billing practices.

Access report   A report of all persons (within the facility) who have had access to a patient's protected health information.

Account (billing) number   A unique number assigned to every new encounter (emergency department visit, outpatient visit, ambulatory surgery visit, inpatient stay, or physician's office visit).

Accountable Care Organization (ACO)   A reimbursement model where hospitals, physicians, and other healthcare providers form partnerships whereby all are accountable for the quality of care, efficiency of medical services (to contain costs), and patient satisfaction; a pay-for-performance model of healthcare reimbursement.

Accounting of disclosures   Providing the patient, upon request, with a listing of all disclosures of his or her health information, both internally and externally.

Accounts payable   Monies being paid from the medical practice—for instance, to pay for supplies, rent, utilities, payroll, etc.

Accounts receivable   Monies coming into a medical practice—for instance, insurance payments or payments made by patients.

Adjudication   The process of reviewing claims by the insurance carrier to determine payment.

Administrative data   Identifying information, insurance-related information, authorizations, and business correspondence found in a patient's health record.

Advancing Care Information Standards   Part of the Merit-based Payment Incentive System (MIPS), the Advancing Care Information performance category supports the **secure exchange** of health information and **encourages use of certified EHR technology**.

Affordable Care Act (ACA)   Signed into law in 2010, the ACA resulted in improved access to affordable healthcare coverage and protection from abusive practices by healthcare insurance companies. Gives consumers more control over their healthcare coverage and ties reimbursement to quality, patient satisfaction, and coordination of care.

Aggregate   The sum total; for instance, the sum total of patients between the ages of 60 and 100 in a practice, as opposed to a separate listing for each patient between the ages of 60 and 100.

American Health Information Management Association (AHIMA)   A professional association for the field of health information management.

American Recovery and Reinvestment Act of 2009 (ARRA)   Signed into law by President Obama on February 17, 2009; this economic "stimulus plan" includes provisions for the Health Information Technology for Economic and Clinical Health (HITECH) Act.

Application   Software that has a special purpose, such as word processing or spreadsheet, or is for a particular industry such as practice management or electronic health record software.

Artificial intelligence (AI)   The use of computer systems that are able to perform tasks that had typically required the use of human intelligence. Examples include the use of robotics to fill prescriptions in pharmacies, the use of natural language processing in speech recognition technology, and facial recognition technology.

Audit trail   A permanent record or accounting of accesses, additions, amendments, or deletions to a health record. Also a report that shows accesses by user to each function of the software.

b

Benchmarking   Comparison of one set of statistics to the overall statistics when the same variables are used for each.

Blockchain   A distributed database that is stored on multiple computers that may or may not be in the same location.

Blog   Ongoing conversations about a topic that take place online via the Internet.

Breach of confidentiality   Releasing information without a required, properly executed authorization or as restricted by law.

c

Care provider   Term used to refer to a physician, physician's assistant, dentist, psychologist, nurse practitioner, or midwife.

Centers for Medicare and Medicaid Services (CMS)   An agency of the Department of Health and Human Services; responsible for administering the Medicare and Medicaid programs.

Certification Commission for Health Information Technology (CCHIT)   A nonprofit, nongovernmental agency whose purpose was to certify electronic health records for functionality, interoperability, and security.

Certified Electronic Health Record Technology (CEHRT)   A complement to Meaningful Use Stage 2; certification by the Office of the National Coordinator (ONC) of EHR software that meets certain standards.

Chargemaster   Lists the services and procedures by CPT® code and description of the service, provided by a healthcare facility along with the charge for each service.

Chief complaint   The reason for which a patient has made an appointment (usually in his or her own words, for instance, "I have a sore throat").

Clearinghouse   A service that processes data into a standardized billing format and checks for inconsistencies or other errors in the data.

Clinical decision support (CDS)   An electronic application that allows access to current treatment options for a disease, through electronic or remote methods. Alerts the care provider to possible medication interactions, gives treatment options based on results of clinical trials or research, and alerts the provider that a patient may have a particular diagnosis based on the data found in the patient's electronic record.

Clinical Documentation Architecture (CDA)   Developed by HL7, a document markup standard that specifies the structure and semantics of clinical documents such as discharge summary, operative report, etc.

Cloning (copy and paste)   Used in an electronic environment, copying similar or identical information from a previous encounter of the same or a different patient.

Cloud computing   The housing of data in a cloud environment, which is a commercially maintained site on the Internet.

CMS-1500   The form used by physicians' offices and other outpatient settings to submit insurance claims.

Co-payment (co-pay)   The amount due from the patient at the time of the office visit; typically a requirement of managed care plans.

Code linkage   On an insurance claim, the relationship between each procedure (CPT® code) and a diagnosis (ICD-10 code) to demonstrate medical necessity.

Coinsurance   A form of cost-sharing in which the insurance carrier pays a percentage of the claim and the patient pays the remaining percentage. Medicare, for example, has an 80-20 coinsurance, in which Medicare pays 80% and the patient pays 20% of the charges.

Compliance plan   A formal, written document that describes how the hospital or physician's practice ensures rules, regulations, and standards are being adhered to.

Computer virus   A deviant program, stored on a flash drive, hard drive, or CD, that can cause unexpected and often undesirable effects, such as destroying or corrupting data.

Computerized physician order entry (CPOE)   Entering physician orders electronically rather than on paper. The order is transmitted directly to the appropriate department; for instance, an order for an x-ray goes directly to the radiology department, and an order for a CBC goes directly to the laboratory.

Confidentiality   The patient's right to expect that his or her health information will not be released to any person or entity without the patient/guardian's written authorization or as required by law or regulation.

Continuity of Care Document (CCD)   A document exchange standard used to share patient summary information, such as in the case of a patient being referred from one healthcare provider to another.

Core objectives   Basic functions or collection of data that should be completed on a patient's visit or hospitalization.

Covered entity   Any healthcare entity that captures or utilizes health information. These include healthcare plans (insurance companies), clearinghouses that process healthcare claims, individual physicians and physician practices, any type of therapist (mental health, physical, speech, occupational), dentists, hospital staffs, ambulatory facilities, nursing homes, home health agencies, pharmacies, and employers.

Credentialing   The process of ensuring a care provider has the proper qualifications (education, experience, malpractice coverage) to practice medicine.

Current Procedural Terminology (CPT®)   Coding system used to convert narrative procedures and services into numeric form. CPT® is used to code procedures and services in a physician's office; in a hospital setting, it is used for outpatient coding (emergency room, outpatient diagnostic testing, or ambulatory surgery, for example).

Custom report   Report that is designed by the office or hospital rather than coming as part of a software package (standard report).

d

Dashboard   A visual comparison of actual performance to required performance.

Data dictionary   A document that specifies the format of each data field as well as a detailed explanation or definition for that field, which allows for consistency of data collection.

Data integrity   Maintaining the accuracy and consistency of data.

Data   A raw fact, or group of facts, such as a patient's name, height, or weight. A health record contains hundreds or thousands of pieces of data. The term *data* is used both as a singular term and a plural term. When pieces of data come together in a meaningful way, information results; thus, the word *data* is often used interchangeably with the word *information*, though they are not synonymous terms.

Decryption   Interpretation of data being received in encrypted (scrambled) form.

Deductible   The out-of-pocket payment amount that a policyholder must meet before insurance covers the service(s).

Default value   A value that automatically appears in a field each time it appears on a screen (e.g., the current date in a date field, the local area code in a home phone number field).

Demographic (identifying) data   Data that identify the patient. Consist of name, date of birth, sex, race, and Social Security number (may vary by facility policy).

Detail report   Any report that includes patient identifying information and lists each case individually rather than as total number of cases.

Directory information   The fact that a patient is an inpatient (or being treated as an outpatient) as well as his or her location within the facility.

Disaster recovery plan   A written document that details an inventory of hardware and software; backup procedure, including location of backup files; the system used to alert users of the disaster; required security training for personnel; and procedure for restoring backup files.

Discharge summary   A report completed by a care provider that summarizes a patient's stay in the hospital. It generally includes the final diagnoses, a summary of the patient's course in the hospital, any procedures performed, a recap of diagnostic results, and discharge instructions.

Drug Enforcement Agency number   A numeric identifier assigned to a health care provider, for instance a physician, optometrist, dentist, or veterinarian, by the United States Drug Enforcement Administration, which allows him/her to write prescriptions for controlled substances.

Drug formulary   A list of provider-preferred generic and brand-name drugs covered under various insurance plans.

e

Electronic claims submission   Submitting insurance claims via wire to a clearinghouse or directly to the insurance carrier.

Electronic health record (EHR)   Comprehensive record of all health records for a patient, which is able to be shared electronically with other health providers as necessary.

Electronic medical record (EMR)   The legal patient record that is created within any healthcare facility (hospital, nursing home, ambulatory surgery facility, physician's office, etc.). The EMR is the data source for the electronic health record (EHR).

Encounter form (Superbill)   A document (paper or electronic) that is used in medical offices to capture the diagnoses and services performed and from which the CMS-1500 billing form is completed. Also known as a routing slip, Superbill, or encounter form.

Encryption   A security method in which words are scrambled and can only be read if the receiver has a special code to decipher the scrambled message.

ePrescribing   Electronically transmitting prescriptions from care provider to pharmacy.

Evaluation and Management (E&M)   The CPT® codes used to capture the face-to-face time between a patient and the care provider; takes into consideration the extent of the history, the extent of the physical exam, and the level of medical decision making required.

Evidence-based medicine   Diagnostic and treatment protocols that are based on proven research and documented best practices.

Explanation of benefits (EOB)   An explanation of the charges for services, the amount paid by the insurance company, and the amount due by the subscriber, which is sent to the subscriber (and to the provider, in some instances).

f

Family history (FH)   Documentation of conditions and diseases found in immediate family members (e.g., diabetes mellitus, cancer, or heart disease).

Fee schedule   The amount charged for services rendered in a physician's office by Current Procedural Terminology (CPT®) code.

Firewall   A system of hardware and/or software that protects a computer or a network from intruders by filtering activity over the network.

Flag   A message that appears on a screen in written form or as an icon to serve as a reminder to staff and care providers.

Fraud   Intentional deception, which in healthcare takes advantage of a patient, an insurance company, Medicare, or Medicaid.

h

Hardware   The tangible items that are used in automation (e.g., the processing unit, screen, keyboard, mouse, laptops, handheld devices).

Health and Medicine Division   As of 2016, Health and Medicine Division is the new name of the Institute of Medicine. The full name is the Health and Medicine Division of the National Academies of Sciences, Engineering, and Medicine.

Health informatics   The management of automated health information; the technological side of managing health information—the design, development, structure, implementation, integration, and management of the technical aspects of electronic (automated) health record-keeping.

Health information exchange (HIE)   The movement or sharing of information between healthcare entities in a secure manner and in keeping with nationally recognized standards.

Health information management (HIM)   A profession that encompasses services in planning, collecting, aggregating, analyzing, and disseminating individual patient and aggregate clinical data (in paper or electronic format).

Health Information Technology for Economic and Clinical Health (HITECH) Act   A portion of the American Recovery and Reinvestment Act (ARRA) that is meant to increase the use of an electronic health record by hospitals and physicians through a monetary incentive program.

Health Insurance Portability and Accountability Act (HIPAA)   Passed in 1996, this act includes regulations that afford people who leave their employment the ability to keep their insurance or obtain new health insurance even if they have a pre-existing medical condition. Also sets standards for storing, maintaining, and sharing electronic health information while ensuring its privacy and security.

Health Level Seven (HL7)   A set of standards that makes sharing of data between or among healthcare entities possible.

Healthcare administrator   A leadership position within a healthcare facility, including chief executive officer, chief operating officer, chief financial officer, chief information officer, or other higher-level management positions. May also be referred to as healthcare manager or health systems manager.

Healthcare Common Procedure Coding System (HCPCS)   Coding system required by Medicare and Medicaid to document services and procedures (Level 1, Current Procedural Terminology, CPT®) and equipment, supplies, and transport (HCPCS Level 2).

Healthcare Information and Management Systems Society (HIMSS)   An association of health informatics and information professionals formed to promote a better understanding of healthcare informatics and management systems.

Healthcare Integrity and Protection Data Bank (HIPDB)   A database of adverse actions related to fraud and abuse; part of the National Practitioner Data Bank (NPDB).

Healthcare systems administrator   A leadership position specifically responsible for the information technology (IT) functions within an organization or facility. May also be known as a chief information officer.

HIPAA Transactions and Code Set Rule (TCS)   Adopted in fiscal year 2003, a set of rules that standardized the electronic exchange of patient-identifiable, health-related information. This rule set is based on electronic data interchange (EDI) standards, and its purpose is to simplify the processes and decrease the costs associated with payment for healthcare services.

History & physical (H&P)   A report completed by a care provider that includes the reason(s) the patient is being seen or admitted; the history of present illness; the pertinent past medical, surgical, social, and family histories; other current conditions/diseases the patient is being treated for; the report of a physical examination; working diagnoses; and plan of care.

History of present illness (HPI)   The patient's description of current complaints such as when the symptoms started, the location of the condition, the quality of the symptoms, the severity of the symptoms, anything that makes the symptoms better or worse, and additional symptoms the patient is experiencing.

i

In-network   Care providers who contract with a managed care plan to offer services to members of the managed care plan at a prenegotiated rate.

Index   A listing—for instance, a Diagnosis Index is a report that is sorted by diagnosis code and includes the total number of patients seen with that disease for a given period of time, and a Master Patient Index (MPI) is a listing of all patients who have ever been seen in a hospital or a practice.

Information governance   As defined by AHIMA, "the enterprise-wide framework for managing information throughout its lifecycle and supporting the organization's strategy, operations, regulatory, legal, risk and environmental requirements."

Information   Raw facts that, when viewed as a whole, have meaning. Example: a report of all patients treated in the emergency department of Memorial Medical Center with a primary diagnosis of streptococcal pharyngitis (strep throat), sorted by patients' age.

Institute of Medicine (IOM)   An independent, nonprofit, nongovernmental organization that works to provide unbiased and authoritative advice to decision makers and the public. Beginning in March 2016, the IOM is the Health and Medicine Division (HDM) of the National Academies of Sciences, Engineering, and Medicine (the National Academies).

Insurance plan   The medical insurance contract under which a patient is covered; the extent to which services are covered. Also referred to as "the plan."

Insurance verification   The process of contacting the insurance carrier and receiving validation of coverage for that patient, deductible status, and co-pay amount.

Interface   The ability of one computer system or component to accept or send data to another system without loss of integrity or meaning.

International Classification of Diseases, 10th revision, Clinical Modification (ICD-10-CM) and Procedure Coding System (ICD-10-PCS)   ICD-10-CM is the classification system used to convert narrative diagnoses into alpha-numeric codes in all healthcare settings.

ICD-10-PCS is the classification system used to convert narrative procedures into alphanumeric codes in hospital settings.

Effective October 1, 2015, these classification systems replaced ICD-9-CM.

Internet   A series of networks that allow instant access to information from around the world.

Interoperability   Many different functions can take place and information can be shared between computer systems, or within applications of the same computer system, which is not possible with a manual or paper record system.

Intranet   A secure environment or private internal network that is available only to a select group (e.g., the staff within an organization).

l

Library   In computer software, a listing or choice of entities, for instance, employers, insurance plans, ICD-10-CM codes, or CPT® codes.

Live   The point at which computer software or systems are put into real-time use within a practice or hospital.

Local area network (LAN)   A network linking computers and related devices that are physically close to one another such as within a building.

m

Malware   Malware is short for malicious software and includes deviant software such as worms, viruses, and Trojan horses, all of which attack computer programs.

Managed care plan   Insurance plan that promotes quality, cost-effective healthcare through monitoring of patients, preventive care, and performance.

Master file   Dataset that provides structure and is the building block for parts of chart notes within an EHR.

Master Patient Index (MPI)/Patient List   A permanent listing of all patients who have received care in a hospital (inpatient or outpatient). In physicians' offices often referred to as a Master Patient List or Patient List. May also be known as a Master Person List or Master Person Index.

Meaningful Use   The use of certified electronic health record technology with the purpose of improving quality, safety, and efficiency, as well as reducing health disparities within healthcare. Meaningful Use is now known as Promoting Interoperability.

Medical necessity   The fact that there is a medical reason to perform a procedure or service. Documentation exists in the patient's record to show there are sufficient signs, symptoms, or history to warrant the services provided.

Medical record number (MRN)   A unique number assigned to a patient that links to all account numbers for that patient in a given healthcare facility or office. Example: A patient is seen for the first time at Memorial Hospital and is assigned medical record number 50801. In the next 10 years the patient has 10 encounters for care at Memorial Hospital. All 10 of those records can be located under medical record number 50801, though all have different account numbers.

Medical record number   A unique number assigned to each patient seen by a facility or an office.

Medicare Access and CHIP (Children's Health Insurance Program) Reauthorization Act (MACRA)   Act that ended the Sustainable Growth Rate formula that had been used to determine payments to providers for healthcare services billed to Medicare beneficiaries. Also known as the Doc Fix Act.

Menu objectives   Additional functions that allow for greater use of EHR functionality.

Merit-based Incentive Payment System (MIPS)   A reimbursement system that replaces the Sustainable Growth Rate formula previously used by Medicare Part B with a value-based system. The value-based system is called the Quality Payment Program (QPP).

Minimum necessary information   As required by the Health Insurance Portability and Accountability Act (HIPAA), releasing the minimum information to satisfy the reason the information is needed or the minimum necessary to perform a job function.

n

National Academies of Sciences, Engineering, and Medicine (the National Academies)   Replaced the Institute of Medicine and provides healthcare-related data at a national level. The specific division of the National Academies that is related to healthcare is the Health and Medicine Division (HMD).

National Practitioner Data Bank (NPDB)   Required by law, a database of malpractice payouts, revocation of privileges, licensure denial or suspension, denial of medical staff privileges, and similar actions.

National Provider Identifier (NPI)   A unique 10-digit identifier, issued by the Centers for Medicare & Medicaid Services (CMS), that must be used on insurance claims to identify the care provider and/or group practice that rendered care to the patient.

Nationwide Health Information Network (NHIN)   A set of standards, services, and policies that enable the secure exchange of health information over the Internet.

Notice of Privacy Practices   A requirement of the Health Insurance Portability and Accountability Act (HIPAA) that patients are made aware (in writing) of their rights under HIPAA, including the fact that the patient has the right to view/receive a copy of his or her own record, the fact that amendment to the documentation may be requested, the ways in which their health information will be used and released to outside entities, and the procedure to file a complaint with the Department of Health and Human Services.

o

Office of the National Coordinator for Health Information Technology (ONC)   The principal federal entity charged with coordination, implementation, and use of health information technology and the electronic exchange of health information.

Optical character recognition (OCR)   Technology that converts a document into a format that is computer readable—that is, into an electronic file.

p

Password   A unique code, known only to the user, that is used to gain access to computer applications.

Past medical history (PMH)   Previous medical condition(s) for which the patient has been treated.

Patient portal   A method of accessing portions of one's own health information from the care provider's or hospital's electronic health record.

Patient-Centered Medical Home (PCMH)   A model that was developed by the American Academy of Family Practitioners to care for patients with chronic conditions, to encourage and facilitate a patient's (and family's) involvement in his or her own care.

Personal digital assistant (PDA)   A mobile device that is small enough to fit in one's hand yet allows access to local area networks (LANs), wide area networks (WANs), and the Internet; may also have telephone capability.

Personal health record (PHR)   A record, kept by the patient, that contains a person's health history, immunization status, current and past medications, allergies, and instructions given by a care provider; it often includes patient education materials as well.

Physical exam (PE)   An examination of the patient's body for signs of disease.

Physician Quality Reporting System (PQRS)   A voluntary pay-for-performance incentive program. Participating care providers submit data on any of the 100 designated quality measures and receive monetary incentives for doing so.

Picture Archiving and Communication System (PACS)   Computerized system for enhanced viewing and sharing of images such as x-rays, scans, ultrasounds, and mammograms.

Point of care (POC)   Documentation, dictation, and ordering of tests and procedures that occur at the same time the patient is being seen.

Practice management (PM)   Software used in physicians' offices to gather data on every patient and perform administrative functions from the time an appointment is made through the time the bill for each visit is paid.

Principal diagnosis   The reason, after study, determined to be chiefly responsible for the patient's admission to the hospital.

Privacy   The right to be left alone; the right to expect that one's personal space is respected while undergoing healthcare.

Problem list   A listing kept in the patient's health record of all of his or her current (active) and resolved medical conditions.

Promoting Interoperability Programs   Formerly known as Meaningful Use, now referred to as Promoting Interoperability, this name change and the provisions of the program were made as a result of the 21st Century Cures Act and the Bipartisan Budget Act of 2018. The goal continues to be the use of certified electronic health record technology to improve quality, safety, and efficiency, as well as to reduce health disparities within the Medicare population.

Protected health information (PHI)   HIPAA defines protected health information (PHI) as "individually identifiable information related to the present, past, or future health status of an individual that is created, collected, or maintained by a HIPAA-covered entity in relation to the provision of healthcare, payment of healthcare services, or use in healthcare operations (PHI business uses)."

q

Qualitative analysis Review of documentation in the health record to ensure the quality of the clinical documentation, that it is timely, not contradictory, complete, and clear.

Quality Reporting Document Architecture (QRDA) Based on HL7's approved Clinical Documentation Architecture (CDA), QRDA is a data standard used for reporting quality measure data and that is EHR compatible across different health IT systems.

Quantitative analysis Review of the health record to ensure that all required documentation is present. Examples include history and physical exam, all entries authenticated (signed) by providers, and operative report present when a procedure has been performed.

Query Searching a database for patients who meet certain criteria.

r

Regional extension center (REC) An organization that assists healthcare providers with the selection and implementation of electronic health record systems.

Regional Health Information Organization (RHIO) Group of healthcare organizations in a geographic area that exchange health information with the goal of improving patient care, reducing duplication, and reducing unnecessary costs.

Registry A listing that is filed in chronological order based on when something occurred. Examples include a birth registry, a death registry, a cancer registry, and a trauma registry.

Remittance advice (RA) A detailed accounting of the claims for which payment is being made by an insurance company. The remittance advice accompanies the payment from the insurance company.

Resolution The quality of a scanned image as it will appear in the record. The higher the resolution, the crisper the image.

Review of systems (ROS) A body-system-by-body-system inventory of any symptoms the patient is having or has had based on a series of questions asked by the care provider.

Routing slip A document (paper or electronic) that is used in medical offices to capture the diagnoses and services or procedures performed and from which the CMS-1500 billing form is completed. Also known as a Superbill or encounter form.

s

Scanner A piece of equipment that digitizes documents into a format that is readable by a computer.

Scribe An assistant who enters data, either in writing or electronically, into the health record as the care provider verbally dictates recent findings.

Smartphone Telephone that allows Internet browsing, audio, video, and camera functionality.

SOAP note An acronym for the documentation used in a care provider's office to record the patient's symptoms, signs, assessment (diagnosis), and plan of care. SOAP stands for Subjective, Objective, Assessment, and Plan.

Social history (SH) Lifestyle or social habits of the patient. Examples include smoking history or current use, use of alcoholic beverages and frequency, and patient's profession.

Social media Interactive communication sites via the Internet. Examples are Facebook, YouTube, Instagram, Snapchat, and Twitter.

Speech recognition technology Software that recognizes the words being said by the person dictating and digitally converts the speech to text; as it is used it "learns" the dictator's voice, and therefore improves the accuracy of the transcription.

Structured data Data that fit a particular model or format, which can be tracked and may be part of a database. Examples include ICD-10-CM/PCS codes, CPT® codes, a patient's temperature, or a patient's age.

Subscriber The primary person covered by an insurance plan.

Summary report A statistical report that includes totals rather than data for individual patients. Examples include a report of the total number of patients seen during a particular time by gender and a report of the total number of patients seen in the office with E&M code 99214.

Superbill A document (paper or electronic) that is used in medical offices to capture the diagnoses and services or procedures performed and from which the CMS-1500 billing form is completed. Also known as a routing slip or encounter form.

Surgical history Previous surgical procedure(s) the patient has undergone, the approximate date(s), the name of the surgeon(s), the reason(s) for the procedure(s), and complications, if any.

t

Tablet computer Computer that is larger than a PDA or smartphone yet smaller than a laptop computer; allows access to local area networks (LANs), wide area networks (WANs), and the Internet.

Telehealth Associated with preventive care, telehealth is the use of audiovisual equipment through which the patient and the care provider or healthcare professional can connect remotely.

Telemedicine The use of technology to remotely monitor a patient's vital signs and perform tests such as an EKG or to forward radiologic images.

Templates Preformatted documents built into practice management and electronic health record systems.

Transactions Posting of charges and the payment of claims in the practice management system to update patients' accounts.

u

UB-04 The form used to submit insurance claims for hospital patients.

Unstructured data Data in the form of words or audio files that cannot be tracked. Examples include emails, written narratives, and audio files from speech recognition technology.

User rights The limitations of one's access to the functionality of the software as defined by one's job description or position within the organization.

Value-based payment modifier program   Part of the Merit-based Incentive Program, payment to solo practitioners (physicians who do not practice as part of a group) and medical practice groups per the Medicare Physician Fee Schedule (PFS) but based on the quality of care furnished compared to the cost of care during a performance period. The Value Modifier was an adjustment made to Medicare payments for items and services.

Variable   In relation to a statistical report, the factor that varies from one patient to the next. Examples include age, ZIP code, and diagnoses.

Virtual private network (VPN)   Software that encrypts (codes) the data being sent as well as interprets the data being received.

Vital signs   Measurements taken (temperature, heart rate, respiratory rate, blood pressure, height and weight, and sometimes Body Mass Index) to determine the status of basic body-system functions.

Voice recognition technology   Software that uses a person's voice to verify that they are who they say they are. A sample of a person's speech is recorded and those speech patterns are tested against a database to verify that their voice matches their claimed identity.

Wi-Fi   Data exchange via high radio frequency.

Wide area network (WAN)   Connects computer networks together that are not physically close.

EHRclinic, 2. *See also specific topics*
  accounts receivable, 141–144
  adding users, 164–165
  applying security measures, 163
  audit trail, 167
  capturing insurance information, 65–66
  care provider set up, 165–166
  chart entries, 173–174
  claims process using, 127–130
  co-pay alert, 128
  customizing Facesheet screen, 198–199
  customizing user preferences in, 199
  dashboard in, 209–220
  demographics, example of, 57
  diagnosis and procedure coding using, 130–133
  documentation of patient's past medical history, 33
  drug allergies, 84–85
  editing demographic data, 63–64
  facesheet, 30–31
  finding status of a claim, 130
  flags, 201–202
  flow of information in, 8–11
  group setup, 169
  Help feature, 11–12, 66–67
  interface capabilities in, 108
  internal communications, 193
  libraries, 52–53
  master files and templates, 197–198
  medication list, 83–84
  past medical history, 82–83
  Patient Information screen in, 58–59
  patient portal, 241
  patient's plan of care, looking up, 96–97
  physical exam, 103
  posting payments, 144
  practice management applications, 2–4
  registering new patient in, 58–62
  registries, 229
  release of information policies/ procedures, 174–176
  restricted access record, 169, 173
  review of systems, 98–102
  scheduling appointments, 62–63
  standard reports, 222–224
  Superbill, 126
  task lists, 199–200
  tracking physicians' orders, 108–111
  user rights for managers, 168–169
  user rights for staff, 166–168
  vital signs, 86–87
Electronic claims submission, 4
Electronic encounter form (Superbill), 126–127
Electronic health (medical) record (EHR/EMR) software
  applications, 7
  barriers to adopting, 239–240

certification of, 163
content, as care provider's responsibility. *See* EHR content, as care provider's responsibility
converting from paper records to, 240
defined, 2
evaluating for HIPAA compliance, 161–163
functions of, 34–35
importing documents to, 194–196
information gathered from, 24
paper records *vs.*, 6
reasons for using, 4–6
Electronic health records systems, 66
Electronic Healthcare Transactions Rule, 36
Electronic medication administration record (eMAR), 218
Electronic prescribing, 7, 106–107
Eligible professionals (EPs), 210
Email policies, 160
eMAR. *See* Electronic medication administration record (eMAR)
Encounter Form, 3, 124–127, 140. *See also* Superbill
  electronic, 126–127
Encryption, 180
  blockchain, 247
  email, 160
  for VPNs, 245
EOB. *See* Explanation of benefits (EOB)
EPs. *See* Eligible professionals (EPs)
Evaluation and Management (E&M) code, 143
Evidence-based medicine, 243
Exchange of health information, 177–179
Explanation of benefits (EOB), 138, 139

f

Facesheet screen, customization, 198–199
FACHE. *See* Fellow of the American College of Healthcare Executives (FACHE)
Family history (FH), 80
FDA Office of Women's Health, 243
Fee schedule, 122
Fellow of the American College of Healthcare Executives (FACHE), 23
FH. *See* Family history (FH)
Financial management
  Accountable Care Organization, 136–137
  accounts payable, 137
  accounts receivable, 137, 141–143
  claims management, 122–124
  claims process with EHRClinic, 127–130
  compliance, 145–146
  diagnosis and procedure coding using, 130–133

  Superbill use, 124–126
Firewall, 160, 245
Flags, 201–202
Flow of information, 8–11
Forms, as data collection tools, 77–79
Formularies, 211
Fraud, 133
Front desk check-in flowchart, 9

g

Garets, D., 34
Group setup, 169

h

Hardware, 160
HCPCS. *See* Healthcare Common Procedure Coding System (HCPCS)
Health and Human Services (HHS), 37
Health and Medicine Division (HMD), 35
Health informatics, 238
Health information exchange (HIE), 34, 177–179
  continuity of care, 177–178
  outside the organization, 178–179
  security measures, 246
Health information management (HIM), 21, 163, 238
  professionals, 26–27
Health information specialty areas, 22
Health information technology (HIT), 163
Health Information Technology for Economic and Clinical Health (HITECH) Act, 36–39, 156
Health information, computer-based media for, 27–30
Health Insurance Portability and Accountability Act (HIPAA), 34, 35–36
  Privacy Rule, 34–35
  Security Rule, 35
Health Level Seven (HL7), 51
Healthcare administrator, 23–24
Healthcare Common Procedure Coding System (HCPCS), 131, 132, 133
Healthcare facility, 2
Healthcare Information and Management Systems Society (HIMSS), 25, 38, 163
Healthcare Integrity and Protection Data Bank (HIPDB), 230
Healthcare professions/professional, 9, 21–25
Healthcare systems administrator, 24
HealthInformation Technology for Economic and Clinical Health (HITECH) Act, 27–30
Help feature (EHRclinic), 11–12, 66–67